Breast Ultrasound

For Elsevier:

Commissioning Editor: Dinah Thom
Development Editor: Catherine Jackson
Project Manager: Jess Thompson
Designer: George Ajayi
Illustrations Manager: Merlyn Harvey
Illustrator: Amanda Williams

Breast Ultrasound
HOW, WHY and WHEN

Anne-Marie Dixon MHSc PGCHEP DMU DCR(R)

Senior Teacher, University of Bradford, Bradford, UK

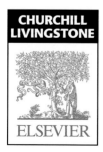

EDINBURGH   LONDON   NEW YORK   OXFORD   PHILADELPHIA   ST LOUIS   SYDNEY   TORONTO   2008

CHURCHILL
LIVINGSTONE
ELSEVIER

First published 2008

ISBN-13: 978 0 443 10076 5

British Library Cataloguing in Publication Data
A catalogue record for this book is available from the British Library.

Library of Congress Cataloging in Publication Data
A catalog record for this book is available from the Library of Congress.

Notice
Knowledge and best practice in this field are constantly changing. As new research and experience broaden our knowledge, changes in practice, treatment and drug therapy may become necessary or appropriate. Readers are advised to check the most current information provided (i) on procedures featured or (ii) by the manufacturer of each product to be administered, to verify the recommended dose or formula, the method and duration of administration, and contraindications. It is the responsibility of the practitioner, relying on their own experience and knowledge of the patient, to make diagnoses, to determine dosages and the best treatment for each individual patient, and to take all appropriate safety precautions. To the fullest extent of the law, neither the Publisher nor the Editor assumes any liability for any injury and/or damage to persons or property arising out or related to any use of the material contained in this book.

The Publisher

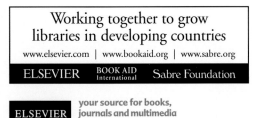

Printed in China

Contents

List of contributors

Caroline Begaj DMU DCR(R)
Clinical Specialist in Ultrasound, Bradford Teaching
Hospitals Foundation NHS Trust, St Lukes Hospital
Bradford, UK

Gillian R. Clough MHSc PGCHEP DCR(R)
University Teacher, University of Bradford, Bradford,
UK

Anne-Marie Dixon MHSc PGCHEP DMU DCR(R)
Senior Teacher, Division of Radiography, University of
Bradford, Bradford, UK

David S. Enion MB ChB FRCS(G) DMRD FRCR
Consultant Radiologist, Royal Blackburn Hospital,
Blackburn, UK

Jacqui Lee MEd BEd (Hons) DMU DCR(R)
Lead Sonographer, Eccleshill NHS Treatment Centre,
Bradford, UK

Mike Stocksley MSc Cert Ed MDCR DMU
Course Leader in Clinical Ultrasound, Department
of Allied Health Professions, Faculty of Health and
Social Care, London South Bank University, London,
UK

Heather Venables BEd (Hons) DMU DCR(R)
Senior Lecturer (Ultrasound), Faculty of Education
Health and Sciences, University of Derby, Derby,
UK

Acknowledgements

I would like to thank all the colleagues and (still, I hope) friends who have helped in the preparation of this book.

Many thanks to Gillian Clough, Heather Venables, Mike Stocksley, David Enion, Caroline Begaj and Jacqui Lee who have formally contributed chapters—thank you for your hard work, your patience and particularly for your good natured response to my relentless editorial demands! I hope you feel, as I do, that it was worth it!

In addition to the co-authors listed above, I would also like to thank the following for their willingness to peer-review chapter drafts, provide helpful and constructive feedback and/or supply illustrations: Dr Peter Britton, Dr Paul Burrows, Dr Pauline Carder, Mrs Linda Clarkson, Dr Barbara Dall, Mrs Daina Dambitis, Dr Erika Denton, Ms Jan Dodgeon, Dr Neelanjana Dutt, Dr Simon Elliott, Dr Tony Evans, Mrs Ann Hampshaw, Ms Dawn Ingham (Toshiba Medical Systems), Dr Joyce Liston, Dr Jan Lowe, Dr Alison Mackie, Mr Tom Skidmore (Agfa-Gevaert Ltd), Mrs Jo Thomas (Philips Medical Systems), Ms Sandra Twardun (GE Healthcare), Mrs Fiona Ware, Dr Anne-Marie Wason, Dr Christian Weismann and Ms Patsy Whelehan.

My thanks also go to Dinah Thom and Catherine Jackson at Elsevier for their persistence and support.

Special thanks to Patricia, Elaine, Gillian Holsey and Gary Culpan for help with the illustrations—you definitely went beyond the call of duty—thank you!

Last but not least, thanks to Martin and Fran for their sufferance and endurance—and yes . . . I have now finished the book!!

Preface

Ultrasound is increasingly being used in breast imaging, both as an additional diagnostic test alongside mammography, and in its own right as the first-line imaging technique when mammography is likely to have reduced sensitivity or when it presents an unacceptable radiation hazard.

The modern breast ultrasound service is invariably located within the context of a multidisciplinary approach to the diagnosis and management of breast disease and, as such, the examination may be performed by a wide range of healthcare professionals. This book therefore is intended to appeal to a wide range of medical, allied health and nursing professionals who wish to practice breast ultrasound. The book aims to provide the student or novice practitioner with a detailed practical guide to the technique of breast ultrasound and the interpretation of images obtained; for the more experienced practitioner, the book describes the application of breast ultrasound to less routine and more complex settings, such as the investigation of the augmented or reconstructed breast and the male breast, and in addition the application and practice of a range of invasive diagnostic and therapeutic applications are also described in detail.

In order that the breast ultrasound practitioner understands the role of breast ultrasound in the overall breast care and management pathway, and to attract a wider breast care team readership, the book considers the relative strengths and limitations of the technique compared with other diagnostic tests, and provides background information about breast disease and breast cancer in particular.

For many of my ex-students who have said 'you should write a book'—here it is! There are several good books already on the market that cover 'breast ultrasound' and I have referred to my own favorites many times. Most of these existing texts are comprehensive, and thus, inevitably, expensive tomes; it is hoped that the majority of those who practice breast ultrasound will find this book readily accessible and affordable, and that they will come to regard it as an invaluable starter manual and practical handbook.

I once naively thought that if I just passed on all that I knew (which I have done in this book)—students would be able to do the job as well as I could. Alas, I now know that this is not true. So, as well as passing on all I know, I hope I have been able to convey some of my passion and enthusiasm for ultrasound and its application in breast disease, and that by reading this book others will come to feel this for themselves. Breast ultrasound is both a science and art: knowledge will allow you to practice the science, but some artistic creativity in the application of this knowledge will also be required to realize the full potential of the technique.

A.-M.D.
2007

List of abbreviations

1.5D	one and a half dimensions (used to indicate multiple row array transducers)	BSc	Bachelor of Science. UK educational degree awarded after 3 years full-time study at University
2DBM	two-dimensional B-mode	CAD	computer-aided/assisted detection
3D	three-dimensional	CASE	Consortium for the Accreditation of Sonographic Education (UK)
AB ratio	peak systolic to end diastolic velocity ratio (Doppler parameter)	ce-MRI	contrast-enhanced MRI scan
ABC	airway, breathing, circulation (resuscitation priorities)	Cerb2	tumor marker indicating overexpression of Her-2 protein
ACR	American College of Radiology	CFM	color flow mapping (Doppler mode)
ADH	atypical ductal hyperplasia	CHE	Certificate of Higher Education. UK educational award made after 1 year's full-time study at university
AIDS	acquired immunodeficiency syndrome		
AIUM	American Institute of Ultrasound in Medicine	CoR	College of Radiographers (UK)
ALARA	as low as reasonably achievable	CR	computed radiography
ALH	atypical lobular hyperplasia	CSL	complex sclerosing lesion
AR-	anti-radial (anatomical plane orientation)	CT	computed tomography
		DCIS	ductal carcinoma in situ
BC	before Christ	DCR	Diploma of the College of Radiographers (UK)
BASO	British Association of Surgical Oncology	DDR	direct digital radiography
BBC	benign breast change	DH	Department of Health (UK)
B-mode	brightness mode	DMU	Diploma in Medical Ultrasound— original ultrasound qualification awarded by the College of Radiographers (UK)
BMUS	British Medical Ultrasound Society		
BRCA-1	breast cancer 1 gene: gene located on long arm of chromosome 17— mutations are associated with increased risk of breast cancer		
		DNA	deoxyribonucleic acid—hereditary material contained in cells
BRCA-2	breast cancer 2 gene: gene located on long arm of chromosome 13— mutations are associated with increased risk of breast cancer	EFSUMB	European Federation of Societies for Ultrasound in Medicine and Biology
		ER	estrogen receptor—protein found in reproductive tissue (and tumors

	thereof)—regulates cell growth when combined with the hormone estrogen
FA	fibroadenoma
FCD	fibrocystic disease
FDG	fluorodeoxyglucose (attached to fluorine 18 for some RNI studies)
FDG-PET	PET scan using FDG
FFD	focus-to-film distance (radiographic exposure parameter)
FNAB	fine needle aspiration biopsy
FNAC	fine needle aspiration cytology
fps	frames per second
FSH	follicle-stimulating hormone
G (or g)	gauge (needle caliber parameter)
Gd-DTPA	gadolinium di-ethylene-triamine-penta-acetic acid (contrast agent used in MRI scanning)
GE	General Electric (ultrasound equipment manufacturer)
GMC	General Medical Council—UK regulatory body for medical practitioners
GnRF	gonadotropin-releasing factor
HE	Higher Education (tertiary or university education)
HER-2	herceptin-2—protein overexpressed by some malignant breast tumors
HIP	Health Insurance Plan (USA)
HIV	human immunodeficiency virus
HRT	hormone replacement therapy
Hz	Hertz (SI unit of frequency)
IBUS	International Breast Ultrasound School
ID	identification
kHz	kiloHertz (10^3 Hertz)
kVp	peak kilovoltage (radiographic exposure parameter)
L or Lt.	left side (of the body)
LCIS	lobular carcinoma in situ
LIQ	lower inner quadrant (anatomical region of breast)
LOQ	lower outer quadrant (anatomical region of breast)
LS	longitudinal scan (anatomical plane orientation)
mAs	milliampere-second (radiographic exposure parameter)
MDA	Medical Devices Agency (UK)
MDT	multidisciplinary team

MHz	megaHertz (10^6 Hertz—typical magnitude of ultrasound transducer frequency)
MI	mechanical index (indicator of ultrasound hazard potential)
MPhil	Master of Philosophy (postgraduate educational award)
MR	magnetic resonance
MRes	Master of Research (postgraduate educational award)
MRI	magnetic resonance imaging
MSc	Master of Science (postgraduate educational award)
NCB	needle core biopsy
NHS	National Health Service (UK)
NHS PASA	National Health Service Purchasing and Supply Agency (UK)
NHSBSP	National Health Service Breast Screening Programme (UK)
NHSCSP	National Health Service Cancer Screening Programme (UK)
NPI	Nottingham Prognostic Index—used to estimate patient prognosis (UK)
NST	no special type (tumor classification)
NVQ3	National Vocational Qualification Level 3—university entry level award (UK)
ONS	Office for National Statistics (UK)
OSCE	objective structure clinical examination
PASH	pseudoangiomatous stromal hyperplasia
PBL	problem-based learning
PBOS	practice-based observation of skills
PD	power Doppler
PET	positron emission tomography
PET-CT	positron emission tomography combined with computed tomography
PGC	postgraduate certificate—university award made after successful study equivalent to one-third of a Master's award (UK)
PGD	postgraduate diploma—university award made after successful study equivalent to two-thirds of a Master's award (UK)
PhD	Doctor of Philosophy—highest UK postgraduate award
PI	pulsatility index (Doppler parameter)
PR	progesterone receptor—a protein found in reproductive tissue (and

	tumors thereof)—regulates cell growth when combined with the hormone progesterone
PRF	pulse repetition frequency (Doppler ultrasound parameter)
PWD	pulsed wave Doppler
PWSD	pulsed wave spectral Doppler
PZT	lead zirconate titanate (piezoelectric material used in ultrasound transducers to generate and detect sound waves)
QA	quality assurance
QAAHE	Quality Assurance Agency for Higher Education (England and Wales, UK)
R or Rt.	right side (of the body)
RAD	radial (anatomical plane orientation)
RCN	Royal College of Nursing (UK)
RCP	Royal College of Pathologists (UK)
RCR	Royal College of Radiologists (UK)
RF	radio frequency
RI	resistance index (Doppler parameter)
RNI	radionuclide imaging
RS	radial scar
SCoR	Society and College of Radiographers (UK)
SDMS	Society of Diagnostic Medical Sonography (USA)
SNB	sentinel node biopsy
SoR	Society of Radiographers (UK)
SPECT	single photon emission computed tomography
SpR	specialist registrar
Tc99m-MDP	Technetium 99m methylene-diphosphonate—radiotracer used for RNI bone scans
Tc99m-MIBI	Technetium 99m sestamibi—radiotracer used for RNI scintimammography
TDLU	terminal duct lobular unit
TGC	time gain compensation
TI	thermal index (indicator of ultrasound hazard potential)
TNM	tumor, node, metastasis (tumor staging system)
TS	transverse scan (anatomical plane orientation)
UIQ	upper inner quadrant (anatomical region of breast)
UKAS	United Kingdom Association of Sonographers
UOQ	upper outer quadrant (anatomical region of breast)
US	ultrasound
VAB	vacuum-assisted biopsy
WBUS	whole breast ultrasound
WDC	Workforce Development Confederation (UK government-funded regional education commissioning body)
WFUMB	World Federation for Ultrasound in Medicine and Biology
Z	acoustic impedance

Chapter 1

Introduction

Anne–Marie Dixon

BACKGROUND

Breast imaging is an exciting and rapidly developing diagnostic specialism, with breast ultrasound having an increasingly important contribution to make. Ultrasound has been used to examine the breast for more than 50 years—in the early years the technique involved whole breast water-path scanners and was essentially limited to the differentiation of cystic and solid masses (Bamber 2005). Today, because of advances in transducer technology and computer processing, high frequency contact breast scanning allows demonstration of fine anatomical detail and appreciation of subtle differences in image contrast—when performed by an experienced practitioner in a multidisciplinary setting, the modern breast ultrasound examination is a highly sensitive and specific diagnostic test.

Ultrasound is classically an operator-dependent technique—despite continual attempts to standardize and quantify breast ultrasound imaging features, in routine practice the diagnostic value of the examination is unavoidably dependent upon the knowledge and skill of the person performing the scan. On modern ultrasound machines there is a range of technological functions, there is also a range of natural biological and physiological variation in breast tissue and a wide range of potential pathological change; given all these variables, some subjectivity in manipulating, optimizing and interpreting breast ultrasound image appearances is unavoidable. Nevertheless, standardization of technique between operators is possible and desirable, and when this is combined with the consistent and accurate application of well-defined interpretation criteria by experienced practitioners, a reasonable degree of objectivity is introduced; as a result, improved diagnostic reliability and accuracy can be achieved.

Breast ultrasound is not practiced in isolation however; the technique is one of several diagnostic tools available for examining the breast, and its full value and potential are only realized when the technique is selected, performed and interpreted within an appropriate context. In the modern healthcare model of provision, the clinical setting is invariably multidisciplinary, with overall service provision influenced by the economic climate and prevailing political agenda as well as pure medical factors. Perhaps as important, whilst the incidence of breast cancer is increasing, so is the likelihood and expectation of timely diagnosis and the potential for 'curative' treatment.

The wide and diverse contextual location of the breast ultrasound examination is reflected in this book. By convention, the person presenting for an ultrasound examination is referred to as 'the patient', since, at the time of writing, and on the basis of the evidence to date, the vast majority of 'appropriate referrals' will be medically indicated.

In Chapter 2, Gillian Clough traces the historical origins of breast cancer and its diagnosis and treatment. She considers the evidence to date that informs our understanding of why some seem more susceptible to the disease than others and outlines the prognostic factors currently used to plan disease management.

Whilst most ultrasound 'textbooks' start off with a general chapter about ultrasound 'physics', Heather Venables has taken an anatomy-specific approach in Chapter 3 and considered the fundamental aspects of ultrasound generation and interaction with tissue, with specific reference to how these affect ultrasound images of the breast. Her application-specific approach limits the content of the chapter to those aspects of underlying physical principles that have a direct impact on diagnostic capability in the breast. The aim of this and the next chapter is that an understanding of such factors enables the ultrasound practitioner to get the most out of the equipment they are using. In Chapter 4, Heather goes on specifically to look at design, choice and use of equipment for breast ultrasound, explaining how the ultrasound practitioner can influence and optimize these—again the application-specific approach is taken, emphasizing how to maximize diagnostic yield in the breast. At the end of Chapter 4, Heather reviews some of the most recent technological developments and their potential use in breast diagnosis.

All ultrasound image interpretation is operator dependent, and a thorough knowledge of what is 'normal' is necessary before an operator can recognize abnormality. In Chapter 5, Mike Stocksley describes the anatomy of the breast and axilla and how to recognize 'normal' anatomical structure in the ultrasound image. Since, the 'normal' ultrasound appearance of the breast varies, the chapter concludes by describing how age- and hormone-related physiological change affects ultrasound appearances.

Chapter 6 is a step-by-step guide of how to perform a breast ultrasound examination. A wide-ranging approach to performance of the examination is taken; the clinical context within which the examination should be undertaken is discussed and the interpersonal, as well as the technical skills of the operator are considered. Chapter 7 is inextricably linked to Chapter 6, as this is where image interpretation, recording and reporting are considered. Chapter 7 describes the sonographic criteria upon which image-based diagnosis is made, explains how and why a visual record of the examination should be made, and most importantly explains how to communicate the findings of the ultrasound examination effectively to other members of the breast care team in the form of an official examination report.

In Chapter 8, David Enion reviews benign breast pathology, with Chapter 9 reviewing malignant disease. In addition to describing the ultrasound appearances, these chapters include background information about clinical signs and symptoms, the correlating mammographic and histological appearances and typical clinical management strategies, to reflect the underpinning multidisciplinary context within which breast ultrasound is practiced.

A substantial number of women have undergone breast augmentation or reconstruction so it is not uncommon to encounter women with breast prostheses in symptomatic and screening populations. Chapter 10 considers the implications for diagnostic imaging in women with breast implants, describing their ultrasound appearance and the resultant impact on evaluation of surrounding breast tissue, the axilla and chest wall structures. Many women experience complications associated with prosthesis implantation; Chapter 10 also describes the use of mammography, ultrasound and magnetic resonance imaging to evaluate and recognize these complications.

Although breast disease is predominantly a female condition, the incidence of male breast cancer is rising and increasing awareness of this is prompting more men to seek diagnostic referral to breast clinics. In Chapter 11, Caroline Begaj explains the principal role ultrasound has in the investigation of the male breast, describes the ultrasound appearances of the most common male breast pathologies, and discusses the need for improvements in diagnostic breast services for men.

Despite the excellent sensitivity and specificity that can be achieved with a breast ultrasound examination, there is an unavoidable need to obtain cellular material or a tissue sample in some cases to confirm the diagnosis and obtain additional prognostic information. In most instances, ultrasound is the technique of choice for guiding minimally invasive percutaneous needle procedures to obtain such samples. Chapter 12 describes how to perform a wide range of currently used needle procedures and includes a thorough discussion of why and when each procedure is appropriate and what the potential complications are.

In a diagnostic breast service, ultrasound is only one of several imaging techniques available; mammography, computed tomography, magnetic resonance imaging and radionuclide imaging can also be used to produce images of the breast, with each technique being based on a fundamentally different physical property of the tissue. Chapter 13 reviews the relative place of these techniques in breast diagnosis and in the staging and follow-up of malignant disease.

Throughout this book, reference is continually made to the need for the ultrasound operator to be well trained and to practice within a coherent multidisciplinary context. In Chapter 14, Jacquie Lee considers the factors that have informed current models of breast imaging service provision and how a multidisciplinary and interprofessional pedagogic approach to ultrasound education and training produces a highly informed and 'reflective' practitioner who is capable of delivering a high quality breast ultrasound service.

SAFETY OF ULTRASOUND

Conspicuous by its absence anywhere in this book is a lengthy discussion of ultrasound safety and consideration of the associated biological risks and hazards. Traditionally ultrasound is promoted as a 'safe and non-invasive' diagnostic test and, particularly when considered with radiation-based diagnostic imaging alternatives such as plain film radiography (mammography), computed tomography and radionuclide imaging, it is usually advocated early in the diagnostic pathway. Lower capital and revenue costs and its accessibility give it an obvious edge over the other 'safe' diagnostic imaging technique, magnetic resonance imaging.

In theory, there is the potential for ultrasound-induced thermal and mechanical tissue damage—several classic ultrasound physics texts explain the underlying physical mechanisms and the conditions for such effects in detail. Of particular interest is the fact that newer image processing developments invariably require higher power outputs than are used for standard traditional imaging formats; the implication thus is that those involved in research and development need to remain mindful of the potential for harm (Duck & Shaw 2003). Fundamentally, ultrasound is a safe imaging test; there is no evidence of a clinically significant adverse bio-effect in routine diagnostic practice (AIUM 1997, EFSUMB

2003). Application of the ALARA principle—to keep exposure 'as low as reasonably achievable', however, applies to ultrasound examinations just as it does to ionizing radiation examinations. As with all requests for imaging investigations, it is important to consider the potential impact of the test results on patient management and only to undertake examinations when the benefit to the patient from the information obtained is likely to outweigh the associated risks of the investigation process (Duck & Shaw 2003, p. 181). When performed inappropriately, the examination may place patients at risk of unnecessary further investigation and/or intervention.

Of the multiple hazards associated with an ultrasound examination, however (Table 1.1), by far the greatest hazard is the potential for misdiagnosis—with the inexperienced or uninformed operator failing to implement the correct technique and/or failing to interpret the image appearances accurately. The ultrasound operator's safety responsibilities are summarized in Table 1.2;

Table 1.1 Hazards associated with ultrasound examinations

Hazard	Risk reduction strategy
Diagnostic error	Use of well-trained competent personnel
Biological	
Cross-infection	Adherence to local infection control policies
Allergic reaction	Use of inert scanning gel; verbal screening when using 'perfumed' gel, transducer covers and examination gloves (latex sensitivity)
Chemical	Use of appropriate transducer cleaning and disinfection materials
Electrical	Electrical insulation of transducer and cables
	Regular electrical safety testing
Mechanical	Physical sealing of transducer mechanism—no risk with electronic arrays
Acoustic	Application of ALARA principle
	Minimize scanning time, dwell time and transducer–skin contact time
	Minimize power output and intensity
	Adhere to safety (TI and MI) limits
	Minimize exposure if pyrexic

Table 1.2 Safety responsibilities invested in the ultrasound practitioner

Be properly trained	Anatomy and physiology
	Strengths and weaknesses of equipment
	Appropriate scanning technique
Keep knowledge up-to-date	
Technology advances	New artifacts
	Safety guidance documents from special interest professional organizations, e.g. AIUM, BMUS, EFSUMB, WFUMB
Changing practice	New applications
Choose and use appropriate equipment and technique for:	
Type of examination to be performed	Breast-specific transducer
	Breast-specific pre-sets
Condition of patient	Few contraindications: in the non-pregnant adult, breast is a 'low-risk' application
Ensure equipment is well maintained and complies with safety standards	Displays TI and MI
	Maintain and repair as per QA protocol
	Liaise with manufacturers and engage in debate to develop industry standards
Follow good practice for reducing risks	Perform examinations only when clinically indicated
	Make sure you have a complete and accurate clinical history
	Keep transducer–skin contact time to minimum required for obtaining information required
	Use Doppler only when likely to add clinically significant additional information

From Duck & Shaw (2003) with permission of Cambridge University Press for Greenwich Medical Media.

this book should help the practitioner meet these responsibilities.

SUMMARY

The provision of high quality breast ultrasound is dependent upon the personnel delivering the service, the equipment available, its utilization and the overall clinical context within which the breast ultrasound service is provided. When all these are optimized, the technique has an invaluable role in the diagnosis and management of patients with breast symptoms.

This book provides a comprehensive introduction to multiple aspects of breast ultrasound service provision. In addition, it signposts the interested reader to relevant primary research reports, reviews by acclaimed breast imaging experts and further classic ultrasound and breast imaging texts.

References

AIUM 1997 Clinical Safety (online) American Institute of Ultrasound in Medicine. Online. Available at: http://www.aium.org/publications/statements/_statement Selected.asp?statement=11 Accessed on 19 March 2006.

Bamber JC 2005 Advances in breast ultrasound. Proceedings of 37th Annual Scientific Meeting of the British Medical UIltrasound Society, Manchester UK. Ultrasound 13(4):269.

Duck FA, Shaw A 2003 Safety of diagnostic ultrasound. In: Hoskins PR, Thrush A, Martin K, Whittingham TA (eds) Diagnostic ultrasound physics and equipment. London: Greenwich Medical Media, pp. 179–203.

EFSUMB 2003 Clinical safety statement for Diagnostic Ultrasound. Copenhagen: European Committee of Medical Ultrasound Safety, European Federation of Societies of Ultrasound in Medicine and Biology. Online. Available at: http://www.efsumb.org/efsumb/committees/Safety_Committee/Safety_Eng/safety_stat2003.htm Accessed on 19 March 2006.

Further reading

Barnett SB 1998 WFUMB Symposium on Safety of Ultrasound in Medicine: conclusions and recommendations regarding thermal and non-thermal mechanisms for biological effects of ultrasound. Ultrasound in Medicine and Biology 24(S1):1–55.

BMUS 2000 Safety of ultrasound. London: British Medical Ultrasound Society. Online. Available: http:// www.bmus.org/safety_of_ultrasoundNF.htm Accessed on 19 March 2006.

ter Haar G, Duck FA (eds) 2000 The safe use of ultrasound in medical diagnosis. London: British Medical Ultrasound Society/British Institute of Radiology.

Chapter **2**

Breast cancer, diagnosis and imaging: a historical perspective

Gillian R. Clough

CHAPTER CONTENTS

INTRODUCTION

What is thought to be the first documented evidence of breast cancer was found on an ancient piece of papyrus originating from Egypt over 3500 years ago (Olson 2002) and in fact may describe a male breast cancer (Boulos 1986). Since that time, physicians have striven to understand, control and cure this disease.

The name 'cancer' first appeared around 200 BC and is a latin translation of *karkinos* a term used in Hippocratic writings to describe both benign and malignant tumors. A demarcation between inflammatory and neoplastic tumors was not made until the second half of the nineteenth century (Rather 1978).

PREVALENCE, INCIDENCE AND RISK FACTORS

Ninety-nine percent of all breast cancers occur in females. In the UK, there are over 41 000 new cases of breast cancer diagnosed, and just under 13 000 deaths attributed to the disease, per year, whilst in North America there are approximately a quarter of a million cases diagnosed, and almost 41 000 deaths per year (Cancer Research UK 2004, Imaginis 2005).

One of the earliest epidemiological studies on the mortality of cancer, conducted by Rigoni-Stern in Verona from 1760 to 1839, found that nuns were five times more likely to die of breast cancer than married women (Greaves 2000), but offered no explanation as to why this might be, although others cited the cause as celibacy.

The epidemiology of breast cancer has proved to be complex. An estimate of global deaths attributed to breast cancer in 2000 was just under half a million (Shibuya et al 2002). The incidence of the disease is five times greater in the developed world than the undeveloped world and Japan (Key et al 2002), and in England and Wales it is estimated that 1 in 9 women will develop breast cancer at some point in their life (National Statistics 1996) whilst in North America the estimated figure is 1 in 7 women (Imaginis 2005).

Areas of the world that have seen rapid development have also seen rapid increases in the incidence of breast cancer (Gao et al 2000), with émigrés from undeveloped countries tending to acquire the incidence rates of their new country (Doll & Peto 1981). Breast cancer has also been shown to be more prevalent in higher social classes (Pukkala & Weiderpass 1999). This evidence points to lifestyle and environmental factors as possible reasons for the pattern of incidence rather than an increased susceptibility by virtue of race. Breast cancer is without doubt a multifactorial disease.

Much research has been undertaken over the last three decades into the causes of breast cancer; much of it is contradictory, but some factors show strong correlation.

The strongest and undisputed risk factor for breast cancer is age. As women get older their risk of developing breast cancer increases, with postmenopausal women being at greatest risk (Botha et al 2003); this pattern is universal.

In addition to age, epidemiologists noted that some families seemed to have significantly higher incidences, and researchers sought the existence of genetic mutations to account for an increased susceptibility. To date, several genes have been identified in which mutations give rise to a predisposition to breast cancer (Box 2.1). The normal function of these genes is associated with control of the cell cycle and/or DNA repair.

It is estimated that familial breast cancer accounts for only about 5–10% of all breast cancers overall (Bennett & Gattas 1999, Olsen et al 1999), with less than half being down to BRCA-1 and BRCA-2 (Greaves 2000). However, in some ethnic populations, the prevalence of mutant genes is much higher, for example 1 in 50 Ashkenazi Jews will have a mutant form of BRCA-1 or BRCA-2 compared with 1 in 800 of the world population (Greaves 2000). The involvement of these genes in DNA repair should be carefully considered before embarking down the route of mammographic screening for individuals with a strong family history of breast cancer, due to the potential for DNA damage from ionizing radiation.

Undisputed as these factors are, none of the above explains the higher prevalence of breast cancer in the developed world. The disparity is thought to be due to lifestyle and/or environmental factors.

A fundamental difference between women in the developed and undeveloped world is their reproduction patterns. Women in undeveloped countries tend to have a greater number of pregnancies, and are far more likely to breastfeed and to breastfeed for longer periods than women in developed countries. Studies have shown that a woman's risk of developing breast cancer decreases with each successive pregnancy and as the total period of time breastfeeding increases (Collaborative Group on Hormonal Factors in Breast Cancer 2002a). Women in developed countries have their first child later in life than women in undeveloped countries and again for each year delay in first pregnancy the risk of developing breast cancer increases. Having said this, there is evidence that in the first years following each pregnancy a woman's risk is slightly elevated (Bruzzi et al 1988). A re-analysis of data linking spontaneous and induced abortions to an elevated risk of breast cancer showed no correlation when confounding factors were removed (Collaborative Group on Hormonal Factors in Breast Cancer 2004).

Interestingly, women who have a late first pregnancy have been shown to be at greater risk of developing breast cancer than women who have never been pregnant. It is believed that in these women, when pregnancy provides the stimulus for ductal epithelial proliferation in the breast, the growth of any existing cancer cells within the breast is also promoted (Greaves 2000).

A relationship between duration of a woman's fertile years and breast cancer has been established. Women who start menstruation at an early age (early menarche) and/or experience a late menopause have an increased risk of developing breast cancer (Collaborative Group on Hormonal Factors in Breast Cancer 2002a, 2004). In societies with a higher calorific intake, the age at menarche is lower (Key et al 2002); women in the undeveloped world are generally older at first menarche than women in the developed world.

Hormonal factors which may account for some of the discrepant incidence between the developed and undeveloped world are the use of oral contraceptives and hormone replacement therapy (HRT). There is strong

---

Box 2.1　Genes associated with increased risk of breast cancer

BRCA-1
BRCA-2
p53　Found in Li–Fraumenei syndrome
PTEN　Found in Cowden's syndrome
ATM　Found in ataxia telangiectasia

Greaves 2000, Ishmail et al 2004,
Thompson et al 2005

evidence that women who are taking combined oral contraceptives or have used them in the last 10 years have an elevated risk of developing breast cancer (Collaborative Group on Hormonal Factors in Breast Cancer 1996). Likewise, women taking HRT have an elevated risk of developing breast cancer which again decreases 5 years after cessation of use (Collaborative Group on Hormonal Factors in Breast Cancer 1997); there is also evidence to suggest that women taking HRT have an increased breast cancer mortality rate (Million Women Study Collaborators 2003). Again, use and/or access to oral contraception and HRT is lower in undeveloped countries than in Western societies.

Diet and exercise have been shown to affect breast cancer risk. Postmenopausal obesity has been associated with an elevated risk of breast cancer, probably by increasing the serum concentration of free estradiol (Key et al 2002). Physical activity has been linked with breast cancer risk, with women who undertake little exercise at increased risk, although separating risk from obesity and risk from low physical activity is difficult as the two factors often coexist (Greenwald 1999).

In terms of lifestyle, alcohol and tobacco use have been studied as possible causal factors for breast cancer. It has been estimated that alcohol accounts for around 4% of breast cancers in the developed world, but no conclusive evidence has been found that smoking increases the risk of developing breast cancer (Collaborative Group on Hormonal Factors in Breast Cancer 2002b).

Environmental factors (such as exposure to ionizing radiation) may increase an individual's risk of breast cancer. There is evidence that women treated with radiotherapy for childhood cancers suffer an increased incidence of breast cancer (Kenny et al 2004) and women exposed to moderate to large doses of radiation in the Japanese atomic bomb blasts or for benign medical conditions such as ringworm, between 1930 and 1960, were found to have an increased incidence of breast cancer (Greaves 2000). The impact of ionizing radiation on a population as a whole will be relatively minor compared with reproductive and hormonal factors; however, it is accepted that diagnostic mammography in all probability induces cancer in a very small proportion of women (Law 1997).

In summary, the factors which predispose women to developing breast cancer can be divided into two categories; those which women have no control over and those which lifestyle choices impact upon (Table 2.1).

TUMOR CLASSIFICATION

Tumors consist of both proliferating neoplastic cells, which characterize the nature of the tumor, and a host-

Table 2.1 Factors influencing risk of breast cancer

Non-controllable factors
  Age
  Genetic mutation
  Length of fertile life
Controllable factors
  Number of pregnancies
  Age at first pregnancy
  Breastfeeding
  Diet and exercise
  Hormonal pharmaceutical use
  Alcohol intake
  Ionizing radiation exposure

derived support stroma of connective tissue and blood vessels that determines the tumor growth pattern (Ibrahim & Tulbah 2001).

Tumor classification is achieved through gross and microscopic histological examination of representative tissue from the tumor and is based on cell histogenesis, differentiation and biological behavior (Ibrahim & Tulbah 2001). A precise histological diagnosis enables healthcare professionals to predict the clinical course of a tumor and is thus required to inform treatment planning and patient counseling.

Whilst benign tumors have well differentiated cells and have characteristics that suggest they will remain localized, malignant tumor cells are enlarged, pleomorphic (varied in shape and size), exhibit a disorganized growth pattern and have features that enable them to breach normal tissue boundaries, invade lymphatic and vascular spaces and allow tumor emboli to be transported to remote sites where they can implant and form new tumor foci (Ibrahim & Tulbah 2001). In addition to abnormalities in cell proliferation, more recently, malignant transformation has also been attributed to aberrations in the control of normal physiological cell death mechanisms resulting in neoplastic extension of the normal life span of ordinary cells (Ibrahim & Tulbah 2001). A similar transformation is sometimes seen with cytotoxic chemotherapy regimes, with a resultant increase rather than reduction in tumor virulence (Greaves 2000).

Tumors are usually given names that pertain to their assumed cells of origin and their predicted behavior, e.g. fibroadenoma, ductal carcinoma, lipoma, fibrosarcoma. Classification of malignant breast disease is discussed further in Chapter 9 where the respective clinical and imaging features are also considered.

TUMOR GRADING

In addition to classifying tumors, the histological features are used to grade the disease, giving a measure of the degree of malignancy, and therefore an indication of disease prognosis, by assessing several tumor cell morphology and function characteristics. Assessment criteria are reasonably well defined, and although grading and tumor typing are inevitably qualitative and subjective due to tumor heterogeneity, sampling error and inherent observer variability, reproducibility is improved with strict adherence to the criteria and the use of well-fixed specimens (Denley et al 2001). Small preoperative (needle core biopsy) samples, however, are particularly vulnerable to sampling error and undergrading (Denley et al 2001).

The modified Bloom and Richardson system is used to grade invasive cancers. Three features of malignant tissue are considered, tubule formation/architecture, nuclear pleomorphism and mitotic count/mitotic index.

Each feature is awarded a score of 1, 2 or 3; all scores are then totaled and the tumor graded accordingly (Elston & Ellis 1991):

- 3–5 grade I well differentiated
- 6–7 grade II moderately differentiated
- 8–9 grade III poorly differentiated.

Tumors exhibiting 'special type' features, i.e. tubular, mucinous, medullary or lobular, often generate low scores and are thus associated with a more favorable prognosis (Allemani et al 2004, Vu-Nishino et al 2005).

TUMOR STAGING AND PROGNOSIS

Tumor staging describes the total anatomical extent of malignant disease and is important for predicting prognosis.

The 'TNM' system is the most widespread system of tumor staging, attributing scores to describe the extent of the primary tumor (T), and the presence or absence of metastases in the regional lymph nodes (N) and at distant sites (M). TNM staging can be carried out on several occasions during the clinical course of a disease to reflect the amount of information available from diagnostic tests and the response of the tumor to therapeutic interventions (Ibrahim & Tulbah 2001). Table 2.2 contains a summarized version of the TNM system.

In 1991, Elston and Ellis demonstrated that there were three features which strongly correlated with breast cancer survival rates: tumor grade, tumor size and the presence or absence of metastatic deposits in the axillary lymph nodes. From their original research, conducted in

Table 2.2 TNM classification of breast cancer

T_{is}	In situ disease
T_1	≤2 cm
T_2	2–5 cm
T_3	>5 cm
T_4	Involvement of one or both of the following 　Chest wall 　Skin Inflammatory cancer
N_0	No regional lymph node metastasis
N_1	Metastasis in movable ipsilateral lymph nodes
N_2	Metastasis in fixed ipsilateral axillary lymph node(s) or in clinically apparent ipsilateral internal mammary lymph node(s) in the absence of clinically evident axillary lymph node metastasis
N_3	Metastasis in ipsilateral infraclavicular lymph node(s) with or without axillary lymph node involvement; or in clinically apparent ipsilateral internal mammary lymph node(s) and when occurring in the presence of clinically evident axillary lymph node metastasis; or metastasis in ipsilateral supraclavicular lymph node(s) with or without axillary or internal mammary lymph node involvement
M_0	No distant metastases
M_1	Distant metastases

T = tumor; N = lymph node; M = metastases.
T, N or M followed by X indicates that the feature could not be assessed.
(NHS Cancer Screening Programmes and The Royal College of Pathologists 2005, National Cancer Institute 2006).

Nottingham, they arrived at a formula that enabled an individual woman's prognosis to be calculated (Box 2.2). The Nottingham Prognostic Index (Table 2.3) is routinely used in the UK as a means of estimating the prognosis of individuals diagnosed with breast cancer and to tailor treatment to individual need.

The size of the tumor at diagnosis depends to a great extent on the method of presentation, i.e. symptomatic or screening, but the aggressiveness of the tumor, i.e. how quickly it grows, and the texture of the surrounding breast tissue, i.e. glandular or fatty, also influence size at diagnosis.

At the time of diagnosis, larger and higher grade tumors are more likely to have metastasized via the lymphatic and vascular systems. This necessitates systemic treatment and is associated with diminished survival

Box 2.2   Nottingham prognostic index formula

NPI = 0.2 × invasive cancer size (cm) + tumor grade + node score
Node score of 1: (no positive lymph nodes), 2 (1–3 positive), 3 (≥4 positive)

Table 2.3   Nottingham prognostic index

EPG	Excellent prognostic group	≤2.4
GPG	Good prognostic group	2.401–3.4
MPG1	Moderate prognostic group 1	3.401–4.4
MPG2	Moderate prognostic group 2	4.401–5.4
PPG	Poor prognostic group	>5.4

(NHS Breast Screening Programme, Association of Breast Surgery at BASO 2005).

rates. Lymphatic spread can be determined by removal and histological examination of ipsilateral axillary lymph nodes at the same time as the therapeutic breast surgery. The presence of vascular space invasion can be seen on microscopic examination of the primary tumor.

In addition to grading and staging, it is now standard practice to establish the hormone receptor status of the tumor in order to identify patients who would benefit from antiestrogen therapy (Denley et al 2001). It is also important to establish a clear surgical margin (usually 1 cm) between the tumor, including any ductal carcinoma in situ, and the excision margins.

Once a diagnosis has been made and the staging process completed, adjuvant therapy such as radiotherapy, chemotherapy and antiestrogen therapy may be given. In approximately 20% of invasive breast cancers there is over expression of the HER-2 protein; in these cases Herceptin has been shown to improve survival rates. However, Herceptin has significant side effects and its use in treating women without metastatic disease is controversial (Priest 2005). Overall, the long-term prognosis for all breast cancer patients continues to slowly improve.

HISTORY OF DETECTION AND TREATMENT

Prior to the mid 1800s, treatment for breast cancer had progressed from a selection of ineffective treatments including the application of noxious poultices, ingestion of various tonics (rhubarb, opium, castor oil and olive oil) and excisions of lumps, to an essentially crude amputation of the breast, with only a minority of patients surviving the ordeal. With the discovery of ether as an anesthetic in 1842, surgeons had more time to perfect their techniques, and in the 1880s William Halstead, using an aseptic technique, pioneered the radical mastectomy—removing the breast en bloc along with the axillary contents and pectoral muscles. Halstead had studied the 3-year survival rates of leading European surgeons prior to developing his technique, and found average survival to be about 20% (Raven 1990). He then carefully audited his patients, on whom he had used his new technique; his 3-year survival rate was almost 40% (Shimkin 1977).

Despite this achievement, many women suffered recurrent disease and endured ever more aggressive surgery before eventually dying of their disease. Into the late twentieth century women continued to fear both the disease and its treatment, and many waited until their cancer was well established before seeking medical help. Even women presenting with relatively small tumors suffered disease recurrence, and surgeons realized they would have to find more effective methods of systemic treatment or detecting tumors earlier in their development, if they were going to make any further impact on achieving a cure.

The discovery of X-rays by Roentgen in 1895 provided medicine with a new diagnostic tool (Beiser 1995). In 1913, the German surgeon Salomon began taking radiographs of amputated breasts and discovered that both palpable and impalpable abnormalities were visible radiographically (Bassett & Gold 1988). In 1930, Warren published the results of radiographic examinations of both normal and symptomatic breasts using a stereoscopic technique on living subjects (Warren 1930). The detail of these early images was restricted by equipment limitations, and mammography did not become more widely practiced until the 1950s following Leborgne and Gershon-Cohen's articles on the radiographic appearances of normal and abnormal breasts (Bassett & Gold 1988).

In the early 1960s, results of studies using mammography for screening asymptomatic women were published, demonstrating that clinically occult disease could be detected (Gershon-Cohen et al 1961, Wolfe 1965). These studies were conducted using conventional X-ray tubes operating at between 28 and 31 kVp, at approximately 30 inches film focal distance (FFD) and using mAs of 1500 per view with direct exposure (non-screen) film. During this period, Stanton and associates investigated the equipment and exposure factors used for mammography and evaluated their effect on radiation dose and image quality (Stanton et al 1963, Stanton &

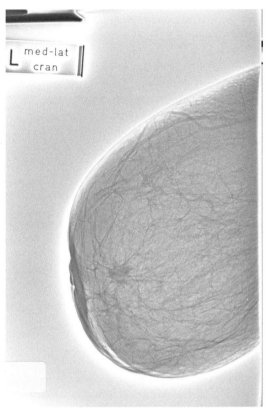

Figure 2.1

Lightfoot 1964). They made recommendations for the required specification of equipment used for mammography (Box 2.3).

The radiation doses received from these early mammographic examinations were high and in some cases resulted in deterministic skin effects including blistering and moist desquamation (Wright et al 1971).

In the mid 1960s, the technique of xeromammography was introduced. Selenium, a semi-conductor, is coated onto a conductive metal plate and, prior to exposure, a uniform positive electrostatic charge is applied to the selenium. Selenium is a photoconductor and, as a consequence, when exposed to X-radiation, charge is conducted from the surface of the selenium plate to the metal substrate leaving a latent image of differential charge on the selenium surface. Negatively charged blue powder is then applied to the surface of the plate and is more attracted to less exposed areas which still hold positive charge. The powder image is fused into coated paper by means of heat (Jenkins 1980). Xeromammography had the advantage of edge enhancement, the electric field distribution produced at tissue boundaries causing extra deposition of powder at these sites, allowing small variations in radiation absorption to be better demonstrated, giving greater contrast compared with the conventional film technique of the day (Figure 2.1). Just as

importantly, xeromammography produced satisfactory images at far higher kVp and much lower mA, thereby reducing the radiation dose significantly (Ruzicka et al 1965).

In the mid 1960s, thermography emerged as a method of imaging the breast. The body emits infrared radiation the intensity of which is determined by body temperature. Thermography units converted infrared radiation into visible light to which Polaroid film was exposed (Gershon-Cohen & Haberman 1964), thereby creating an image. Any breast abnormality with increased blood supply will emit more infrared radiation than surrounding normal tissue and would therefore be seen on the resultant thermogram. Thermal imaging was, and to this day is, an attractive imaging modality because it does not involve ionizing radiation or require the breast to be compressed; however, its significant limitation is that it does not demonstrate morphological features and therefore allow characterization of abnormalities. Thermography's reliance on vascularity alone as a means of detection does not allow differentiation between vascular abnormalities with morphologically malignant and benign features whilst avascular pathology remains occult; this gives the technique somewhat reduced sensitivity when compared with X-ray mammography (Williams et al 1990).

The first dedicated mammography unit was developed in the mid 1960s incorporating a molybdenum, rather than tungsten, target to maximize radiation contrast. The unit also had a breast compression device and a smaller focal spot (0.7 mm), resulting in decreased movement and geometric unsharpness in the image (Bassett & Gold 1988).

The first large-scale randomized controlled mammography screening trial, with the effect on mortality in the interventional group as a major outcome measure, took place in New York. The results of this Health Insurance Plan (HIP) study were published in 1977 (Shapiro 1977). This was followed in 1979 by the results of the Swedish two-counties trials (Andersson et al 1979, Lundgren 1979) which were again randomized controlled trials but focused on comparing the etiology of the cancers detected in the screened and control groups, as well as attendance rates and the cost effectiveness of screening a population. The HIP study used both clinical breast examination and mammography to screen women aged 40–64 years in the intervention group and found that both contributed equally to the detection of cancer overall, but that mammography was of little value in women younger than 50 years of age. The mortality rate of women undergoing screening was a third less than in the control group. In Sweden, Lundgren's study used single view (oblique) mammography to screen women aged over 35 years, whilst Andersson used two-view mammography to screen women aged 50–64 years; both studies recalled subjects with abnormalities for further tests. Both studies provided detailed costings and demonstrated that fewer cancers were detected in younger women. All three studies found that the cancers detected through screening were less advanced than cancers presenting symptomatically in the control groups.

By the mid 1970s, X-ray film manufacturers had developed dedicated single emulsion mammography film to be used in conjunction with a single intensifying screen; these together with the advantages of a dedicated mammography unit meant that radiation dose could be significantly reduced when compared with both direct exposure film and xerographic plates, whilst still maintaining good contrast and resolution (Haus et al 1975, Chang et al 1976).

In 1985, Professor Sir Patrick Forrest chaired a working party investigating the efficacy of a national breast screening program in the UK. The subsequent report published in 1986 (Forrest et al 1986) stated

'high quality single medio-lateral oblique view mammography has been shown to be an effective method of reducing mortality from breast cancer and we conclude that this is the preferred option for the development of mass population screening'. In 1988 the National Health Service breast screening programme (NHSBSP) was established as a result of the Forrest report, and national coverage was achieved by the mid 1990s.

The NHSBSP is comprised of approximately 90 screening units utilizing both mobile and static screening facilities in order to ease access for the target population and maximize attendance rates. It is centrally coordinated and sets national targets and standards which are monitored through the national quality assurance network (Caseldine & Pearce 1992). Training for staff is provided at five centers in the UK and, once staff have reached the desired competence level, their performance is continually reviewed thereafter (Caseldine et al 1994).

Originally the screening program used single oblique view mammography to screen women aged 50–64 every 3 years. This changed, following publication of the NHS Cancer Plan in 2000, to two-view mammography, as subsequent research found that 24% more women with cancer were detected with two-view mammography (Wald et al 1995). The age range has been extended to 70 years in response to pressure groups representing the elderly (Greengross 1996). Patients who are found to have a suspicious abnormality on initial screening are recalled to an assessment center for 'triple assessment'— further imaging, clinical examination and needle biopsy if required (Vetto et al 1995). Following a positive biopsy result, women requiring treatment are given an appointment to see a breast surgeon within 5 days (Wilson et al 2001).

In light of the success of the breast screening program and the consistently high standards it achieves, the Royal College of Radiologists produced the *Guidance on Screening and Symptomatic Breast Imaging* in 1999 (RCR 1999). This document explicitly states that equipment and services for symptomatic breast imaging should meet the requirements laid down by the NHSBSP. As a result, symptomatic breast imaging services have improved and in some areas have merged with the screening services.

Thanks to pioneering work by oncologist Robert McWirter in the 1930s, women diagnosed with breast cancer no longer have to face the radical Halstead mastectomy; instead they are offered morbidity-reducing breast-conserving surgery with radiotherapy, or simple mastectomy with or without radiotherapy (Olsen 2002). Although the incidence of breast cancer is rising in the UK, early diagnosis and intervention, prompted by the introduction of performance targets by the government

(National Institute for Clinical Excellence 2002), good surgical techniques and improved cytotoxic and antiestrogen regimes have ensured that mortality rates are falling (Botha et al 2003).

ULTRASOUND IMAGING OF THE BREAST

B-mode ultrasound of palpable breast masses was performed in the mid 1970s using relatively low (2.5 MHz) transducer frequencies by today's standards. However, Cole-Beuglet and Beique failed to demonstrate 20% of palpable lesions in their ultrasound study, all of which were less than 2 cm in size (Cole-Beuglet & Beique 1975).

Ultrasound, like thermography, does not utilize ionizing radiation or require the breast to be compressed. Ultrasound, however, is able to delineate morphological features and internal architecture, allowing some characterization and the accurate measurement of abnormalities. Its use in imaging palpable abnormalities increased in the early 1980s and it was found to be a useful adjunct to mammography, increasing the preoperative diagnostic accuracy (Guyer et al 1986) in particular in the dense breast (Guyer & Dewbury 1985).

As ultrasound technology improved and higher frequency transducers became available, smaller structures within the breast were visualized. From its inception, the UK breast screening program included breast ultrasound as part of the triple assessment of recalled patients. The quality assurance body of the screening program originally advocated a minimum transducer frequency of 7.5 MHz for all assessment centers (Wilson et al 2001), and in 2005 this increased to 10 MHz (Wilson et al 2005).

In addition to improvements in transducer frequency, Doppler ultrasound started to be employed to interrogate breast abnormalities, particularly color flow Doppler. In order to thrive, malignant cells secrete angiogenic factors which enable tumors to grow their own blood vessels which in turn connect with the normal circulatory system. Malignant tumors are therefore more likely to have increased vascularity when imaging with color flow Doppler than benign lesions, although there is significant overlap.

With improvements in ultrasound image quality, screening ultrasound became more feasible and more desirable in view of raised anxiety over the possible induction of malignant breast lesions with the increasing popularity and availability of mammography. However, it is still not possible to reliably detect small clusters of microcalcification, an indicator of ductal carcinoma in situ, with ultrasound unless it is associated with a mass. Screening bilateral whole breast ultrasound is also

more time consuming than screening mammography. The Royal College of Radiologists recommended ultrasound as a first-line investigation in symptomatic women under the age of 35 as they are more likely to have benign abnormalities and mammography has lower sensitivity in younger women (RCR 1999).

The ultrasound technique used to interrogate the breast has been debated over recent years, with some advocating simple target scanning of an abnormality, to avoid detection of incidental, clinically insignificant longstanding, benign and clinically occult solid lesions, whilst others favor the possibility of detecting clinically and mammographically occult malignant disease by performing whole breast ultrasound. As yet there are no national guidelines as to which technique should be adopted.

CURRENT IMAGING REGIMES

Although the technologies available to image the breast have increased, the gold standard and first-line investigation for the majority of women remains mammography. The latest generation of mammography units incorporates dual targets and filters enabling the tube to produce X-ray beams of different qualities to cater for the range of breast densities encountered. Both CR (computed radiography) and DDR (direct digital radiography) are now available for mammography together with CAD (computer-aided detection) to improve the detection rate for cancer.

Mammography is used to evaluate the breasts of symptomatic patients aged 35 years or over and to screen high risk groups (familial or genetic predisposition and women aged 50 years or older), monitor tumor response to primary chemotherapy and for surveillance of the treated breast. It can be used to localize abnormalities for biopsy.

It is now generally acknowledged that ultrasound should be used as a first-line investigation in women aged under 35 years and to further assess palpable and mammographically detected abnormalities in all patients. Ultrasound is also useful in assessing the response of both benign and malignant lesions to treatment. It can be used to localize abnormalities for aspiration and biopsy.

Other imaging techniques that have niche roles in the diagnosis and management of breast disease are more fully discussed in Chapter 13. Magnetic resonance imaging and radionuclide imaging are valuable adjuncts for a small number of cases; however, the vast majority of cancers are still currently detected and diagnosed using a combination of X-ray mammography, ultrasound, clinical examination and tissue biopsy.

References

Allemani C, Sant M, Berrino F et al 2004 Prognostic value of morphology and hormone receptor status in breast cancer—a population-based study. British Journal of Cancer 91:1263–1268.

Andersson I, Andren L, Hildell J et al 1979 Breast cancer screening with mammography: a population based, randomised trial with mammography as the only screening mode. Radiology 132:273–276.

Bassett W, Gold RH 1988 The evolution of mammography. American Journal of Roentgenology 150:493–498.

Beiser A 1995 Concepts of modern physics. 5th edn. New York: McGraw-Hill.

Bennett IC, Gattas M 1999 The genetic basis of breast cancer and its clinical implications. Australian and New Zealand Journal of Surgery 69:95–105.

Botha JL, Bray F, Sankila R et al 2003 Breast cancer incidence and mortality trends in 16 European countries. European Journal of Cancer 39:1718–1729.

Boulos FS 1986 Oncology in Egyptian Papyri. In: Retsas S (ed.) Palaeo-oncology: the antiquity of cancer. London: Farrand Press, p. 38.

Bruzzi P, Negri E, Vecchia CL et al 1988 Short term increase in risk of breast cancer after full term pregnancy. British Medical Journal 297:1096–1098.

Cancer Research UK 2004 Information resource centre. Online. Available at: http://info.cancerresearchuk.org/cancerstats/types.breast/ Accessed on 21 December 2005.

Caseldine J, Pearce P 1992 A radiographic quality control manual for mammography. Sheffield: NHSBSP Publications.

Caseldine J, Cush S, Rossiter T et al 1994 Quality assurance guidelines for radiographers. Publication 30. Sheffield: NHSBSP Publications.

Chang CHJ, Sibala JL, Martin NL et al 1976 Film mammography: new low radiation technology. Radiology 121:215–217.

Cole-Beuglet C, Beique RA 1975 Continuous B-scanning of palpable breast masses. Radiology 117:123–128.

Collaborative Group on Hormonal Factors in Breast Cancer 1996 Breast cancer and hormonal contraceptives: collaborative reanalysis of individual data on 53297 women with breast cancer and 100239 women without breast cancer from 54 epidemiological studies. Lancet 347:1713–1727.

Collaborative Group on Hormonal Factors and Breast Cancer 1997 Breast cancer and hormone replacement therapy: collaborative reanalysis of data from 51 epidemiological studies of 52705 women with breast cancer and 108411 women without breast cancer. Lancet 350:1047–1059.

Collaborative Group on Hormonal Factors in Breast Cancer 2002a Breast cancer and breastfeeding: collaborative reanalysis of individual data from 47 epidemiological studies in 30 countries, including 50302 women with breast cancer and 96973 women without the disease. Lancet 360:187–195.

Collaborative Group on Hormonal Factors and Breast Cancer 2002b Alcohol, tobacco and breast cancer—collaborative reanalysis of individual data from 53 epidemiological studies, including 58515 women with breast cancer and 95067 women without the disease. British Journal of Cancer 87:1234–1245.

Collaborative Group on Hormonal Factors in Breast Cancer 2004 Breast cancer and abortion: collaborative reanalysis of data from 53 epidemiological studies, including 83000 women with breast cancer from 16 countries. Lancet 363:1007–1016.

Denley H, Pinder SE, Elston CW, Lee AHS, Ellis IO 2001 Pre-operative assessment of prognostic factors in breast cancer. Journal of Clinical Pathology 54:20–24.

Doll R, Peto R 1981 The causes of cancer: quantitative estimates of avoidable risks of cancer in the United States today. Journal of the National Cancer Institute 66:1191–1308.

Elston CW, Ellis IO 1991 Pathological prognostic factors in breast cancer. The value of histological grade in breast cancer: experience from a large study with long term follow up. Histopathology 19:403–410.

Forrest P, Chamberlain J, Elton A et al 1986 Breast cancer screening: Report to the Health Ministers of England, Wales, Scotland & Northern Ireland. London: Her Majesty's Stationery Office.

Gao YT, Shu X O, Dai Q et al 2000 Association of menstrual and reproductive factors with breast cancer risk: results from the Shanghai breast cancer study. International Journal of Cancer 87:295–300.

Gershon-Cohen J, Haberman JD 1964 Thermography. Radiology 82:280–285.

Gershon-Cohen J, Hermel MB, Berger SM 1961 Detection of breast cancer by periodic X-ray examinations. A five-year survey. Journal of the American Medical Association 176:1114–1116.

Greaves M 2000 Cancer the evolutionary legacy. Oxford: Oxford University Press.

Greengross S 1996 Breast screening has failed older women. British Medical Journal 313:559.

Greenwald P 1999 Role of dietry fat in the causation of breast cancer. Cancer Epidemiology, Biomarkers and Prevention 8:3–7.

Guyer PB, Dewbury KC 1985 Ultrasound of the breast in the symptomatic and X-ray dense breast. Clinical Radiology 36:69–76.

Guyer PB, Dewbury KC, Warwick D et al 1986 Direct contact B-scan ultrasound in the diagnosis of solid breast masses. Clinical Radiology 37:451–458.

Haus AG, Doi K, Chiles JT et al 1975 The effect of geometric and recording system unsharpness in mammography. Investigative Radiology 10(1):43–52.

Ibrahim EM, Tulbah AM 2001 Basic principles of tumour pathology and biology. In: Elgazzar A (ed.) The pathophysiological basis of nuclear medicine. Berlin: Springer-Verlag, pp. 170–178.

Imaginis 2005 The breast cancer resource. Online. Available at: http://imaginis.com/breasthealth/statistics.asp#1 Accessed on 21 December 2005.

Ismail SM, Buchholz TA, Story M et al 2004 Radiosensitivity is predicted by DNA end-binding complex density, but not by nuclear levels of band components. Radiotherapy and Oncology 72(3):325–332.

Jenkins D 1980 Imaging techniques and processes. In: Radiographic photography and imaging processes. Lancaster: MTP Press.

Kenny LB, Yasui Y, Inskip PD et al 2004 Breast cancer after childhood cancer: a report from the Childhood Cancer Survivor Study. Annals of Internal Medicine 141(8):590–597.

Key TJ, Allen NE, Spencer EA et al 2002 The effect of diet on risk of cancer. Lancet 360:861–868.

Law J 1997 Cancers detected and induced in mammographic screening: new screening schedules and younger women with family history. British Journal of Radiology 70:62–69.

Lundgren B 1979 Population screening for breast cancer by single view mammography in a geographic region of Sweden. Journal of the National Cancer Institute 62(6):1373–1379.

Million Women Study Collaborators 2003 Breast cancer and hormone-replacement therapy in the Million Women Study. Lancet 362:419–427.

National Cancer Institute 2006 TNM definitions. US National Institute of Health. Online. Available at: http://www.nci.nih.gov/cancertopics/pdq/treatment/breast/HealthProfessional/page3 Accessed on 17 January 2006.

National Institute for Clinical Excellence 2002. Guidance on cancer services: improving outcomes in breast cancer: manual update. Online. London: National Institute for Clinical Excellence. Available at: http://www.nice.org.uk/pdf/Improving_outcomes_breastcancer_manual.pdf Accessed on 2 February 2006.

National Statistics 1996 Cancer trends in England and Wales Appendix 1. Online. Available at: http://www.statistics.gov.uk/StatBase/xsdataset.asp?More=Y Accessed on 15 June 2005.

NHS Breast Screening Programme, Association of Breast Surgery at BASO 2005 An audit of screen detected breast cancers for the year of screening April 2003 to March 2004. Sheffield: NHS Cancer Screening Programmes.

NHS Cancer Screening Programmes, Royal College of Pathologists 2005 Pathology reporting of breast disease: a joint document incorporating the third edition of the NHS Breast Screening Programme's Guidelines for Pathology reporting in breast cancer screening and the second edition of the Royal College of Pathologists minimum dataset for breast cancer histopathology. Publication 58, Sheffield: NHS Cancer Screening Programmes.

Olsen JH, Seersholm N, Boice JD et al 1999 Cancer risk in close relatives of women with early-onset breast cancer—a population-based incidence study. British Journal of Cancer 79(3/4):673–679.

Olson JS 2002 Bathsheba's breast: women, cancer and history. Baltimore: Johns Hopkins University Press.

Priest L 2005 Herceptin debate comes amid scepticism about all drugs. The Globe and Mail November 24. Online. Available at: http://www.theglobeandmail.com/servlet/ArticleNews/TPStory/LAC/20051124/HHERCEPTIN24/TPHealth/ Accessed on 25 November 2005.

Pukkala E, Weiderpass E 1999 Time trends in socio-economic differences in incidence rates of cancer of the breast and female genital organs (Finland, 1971–1995). International Journal of Cancer 81:56–61.

Rather LJ 1978 The genesis of cancer: a study in the history of ideas. London: Johns Hopkins University Press.

Raven RW 1990 The theory and practice of oncology: historical evolution and present principles. Carnforth: Parthenon Publishing Group.

RCR 1999 Guidance on screening and symptomatic breast imaging. BFCR(99)12. London: The Royal College of Radiologists.

Ruzicka FF, Kaufman L, Shapiro G et al 1965 Xeromammography and film mammography: a comparative study. Radiology 85:260–269.

Shapiro S 1977 Evidence on screening for breast cancer from a randomised trial. Cancer 39(6 Suppl):2772–2782.

Shibuya K, Mathers CD, Boschi-Pinto C et al 2002 Global and regional estimates of cancer mortality and incidence by site: results for the global burden of disease 2000. British Medical Council Cancer 2:37. Online. Available at: http://www.biomedcentral.com/1471-2407/2/37 Accessed on 15 June 2005.

Shimkin MB 1977 Contrary to nature. Washington DC: US Department of Health, Education and Welfare.

Stanton L, Lightfoot DA 1964 The selection of optimum mammography technique. Radiology 83:442–454.

Stanton L, Lightfoot DA, Boyle JJ et al 1963 Physical aspects of breast radiography. Radiology 81(1):1–16.

Thompson D, Antoniou AC, Jenkins M et al 2005 Two ATM variants and breast cancer. Human Mutation 25(6):594–595.

Vetto J, Pommier R, Schmidt W et al 1995 Use of the 'Triple Test' for palpable breast lesions yields high diagnostic accuracy and cost savings. American Journal of Surgery 169:519–522.

Vu-Nishino A, Tavassoli FA, Ahrens WA et al 2005 Clinopathologic features and long term outcome of patients with medullary breast carcinoma managed with breast conserving therapy. International Journal of Radiation Oncology, Biology and Physiology 62(4):1040–1047.

Wald NJ, Murphy P, Major P et al 1995 UKCCCR multicentre randomised controlled trial of one and two view mammography in breast cancer screening. British Medical Journal 311:1189–1193.

Warren SL 1930 A roentgenologic study of the breast. American Journal of Roentgenology and Radium Therapy 24(2):113–124.

Williams KL, Phillips BH, Jones PA et al 1990 Thermography in screening for breast cancer. Journal of Epidemiology and Community Health 44(2):112–113.

Wilson R, Asbury D, Cooke J 2001 Clinical guidelines for breast cancer screening assessment. Publication 49. Sheffield: NHS Cancer Screening Programmes.

Wilson R, Liston J, Cooke J 2005 Clinical guidelines for breast cancer screening assessment. Publication 49. 2nd edn. Sheffield: NHS Cancer Screening Programmes.

Wolfe JN 1965 Mammography as a screening examination in breast cancer. Radiology 84:703–708.

Wright DJ, Nichini FM, Stauffer HM 1971 Beryllium window tubes for mammographic examinations. British Journal of Radiology 44:480.

Chapter **3**

Principles of diagnostic medical ultrasound

Heather Venables

INTRODUCTION

It is widely acknowledged that ultrasound is the most operator dependent of all imaging modalities. In the hands of an expert, the production of a diagnostic ultrasound image looks easy. However, both image acquisition and interpretation are hugely reliant on a reasonable depth of understanding of 'how ultrasound works.' Where this is lacking, there is considerable scope for confusion and thus misdiagnosis.

The aim of this chapter is to introduce enough of the underlying physical principles of ultrasound to enable the reader to make sense of image appearances specifically in relation to ultrasound of the breast. This chapter, and the next, which looks at ultrasound equipment and how to use it, are not intended as a substitute 'physics text book'. A number of other authors (Hedrick et al 1994, Zagzebski 1996, Hoskins et al 2003) have produced clear and 'readable' ultrasound physics and equipment texts, and the interested reader is referred to these for further detail and explanation. Chapter 4 should be read in conjunction with this chapter as it provides guidance, again which is breast ultrasound application specific, on equipment requirements, initial set-up, subsequent optimization of controls and quality assurance procedures. Chapter 4 also gives an overview of the relevance of some of the more recent technical developments in breast imaging.

GENERATION AND DETECTION OF ULTRASOUND

Sound of any description is simply the transfer of mechanical energy from a vibrating source through a medium. *Ultra*sound is defined as sound of a frequency above the human audible range, i.e. above 20 kHz. For the purposes of breast imaging, frequencies in the region of 7–15 MHz (7–15 million cycles per second) are required. Utilization of the piezoelectric effect enables the production of controlled vibrations within this frequency range.

The term *transducer* is used to describe a device that converts energy from one form to another. In the case of an ultrasound transducer, a device that is capable of converting both electrical energy into mechanical energy (sound generation) and mechanical energy into electrical energy (detection of return echoes from within the patient) is required.

Piezoelectric materials contract or expand when a voltage is applied across them; quartz crystal is a naturally occurring example. Manufactured piezoelectric materials include lead zirconate titanate (PZT), a synthetic ceramic used in the manufacture of diagnostic ultrasound transducers. Thin layers of such materials can be constructed to vibrate at a resonant frequency within the required range—these act as a source of ultrasound. Conversely, pressure or strain applied to the surface of the piezoelectric material will generate a positive or negative voltage. As the pressure wave of a returning 'echo' hits the transducer surface, a voltage is registered. The magnitude of this voltage is related directly to the amount of energy carried by the returning echo. The use of piezoelectric ceramics provides both controllable generation of high frequency sound and efficient detection of small returning pressure changes.

THE PULSE–ECHO PRINCIPLE

Diagnostic medical ultrasound utilises the pulse-echo principle to construct a two-dimensional image of anatomical structures within a patient. This is essentially the same principle bats use to catch insects through echolocation. A pulse of sound leaving the transducer will travel into the patient until it encounters an 'acoustic' interface. At such an interface, a proportion of the sound energy is reflected back to the transducer and this return echo is detected. If the speed of sound is known and the time taken for the echo to return is measured, the depth of the reflecting interface can be calculated (Fig. 3.1).

IMAGE FORMATION

Each pulse of sound transmitted into the patient will generate a stream of returning echoes from multiple reflecting interfaces at various depths within the tissue. The mechanical energy carried by each echo is converted into electrical energy by the piezoelectric crystals within the transducer, the magnitude of the voltages being proportional to the energy carried by each echo. In simple terms, these values are then stored within the

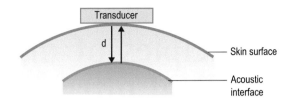

Depth of interface (d) = $\dfrac{\text{speed of sound} \times \text{time for echo to return}}{2}$

Figure 3.1   Diagram to illustrate how the depth of the reflecting interface is calculated from the sound pulse 'go–return' time.

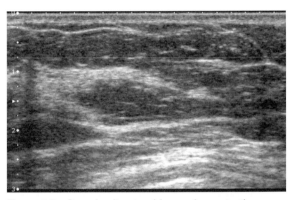

Figure 3.2   B-mode ultrasound image demonstrating a two-dimensional anatomical cross-section of breast tissue.

ultrasound machine's digital computer memory as a single 'scan line' of information; the voltage values are used to determine the brightness levels allocated to points in a vertical line on the image to represent the interfaces at corresponding depths in the patient. By firing pulses of sound in sequence from multiple adjacent piezoelectric crystals across the face of the transducer, numerous contiguous scan lines can be generated and a single *brightness mode* (B-mode) 'frame' of information produced to represent a two-dimensional anatomical cross-section (Fig. 3.2).

If performed fast enough, rapid update of frames can create a 'real time' image. The frame rate, however, is limited by several factors. The system must wait for echoes to return from the maximum depth of interest along each scan line before that line's next pulse is sent out. The time taken to produce each frame will depend on the depth of interest and the total number of scan lines in each frame. Frame rate is therefore limited by the width of the *field of view* (how many scan lines are required across the image), the *line density* (the number of lines per mm width in the image) and the *depth of view* selected (the deepest location from which echoes are displayed)—operator control of these features is discussed in Chapter 4.

The range of returning echo signal values arriving at the transducer is in the region of 1 000 000 : 1, from the strongest to the weakest. Due to the finite memory capacity of the computer, and the limited range of brightness levels available on the display monitor, it is impossible either to store or to display the whole range of values. Significant 'compression' of the returning signals is necessary. Initially this is achieved by rejecting the very weakest and the highest signals. The number of values between these extremes is further reduced by the use of *compression curves*. These allocate a single stored value to a range of similar returning signal values, thus reducing the total range of stored values. A similar process, the application of *gray-scale transfer curves*, is used to manipulate and compress the stored values further before they are displayed on the viewing monitor.

A significant amount of detail is lost from the returning signal through this processing, so it is essential that the equipment is programmed to apply compression and gray-scale transfer curves that maintain the range of signals of interest within the breast. Application-specific pre-sets are used to achieve this, but can, and in some circumstances should, be adjusted by the operator—Chapter 4 discusses how this is done in practice.

THE INTERACTION OF SOUND WITH BREAST TISSUE

During an ultrasound examination of the breast, most of the diagnostic conclusions about both normal and abnormal appearances are based upon four key observations:

- the spatial definition of tissue boundaries
- relative tissue reflectivity
- echo-texture

- the effect of tissue on the through transmission of sound.

All of these observations are based not just upon the anatomical structure of the breast, but also upon appearances within the image that are the result of how sound waves interact with breast tissue. A great deal of potentially useful diagnostic information can be inferred from these observations, but some understanding of how sound behaves is required to appreciate why the appearances arise.

ACOUSTIC IMPEDANCE

Acoustic impedance (Z) is a measure of the response that particles within a specific tissue will make as sound waves pass through it. Changes in pressure associated with transmission of the sound wave give rise to particle displacement. The acceleration and degree of this displacement depend on the impedance of the tissue; impedance is determined by tissue density and compressibility. Tissues that are dense and have low compressibility, e.g. dense glandular tissue, will have high impedance, and tissues that are less dense and have greater compressibility, e.g. fat, will have low impedance (Table 3.1).

The fundamental basis of ultrasound imaging is that some sound energy is reflected at interfaces across which there is a change in acoustic impedance. If there is sufficient difference between the density and compressibility of a breast 'lesion' compared with surrounding breast tissue, the lesion is potentially visible on ultrasound.

SOUND BEHAVIOR AT ACOUSTIC BOUNDARIES

In many ways, sound and light behave in a similar fashion. Concepts such as reflection, scattering and refraction are common to both.

Table 3.1   Acoustic impedance values

Tissue	Average speed of sound (ms^{-1})	Average density (kg m^{-3})	Acoustic impedance (kg m^{-2} s^{-1} × 10^{-6})
Breast fat	1470[a]	928[c] (range 917–939)	1.36
Breast tissue		1020[c] (range 990–1060)	
Premenopausal	1510[b] (range 1450–1570)		1.54
Postmenopausal	1468[b] (range 1430–1520)		1.49

[a]Scherzinger et al (1989).
[b]Kossoff G et al (1973).
[c]Duck (1990).

Reflection and lesion margin definition

Reflection of the ultrasound pulse occurs when there is a change in acoustic impedance across a boundary between tissues, i.e. if Z_1 and Z_2 are different in Figure 3.3. At such an acoustic interface, a proportion of the sound energy is reflected and the remaining sound energy is transmitted beyond the boundary.

If the boundary is smooth and large compared with the wavelength of the sound, *specular reflection* occurs. This is similar to when light is reflected from a smooth surface, and the laws of optical reflection can be used to predict the path that the reflected sound pulse (or 'echo') will follow. At 90° or *normal* incidence, a proportion of the sound pulse energy will be reflected directly back towards the transducer.

The relative proportions of reflected and transmitted energy are determined by the magnitude of the difference between the acoustic impedance on each side of the boundary. If the difference between Z_1 and Z_2 is small, most of the pulse energy will be transmitted and only a weak reflection occurs. If the difference is large, a high proportion of the energy will be reflected back to the transducer and the boundary will appear prominent (brighter) in the image.

As with light, where the sound pulse hits a boundary at an angle other than 90° it will be reflected at an equal and opposite angle, where the angle of incidence equals the angle of reflection (Fig. 3.4). This equates to the basic 'law of reflection' that we observe when light hits a highly reflective surface. If the angle at which the sound hits a boundary is sufficiently steep, the reflected echo may not be detected by the transducer (Fig. 3.5).

Reflection at a boundary is further complicated since the angle of incidence affects not only the direction of the reflected pulse, but also its intensity and the degree

of refraction that occurs in the transmitted component. In practice, boundaries will be detected most clearly if insonated at 90°—for this reason it is important to scan the breast using a variety of different transducer angulations.

Diffuse reflection occurs where irregularities in the tissue boundary exist that are small compared with the wavelength of the sound: at 10 MHz the wavelength is approximately 0.15 mm. These irregularities cause the sound energy to be reflected in multiple directions—an optical analogy would be to consider the difference between gloss and matt paint. In practice, most natural soft tissue boundaries are irregular and produce diffuse reflection to some degree.

In clinical breast ultrasound practice, the boundaries of breast lesions that have a smooth thin capsule, such as those of a cyst or fibroadenoma, act as specular reflec-

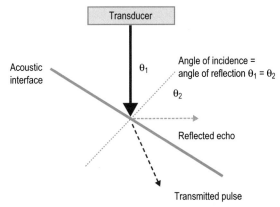

Figure 3.4   Diagram to illustrate that the angle of the reflected ultrasound beam is equivalent to the angle of the incident ultrasound beam.

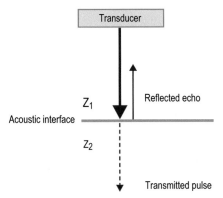

Figure 3.3   Diagram illustrating how an ultrasound 'echo' (or 'reflection') occurs when there is a boundary between tissues of different acoustic impedance.

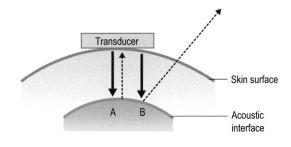

A pulse hitting the interface at A will be partially reflected directly back to the transducer. A pulse hitting the interface at B will be partially reflected back at an angle and may not be detected.

Figure 3.5   Diagram to illustrate how the reflected ultrasound pulse may not be detected at the transducer when the beam is directed obliquely at an acoustic interface.

tors and are clearly defined if insonated at 90° (Fig. 3.6). However, lesion margins that lie at more acute angles to the ultrasound beam, i.e. the lateral borders, are not well visualized and may even show some degree of posterior edge shadowing (see below—critical angle shadowing). The boundaries of lesions that lack a smooth capsular margin, such as those of an infiltrating carcinoma, act as diffuse reflectors and thus appear more ill defined in the image (Fig. 3.7).

Scattering and echo texture

Acoustic impedance changes occur at large-scale boundaries but are also present throughout soft tissue struc-

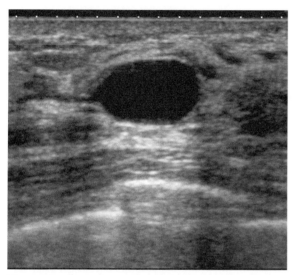

Figure 3.6 A cyst has a smooth thin capsule, its anterior and posterior surfaces are well defined.

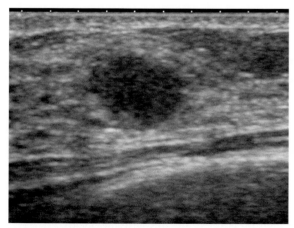

Figure 3.7 Lesions such as carcinomas are not so well defined if they have an irregular margin.

tures. Small-scale localized changes in acoustic property act as tiny reflecting targets that *scatter* the sound in many directions. If these targets are small compared with the wavelength of the sound, this is known as *Rayleigh scattering*.

The net effect of multiple scattering within the width of the ultrasound beam produces the characteristic echo texture (graininess) associated with soft tissue structures and their gray-scale shading. Scattering is highly frequency dependent and contributes to the overall loss of energy (attenuation) from the transmitted beam (see below).

Refraction

Refraction occurs when the ultrasound beam crosses a boundary between tissues that have different speeds of sound propagation; the term describes the phenomenon whereby the sound beam 'bends' from its original path. The effect of light refraction is seen clearly if a straw is placed in a glass of water (Fig. 3.8).

A similar effect occurs, for instance, when a sound beam travels from a region of low propagation speed, e.g. a fluid structure, into a region of higher speed, e.g. solid tissue. As the wave front crosses the boundary, the leading edge speeds up relative to the trailing edge and the transmitted wave front is deviated from its original path. The effects of refraction in the image are considered later in this chapter under 'artifacts'.

Attenuation

As sound travels through breast tissues, it will lose energy. A number of interactions contribute to this process of *attenuation* including reflection, scattering and absorption. This results in the sound pulse becoming

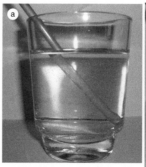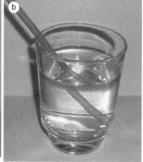

Figure 3.8 (a) Refraction of light—misregistration of the true position of the straw immersed in water. (b) The straw appears to bend as it enters the water because the speed of light in water and the speed in air are different.

progressively lower in energy (and therefore producing weaker echo signals) the deeper it travels into the patient.

If some sound energy is reflected at an interface, the intensity of the transmitted pulse is reduced. If the impedance difference is high enough, for example at a soft tissue–calcification interface, total attenuation occurs—all of the sound energy will be reflected and none transmitted to deeper structures.

If the reflecting target is small compared with the wavelength, Rayleigh scattering occurs; a small proportion of the total sound energy is scattered in all directions into the surrounding tissue, some of which will reach the transducer. Although most of the incident energy is transmitted, the scattered energy contributes to overall attenuation. Rayleigh scattering is highly frequency dependent (to the fourth power). This results in increased attenuation, and thus reduced *penetration* of the sound beam to deeper structures, when higher transmit frequencies are selected.

Absorption

Absorption is the process by which the mechanical energy carried by the sound pulse is converted into heat within the tissues. The exact mechanisms for energy loss are not fully understood, but absorption is the most significant form of attenuation in many tissues.

As the sound wave passes through tissue, the tissue particles oscillate back and forth creating regions of compression and rarefaction, and must both acquire and then release energy. At lower frequencies, there is efficient release of energy as the wave passes. At higher frequencies, there is insufficient time between wave fronts for this to occur, and particle displacement becomes out of phase with the passing wave. Some energy carried by the particles is then dissipated as heat. The degree of absorption is also determined by the structure and composition of the tissue (Hoskins et al 2003); absorption is therefore both tissue and frequency dependent.

Loss of energy through scattering and absorption is exponential, i.e. the energy is reduced by the same fraction for each unit distance traveled. Thus the sound beam is gradually reduced in intensity as it passes deeper into the tissue. The operator can compensate for this reduction in signal strength and *amplify* weaker signals from deeper tissues by using the time gain compensation (TGC) control (Fig. 3.9).

Beam penetration

The frequency-dependent nature of both absorption and scattering results in limited ability to penetrate to deeper tissues when using high frequency transducers. The high

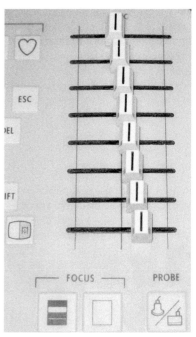

Figure 3.9 TGC slider controls that allow the operator to increase amplification of echoes from deeper structures to compensate for increased attenuation.

spatial and contrast resolution important for breast imaging is achieved at high frequency (see Ch. 4), but the ability to utilize a high frequency is limited by the requirement for adequate depth penetration. Fortunately, the breast is a superficial structure and rarely exceeds an antero-posterior depth greater than 4 cm; this routinely allows high resolution clinically useful images to be obtained at frequencies up to 15 MHz.

ULTRASOUND ARTIFACTS IN THE BREAST

In any diagnostic application of ultrasound, the recognition of what is 'real' in the image and what is '*artifact*' is an important part of the image interpretation process.

In the context of clinical imaging, artifacts are appearances within the image that do not correspond directly to the reality of structures within the patient. The structure of the breast is such that many artifacts are generated as sound travels through the different tissues. Appearances and relationships of real structures can be misrepresented, misplaced or absent, and spurious appearances can be generated within the image that simply do not have any true anatomical correlate.

However, artifacts are not always undesirable, indeed pathological lesions are often recognized and characterized by the artifacts they produce. To help distinguish between 'normal' and true pathological appearances, it is necessary to have a clear understanding of how ultrasound artifacts originate.

False assumptions

In ultrasound imaging, most artifacts arise because of one or more false assumptions that are basic design features of all ultrasound equipment. These assumptions include that:

- the speed of sound is constant
- sound always travels in a straight line along the axis of the beam
- the beam has negligible thickness
- the rate of attenuation in tissue is constant.

There are a number of features of both ultrasound transducer design and sound propagation that violate these basic assumptions and result in image artifacts. The origin of some of the more common artifacts is outlined here, whilst their operational and clinical significance is considered under technique and image interpretation in Chapters 6 and 7.

Variation in the speed of sound

The basic principle used in the scanner to calculate the depth of a reflecting interface, and thus the position of the body structures to be represented in the image, is that sound travels at a constant, known velocity. In practice, the *average speed of sound in soft tissue* is assumed to be 1540 ms^{-1} and ultrasound equipment is calibrated at this value. Where the true speed of sound in a structure is significantly different, for example within a breast implant, basic calculations of the depth of the reflecting surface will be inaccurate, resulting in misrepresentation of the size of the structure and its relationship to adjacent anatomic structures (Fig. 3.10).

The actual speed of sound in any particular tissue is determined by its density and compressibility. Generally, denser tissues are less compressible and sound will travel through them faster. Throughout its development and involution, the normal breast contains varying proportions of dense glandular tissue, fibrous connective tissue and fat. Kossoff et al (1973) measured the speed of sound in normal breast tissues (Table 3.2). There is therefore considerable scope for the subtle misregistration of structures that may not necessarily be obvious in the final image. The clinical significance of this degree of misregistration is difficult to determine and it is rarely apparent, other than when seen distal to an implant.

Refraction artifacts

Ultrasound equipment is programmed to assume that sound travels in straight lines and that received echoes have come from a source directly in line with the transmitted sound pulse. This is not always a correct assumption.

Table 3.2 Speed of sound in soft tissue

Tissue type and physiological state	Mean value—speed of sound
Normal premenopausal breast	1510 ms^{-1} (range 1450–1570 ms^{-1})
Normal postmenopausal breast	1468 ms^{-1} (range 1430–1520 ms^{-1})
Fat	1470 ms^{-1}

From Kossoff et al (1973), with permission of the American Institute of Physics.

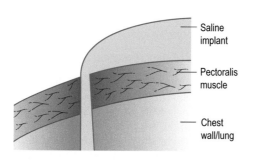
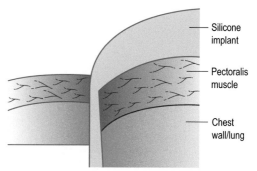

Figure 3.10 Diagram to show how the slower speed of sound in a silicone breast implant results in misregistration of the position of structures lying deep to the implant. No such artifact occurs with saline implants because the speed of sound in saline is similar to that in soft tissue.

As explained above, when the sound beam travels from a region of low propagation speed into a region of higher speed it is *refracted*, with the transmitted portion of the beam displaced from its original path. Echoes generated from this transmitted beam as it continues its journey beyond the boundary will therefore be misplaced in the image. The equipment will assume that these echoes originated along the original beam pathway—echoes are therefore picked up (and displayed in the images) from 'off-axis' structures (Fig. 3.11).

The effects of refraction within the breast are difficult to appreciate in practice, but they certainly do exist. The speed of sound in the normal breast varies considerably—sound traveling much faster through dense connective and glandular tissue than through the surrounding fat. The lobular structure of the breast also provides numerous curved interfaces at which refraction occurs. This leads to distortion of the beam and displacement of structures within the image. In vivo measurements have demonstrated deviations of the main beam by up to 10–15 mm for a 10 cm depth of breast tissue (Teboul 1995, p. 12). The failure of early water-path scanners in which the breast is dependent has been attributed largely to beam distortion due to refraction within fat lobules (Teboul 1995, p. 12).

In practice, if the ultrasound beam hits a boundary at 90°, no refraction occurs as there is no relative increase in the speed of either edge of the wave front. Refraction artifact can therefore be reduced considerably by applying gentle compression as the breast is scanned. By flattening the tissue against the chest wall, the normal breast tissue boundaries will be brought to lie approximately parallel to the face of the transducer (Fig. 3.12). This will also result in a reduction of Cooper's ligament shadowing artifact (see below) and should improve visualiaation of the ductal/lobular anatomy. Care needs to be taken, however, not to use excessive pressure as this can distort anatomical relationships and may mask the appearance of subtle abnormalities; in particular, intra-duct pathology may be missed if small ducts are compressed.

Reverberation

Sometimes, particularly just below a strongly reflecting superficial interface that lies parallel to the transducer face, multiple horizontal linear echoes are displayed that do not represent real tissue boundaries (Fig. 3.13). This *reverberation* artifact is due to multiple sound reflections between the interface and the transducer. When a sufficiently large amplitude echo reaches the transducer, some of the sound energy may be re-reflected back into the patient. This then acts as if it were an additional transmitted pulse and can thus give rise to further echo signals from the original interface. When these arrive back at the transducer, however, they are assumed to have resulted from the original transmitted pulse. Since the reverberation echo signal information has taken twice as long to arrive, the scanner assumes that the reflecting interface is at twice the depth. Further re-reflection gives rise to additional echo signals, and spurious equidistant parallel horizontal lines in the image corresponding to equal multiples of time/depth. As the reverberating pulse–echo travels increasing distances through tissue, it undergoes corresponding attenuation; the reverberation lines thus characteristically diminish in brightness with depth.

Finite thickness of the ultrasound beam

The signal value stored in the scanner's digital memory for any single location (pixel) within the image actually represents the total sound energy returning from a small volume of tissue. The size of this volume—the *resolution cell*—is determined by the lateral width of the beam, the slice thickness and the pulse length. Echoes generated by all structures lying within the resolution cell at a specific depth will be displayed as a single brightness value in the image. This 'volume averaging' results in loss of both spatial and contrast resolution (see Ch. 4).

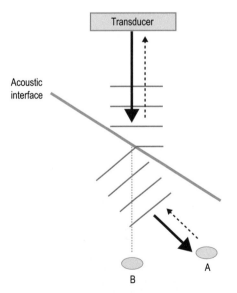

Target A will be displayed in the final image in position B

Figure 3.11   Diagram to show how 'off-axis' structures beyond an oblique boundary are represented in the image because of refraction of the ultrasound beam.

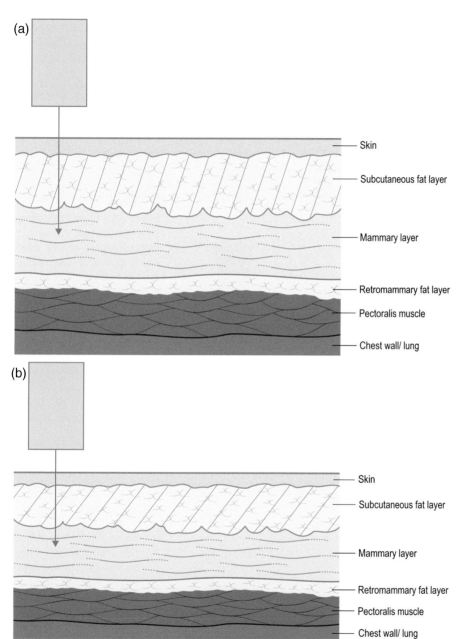

Figure 3.12 (a) Diagram to show how tissue interfaces such as Cooper's ligaments, tend to lie obliquely if minimal transducer pressure is used. (b) With additional transducer pressure, oblique interfaces can be brought to lie more horizontally.

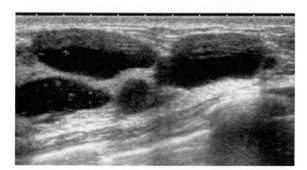

Figure 3.13 Reverberation artifact seen deep to the anterior surfaces of superficial cysts.

Beam width artifact

In the lateral (long axis) direction, the width of the ultrasound beam is controlled by the use of electronic focusing. A single small reflective target within the field of view (such as a microcalcification) will appear as a linear or tiny ovoid structure that is approximately the same width as the beam (Fig. 3.14).

Small structures situated side by side within the field of view will be seen as two separate structures only if their separation is greater than approximately half the beam width. Where the structures are closer together, they will be merged into one in the image (Fig. 3.15).

Slice thickness artifact

Since ultrasound images are viewed as a series of two-dimensional images, it is easy to think of them representing anatomy in two dimensions only. In reality, the ultrasound beam is three-dimensional and the tissues imaged are interrogated in slices of finite width (Fig. 3.16).

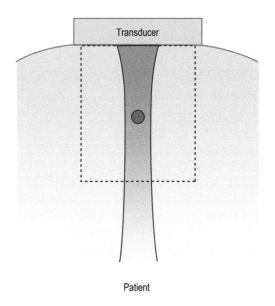

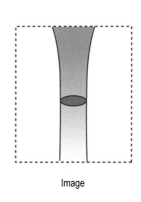

Figure 3.14 Small anatomical structures that are narrower than the beam width are displayed as linear or ovoid structures of beam width magnitude in the image.

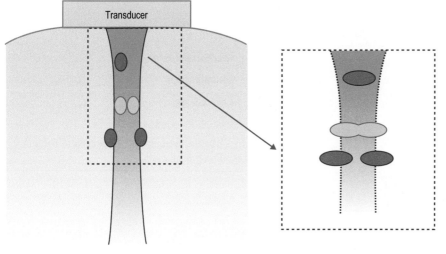

Figure 3.15 When adjacent anatomical structures are separated by distances smaller than half the beam width, they are not resolved as separate structures in the image.

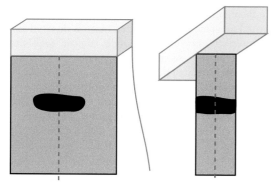

Figure 3.16 The ultrasound image is a two-dimensional representation of a three-dimensional slice of tissue of finite thickness.

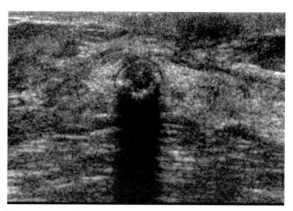

Figure 3.18 Total acoustic shadowing prevents visualization of anatomical structures deep to this calcified oil cyst. (Image courtesy of Philips Medical Systems.)

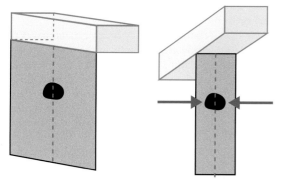

Figure 3.17 Due to slice thickness artifact, tiny cysts of smaller diameter than the slice thickness will not be displayed as truly echo free. Scatter from soft tissue adjacent to a cyst that is small compared to the slice thickness will be displayed as low level echoes within the cyst.

Focusing of the beam in this 'elevation' plane is achieved by use of a mechanical lens attached to the face of the transducer and is normally limited to one specific depth. The operator has no control of this and simply needs to be aware of resultant image appearances.

The scattered echoes from targets lying at the same depth within this slice will be averaged, stored and displayed as a single pixel value within the image. The effect of slice thickness artifact is most commonly appreciated within the breast when imaging small cysts—a cyst that is small enough to sit wholly or partially within the beam will appear to contain low-level echoes (Fig. 3.17).

Slice thickness is one of a number of key features of an ultrasound system that have a significant impact on our ability to detect and characterize breast pathology. Recommendations for optimizing equipment selection, initially setting up and subsequently manipulating operator controllable features are considered further in Chapter 4.

Acoustic shadowing

Shadowing from structures within the breast can be a source of confusion to the image observer. Technological advances such as 'compound imaging' reduce the effect of shadowing artifact (see Ch. 4), but the ability to distinguish between pathological and 'normal' artifact appearances, and an awareness of the potentially useful information that is lost from the image on activating features such as compound imaging, require a clear understanding of why different types of shadowing occur.

Acoustic shadowing occurs when the proportion of sound energy transmitted beyond a specific target is too small to produce detectable echo signals and thus contributes no further useful information to the image. This occurs when the target attenuates a high proportion of the ultrasound beam energy through *reflection* or *absorption*.

Since reflection of the sound beam occurs at an interface across which there is a difference in acoustic impedance, when there is a large change in impedance a high proportion of sound energy is reflected back to the transducer. This greatly reduces the energy transmitted beyond the reflecting boundary and may render it insufficient for imaging distal structures. This feature can be used to characterize calcification within lesions such as oil cysts or hyalinized fibroadenomas (Fig. 3.18).

For very small structures, however, such as microcalcifications within the breast, even a very large change in impedance may not produce convincing shadowing.

Since the area of calcification is small compared with the effective width of the ultrasound beam, not all of the sound energy will be reflected. Sound energy will pass to each side of the calcification and continue into the deeper tissues (Fig. 3.19). As the scanner assumes all echoes return from structures along the central axis of the beam, echo information obtained from tissue adjacent to the area of calcification will register in the same axis location. If the calcification is sufficiently small, it will not be seen within the final image due to volume averaging.

Even areas of calcification that are large enough to be clearly visible in the final image may demonstrate no convincing shadow. Echo information from distal and adjacent structures may be represented in the image immediately behind the calcification, reducing or eliminating any shadowing effect.

Critical angle shadowing

Simple physical laws of reflection dictate that when an ultrasound pulse hits an interface at an oblique angle, the reflected pulse will be directed at an equal and opposite angle (Fig. 3.20).

At any angle other than near normal incidence, there will be some loss of image information as the reflected pulse either hits the transducer at an angle, or misses the transducer completely. Interfaces that are at a steep angle relative to the direction of the ultrasound beam, such as the lateral margins of a focal lesion, can therefore be difficult to demonstrate.

In addition, where there is a change in the speed of sound across the boundary, as the obliquity of the inter-face increases, Snell's law predicts that a *critical angle* is reached at which the transmitted beam is directed along the interface. Beyond this angle, almost total beam reflection occurs. As no sound energy is transmitted beyond the interface, this results in an area of shadowing where no distal information is obtained.

Critical angle shadowing is characteristic at the lateral margins of a well-defined fibroadenoma, but is also seen deep to steeply oriented structures such as Cooper's ligaments (Fig. 3.21). Critical angle shadowing makes visualization of deep structures difficult. It can also mimic the attenuation shadowing associated with the desmoplastic reaction seen with invasive malignancies (see below).

Pathological shadowing

Shadowing is an important diagnostic feature of breast lesions and is often the feature most likely to alert the operator to the presence of pathology.

One of the features of many breast carcinomas is the desmoplastic response that results in the lesion presenting as a palpable lump (Walker 2001). An increasing degree of desmoplasia (development of fibrous tissue) results in the typical malignant sonographic appearance of a hyporeflective lesion with dense posterior acoustic shadowing and varying degrees of margin spiculation (Fig. 3.22). Since fibrous tissue in the normal breast appears hyper-reflective in comparison with fat, it is somewhat paradoxical that desmoplastic malignant lesions appear hyporeflective or almost echo free in extreme cases.

Desmoplasia results in an increase in the density of the lesion and a decrease in its compressibility. This has

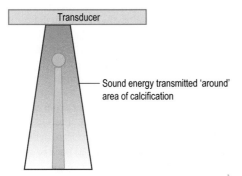

Figure 3.19 Microcalcifications smaller than the beam width will not exhibit posterior shadowing since they do not completely stop the sound reaching structures behind them.

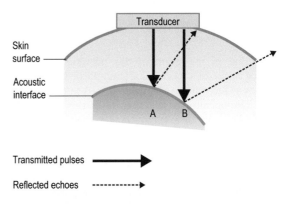

Figure 3.20 The direction in which the sound beam is reflected from an anatomical surface is equal and opposite to that of the incident sound beam.

(a)

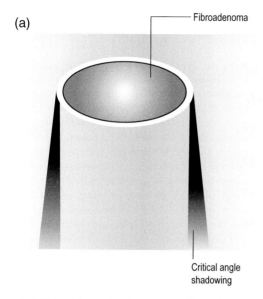

Fibroadenoma

Critical angle
shadowing

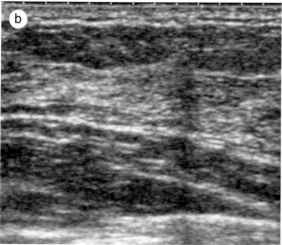

Figure 3.21   (a) Diagram to show how 'critical angle' artifact occurs at the edges of steeply curved structures such
as the lateral margins of a fibroadenoma. (b) Ultrasound
image demonstrating the 'critical angle' shadowing artifact
associated with Cooper's ligaments.

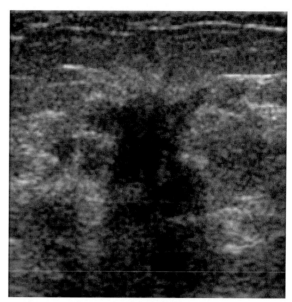

Figure 3.22   Ultrasound image showing the typical spiculated margin and posterior shadowing associated with a
breast carcinoma.

a significant impact on the through transmission of
sound, the relative reflectivity of the lesion and associated
artifacts. Absorption of sound within the lesion is
increased and the ultrasound beam markedly attenuated,
thus limiting through transmission of sound. This effect
is more marked at higher frequencies since absorption is
frequency dependent. In addition, unlike the smooth
interfaces of normal fibrous connective tissue, the boundaries of malignant lesions are irregular and act as diffuse
rather than specular reflectors. The net result of these

effects is a hyporeflective area in the image that has ill-
defined boundaries and is associated with an intense
posterior acoustic shadow.

Shadowing from anatomically normal structures can
be reduced by altering the orientation of the transducer
to the breast surface and scanning from different angles,
altering patient position to flatten the breast tissue interfaces or by using moderate transducer pressure to compress the breast tissue against the chest wall. These
maneuvers can reduce the angle between the ligaments
to near perpendicular to the beam, thus reducing critical
angle shadowing—true pathological shadowing will
invariably persist.

Increased through transmission

Cystic structures appear echo free or anechoic within the
image, i.e. they are displayed as uniformly black. As the
sound pulse travels through homogeneous cyst fluid, it
encounters no changes in acoustic impedance; since the
cyst contains no scattering targets, no reflected echoes
are returned to the transducer for the corresponding
position in the image. Features that enable us to identify
a cyst with confidence include this anechoic appearance
and the presence of increased through transmission.

As sound travels through solid tissue, it is attenuated
as a result of absorption and scattering. TGC is used to
compensate for this attenuation by gradually increasing
the amplification of echoes with increasing depth.

Attenuation within a fluid-filled structure, such as a simple serous cyst, is minimal. Since the scanner is calibrated to assume uniform attenuation throughout body, there will be an area of 'overcompensation' distal to such a lesion. Echoes arising from tissues within this region are thus overamplified; they will be stronger that those from adjacent areas at a similar depth and will therefore appear brighter than similar adjacent areas within the final image (Fig. 3.23).

This increase in through transmission is not confined to fluid-filled structures and may be seen, albeit to a lesser extent, posterior to solid lesions such as a fibroad-

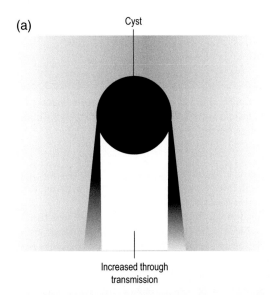

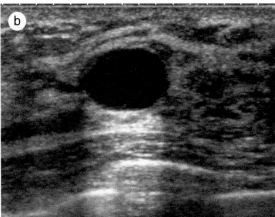

Figure 3.23   (a) Diagram illustrating increased posterior through transmission deep to a low attenuating lesion. (b) The structures deep to a simple cyst look characteristically 'brighter' because of increased through transmission of sound.

enoma. The key causative mechanism is that attenuation within the lesion is less than that of surrounding tissue.

PRINCIPLES OF DOPPLER IMAGING

When transmitted pulses of ultrasound are reflected from targets that are moving either towards or away from the transducer, the reflected echo signals have a different frequency from that of the transmitted pulses. If the reflecting target is moving towards the transducer, the echo frequency will be higher than the transmitted frequency, if the target is moving away the echo frequency, will be lower (Fig. 3.24). This *Doppler effect*, after Christian Andreas Doppler (1803–1853) the Austrian mathematician who first described it, is essentially the same phenomenon that causes the stationary observer to perceive a change in the pitch of a police siren or train whistle as it speeds past them. The effect is used in medical ultrasound particularly to detect and evaluate blood flow.

When Doppler mode is activated, the frequency of the received echoes is compared with the frequency of the transmitted pulses, and any difference—the *Doppler shift frequency*—is extracted. By virtue of the mathematical relationship between the Doppler shift frequency and the velocity of the reflecting target, i.e. the red blood cells, once the frequency and the direction of flow with reference to beam axis are known, the blood flow velocity can be calculated (Fig. 3.25). This information can then be displayed as either a color-coded overlay on the B-mode image—*color flow mapping*, or as a graphical representation of the velocity profile over time at a specific operator-selected anatomical location—*spectral Doppler* (Fig. 3.26).

In *power Doppler* mode, colors are allocated to a B-mode image overlay to represent the amplitude (strength) of the frequency-shifted signal, rather than the actual frequency shift itself. As such, velocity and directional information is lost, but the technique is more sensitive to weaker signals from smaller vessels than conventional color flow Doppler.

CONTRAST AGENTS

Over the last few years, pharmaceutical ultrasound *contrast agents* have been developed. In essence, these are solutions of tiny (2–8 μm) encapsulated gas microbubbles that are injected into the bloodstream, usually through a peripheral intravenous injection. The presence, constitution and resonant activity of these microbubbles in the bloodstream increases echo signal strength—the effect being known as *contrast enhancement*. The effect is observable in the B-mode image, but particularly improves sensitivity of Doppler imaging. Contrast agents allow improved interrogation of the per-

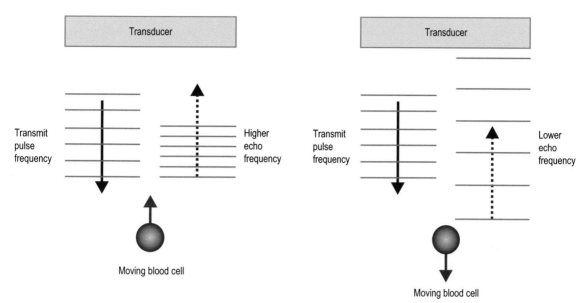

Figure 3.24 The Doppler effect—as blood cells move towards (and away from) the transducer, the frequency of the returned echoes is correspondingly increased (and decreased).

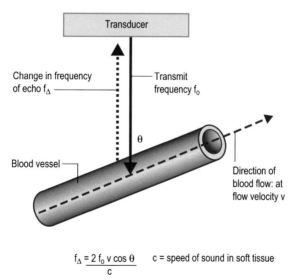

$$f_\Delta = \frac{2 f_0 v \cos \theta}{c} \qquad c = \text{speed of sound in soft tissue}$$

Figure 3.25 The relationships of frequency and velocity are described in the Doppler equation.

fusion characteristics of the breast, with additional software processing allowing the monitoring of arrival and transit times of the contrast agent through a lesion and thus enabling some assessment of physiological and pathophysiological function. It is possible that use of ultrasound contrast agents might enable more accurate discrimination of benign and malignant lesions, particularly if contrast enhancement can be quantified rather

than assessed subjectively. In practice, however, the value that ultrasound contrast agents add to the routine 'triple assessment' diagnostic approach is not yet established. More promising potential applications are the accurate assessment of tumor size and extent, evaluation of tumor response to neoadjuvant chemotherapy and targeted delivery of drug or gene therapy (Hoskins et al 2003, Svenssen 2006).

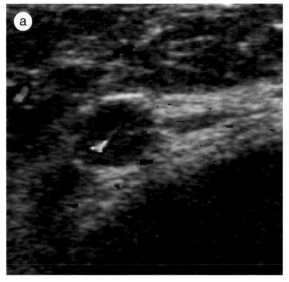
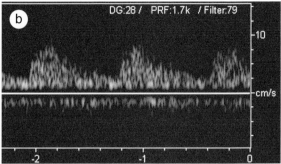

Figure 3.26 (a) The color flow mapping function overlays Doppler (perfusion) information on the two-dimensional B-mode gray-scale image. (b) The spectral Doppler function displays a graph of change in blood flow velocity (vertical axis) over time (horizontal axis).

References and further reading

Duck F (ed.) 1990 Physical properties of tissue: a comprehensive reference book. London: Academic Press Harcourt Brace Jovanovich.

Hedrick WR, Hykes DL, Starchman DE 1994 Ultrasound physics & instrumentation. 3rd edn. Edinburgh: Mosby.

Hoskins PR, Thrush A, Martin K, Whittingham TA 2003 Diagnostic ultrasound physics and equipment. London: Greenwich Medical Media.

Kossoff G, Fry EK Jellins J 1973 Average velocity of ultrasound in the human female breast. A technique for measuring the in vivo average velocity of ultrasound in the human female. Journal of the Acoustical Society of America 53(6):1730–1736.

Scherzinger A, Belgam R, Carson P et al (1989) Assessment of ultrasonic computed tomography in symptomatic breast patients by discriminant analysis. Ultrasound in Medicine and Biology 15(1):21–28.

Svenssen WE 2006 Breast ultrasound update. Ultrasound 14(1):20–33.

Teboul M, Halliwell M 1995 Atlas of ultrasound and ductal echography of the breast. Oxford: Blackwell Science.

Walker R 2001 The complexities of breast cancer desmoplasia. Breast Cancer Research 3(3):143–145.

Zagzebski JA 1996 Essentials of ultrasound physics. Edinburgh: Mosby.

Chapter 4

Equipment for breast ultrasound

Heather Venables

INTRODUCTION

As in any other area of ultrasound practice, both the specification of the equipment used and the operator's use of relevant equipment controls have a profound effect on the quality of images produced. In addition to this, there has been phenomenal development in ultrasound technology over the last decade. It is not always easy to define which features of a machine are essential for a specific application and which should be considered as complementary or investigational. It may be even harder to justify these at the time of purchase.

This chapter outlines the key features that need to be considered when choosing ultrasound equipment for breast imaging; it discusses optimization of equipment settings, addresses quality assurance issues and gives a brief overview of some of the more recent technical developments.

CHOOSING A MACHINE FOR BREAST ULTRASOUND

There is a huge range of ultrasound machines on the market ranging in price from a few thousand pounds to well in excess of £100 000. There is no doubt that breast ultrasound requires the best that you can afford—more expensive machines are able to produce images of higher quality and are therefore more likely to have improved diagnostic capability (Madjar 2000). Cost is usually the predominant factor affecting equipment choice (Miles 2005), and an understanding of the imaging objectives and how these are met by equipment performance will help to justify significant financial outlay. When selecting ultrasound equipment for any clinical context, there are a number of general factors that need to be considered (Box 4.1).

Box 4.1   General considerations when purchasing ultrasound equipment

- Clinical application(s) for which equipment will be used
- Relative workload in (each) application
- Transducer requirements
- Scanning capabilities required
- Measurement and analysis facilities required
- Physical size and maneuvrability
- Ultrasound controls/settings—availability, ease of location and operation
- Annotation and documentation—availability, ease of operation
- Facility for permanent recording of images
- Safety compliance, quality assurance
- Equipment trials and training
- Equipment review and replacement

Summarized from RCR (2005)

Table 4.1   Work related musculoskeletal injury reduction

Issues to consider	Risk reduction strategies
Service provision/ professional issues	
Education	Ergonomics
	Health and safety
	Risk assessment
Workload scheduling	Caseload rotation
	Reducing overtime
	Restricting addition of 'extras' to lists
	Ensuring regular breaks
Environment	Large room
	Adequate ventilation and heating—air conditioning
	Ambient lighting—dimmer switches
Equipment	Selection of good ergonomic design
	Maintenance and quality assurance programs

Helpful guidelines on ultrasound equipment procurement have been produced by a number of agencies and professional bodies, e.g. NHS PASA (2005) and RCR (2005). It is important that personnel who will be using the equipment in clinical practice are involved in the selection process; they should contribute to development of the equipment specification and have the opportunity to test, evaluate and compare a range of potentially suitable machines.

ERGONOMIC CONSIDERATIONS

Before looking at the diagnostic requirements of the ultrasound machine, it is important to consider the interrelationship between the scanning machine and the operator—even the most highly sophisticated machine is of no value if it is not being used.

It is estimated that more than 80% of ultrasound professionals sustain some level of work-related injury during their professional careers; 20% of sonographers ultimately retire from their profession due to physical incapacity directly related to musculoskeletal injury (SDMS 2003). Sonographers complain of pain, discomfort, tenderness, swelling, aching and stiffness, particularly in the shoulder joints and the neck (Miles 2005). Such symptoms are not limited to the sonography profession but are very common in workers whose daily tasks involve repetitive, awkward or forceful movements that

result in tendon and ligament microtrauma; eventually this can lead to disabling inflammation, scarring and contracture (Miles 2005).

Risk of work-related musculoskeletal disorder can be reduced by educating personnel, making changes to workload scheduling and by ensuring that good ergonomic design is an integral part of the whole scanning environment (Table 4.1). Consideration should be given to the size and layout of the scanning room, particularly the design and positioning of the patient table and operator chair, as well as features of the ultrasound machine itself (Table 4.2). Any ultrasound equipment purchase should be made with reference to current guidance on optimal ergonomic features (Dodgeon & Newton-Hughes 2003, SDMS 2003). In particular, good ergonomic design should encourage a balanced, upright operator posture and minimize the strain on the joints of the neck and upper limb (see Ch. 6).

EQUIPMENT PERFORMANCE—WHAT DOES THE EQUIPMENT NEED TO DO WELL?

To produce high quality ultrasound images of the breast, it is essential that the equipment used is of high specification and that the specification is purposely tailored to breast imaging. A number of professional organizations have produced guidelines that include breast ultrasound

Table 4.2 Key ergonomic design features to consider when selecting equipment for breast imaging

Scanning practice	Features required
Many practitioners stand to scan the breast	Adjustable height and tilt keyboard
	Adjustable height and tilt monitor
	Adjustable height patient couch
If seated	Footrest
	Adjustable height chair
Importance of reducing transducer pressure	
During Doppler examinations	Lightweight transducer and cables
To reduce operator fatigue	
	Adequate size and shape to allow a dynamic grip
	Cable tidy/arm supports
Need for hands-free manipulation of controls	
Simultaneous scanning and palpation	Footswitch controls
	Voice activation
Undertaking interventional procedures	

Box 4.2 Clinical capabilities required of breast ultrasound equipment

- Display normal and pathological breast tissue detail
- Differentiate between solid and cystic lesions down to 2 mm diameter
- Image a 22-gauge needle in the breast
- Measure the dimensions of breast lesions
- Penetrate breast thickness of at least 40 mm
- Demonstrate irregularities in lesion margins and perturbations in surrounding tissue layers

MDA (1998a)

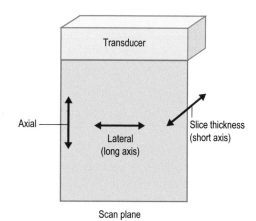

Figure 4.1 Diagram illustrating axial, lateral (long axis) and slice thickness (short axis) plane orientation.

equipment specifications (Madjar et al 1998, MDA 1998a, UKAS 2001, ACR 2002, AIUM 2002, RCR 2003).

KEY IMAGING OBJECTIVES

Before attempting to define the essential features of a system for breast imaging, it is worth pausing to consider what the imaging objectives are. Guidance notes on ultrasound equipment for breast imaging within the context of the United Kingdom National Health Service Breast Screening Programme (NHSBSP) were produced by the Medical Devices Agency (MDA) in 1998 (MDA 1998a). This guidance details the clinical capabilities required for breast ultrasound (Box 4.2), and the same key capabilities are assumed in the most recent guidance document from the Royal College of Radiologists (RCR 2005).

Cancer detection is the raison d'être for breast imaging. When considering the ability of ultrasound to detect breast cancer, it is important to remember that not all breast cancers are the same (Stavros 2005). Lesions may have spiculate or smooth margins, be small and focal or diffuse, they may lie deep within a large breast or within a few millimeters of the skin surface.

Against a widely varying background of breast size, normal age- and hormone-moderated physiological change and the presence of benign disease, the specific imaging objectives will change from patient to patient. Nevertheless, the nature of normal breast tissue and the spectrum of potential pathological change are such that, in all cases, excellent spatial and contrast resolution are required throughout the full depth of the breast as well as very close to the skin.

SPATIAL RESOLUTION

This is the ability of the ultrasound system to detect and display two closely associated reflectors as separate structures; it can be considered in three distinct planes (Fig. 4.1):

- axial resolution
- lateral resolution (long axis)
- slice thickness (short axis).

Axial resolution

Axial resolution is the ability of the system to distinguish reflectors that lie along the axis of the beam. In the standard breast ultrasound patient position (supine oblique), this relates to the anterior–posterior direction. Axial resolution limits the ability of the system to demonstrate breast tissue planes that lie parallel to the skin surface, i.e. normal ductal anatomy and the pseudocapsule that is an important diagnostic feature of some benign lesions (Stavros 2004, p. 24).

The limit of axial resolution of a system is approximately half the ultrasound pulse length (Hoskins et al 2003). Since pulse length is inversely related to transducer frequency, axial resolution is improved at higher frequencies when the wavelength is smaller; the wavelength at 5 MHz is approximately 0.31 mm, at 10 MHz the wavelength is 0.15 mm (Hoskins et al 2003, p. 12).

Lateral resolution (long axis)

Lateral resolution is the ability of the system to distinguish reflectors that are closely spaced and situated side by side within the image plane, i.e. in a plane parallel to the transducer surface. As the spacing between reflectors approaches the width of the beam at this depth, they are no longer visualized as entirely separate structures (see Ch. 3). Lateral resolution is therefore limited by beam width and is, at best, equal to half the width of the beam. For an array transducer, the width of the beam is reduced by means of electronic focusing techniques.

Transducer focusing

Electronic focusing of the transmitted pulse allows the operator to select the depth to which the beam is focused, i.e. at its narrowest. Groups of elements across the face of the transducer are fired in a staggered sequence to achieve focusing to a specific depth. This ensures that a high amplitude pulse with limited beam width arrives at a particular depth of interest. As the distance from the outer elements to the focus is greater than for the central elements, the outer elements are fired first (Fig. 4.2). The more elements that are active for any given pulse transmission, the greater the effective aperture and the tighter the focusing that can be achieved (Hoskins et al 2003). The operator has control over the depth to which the beam is focused in transmission. By placing the *focal zone* (usually annotated by a small arrowhead on one of

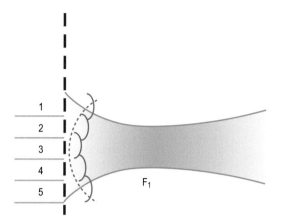

Transducer elements are activated in sequence
Elements 1 and 5 are activated first
Element 3 is activated last
This produces a beam that is focused to depth F_1

Figure 4.2   Diagram illustrating how electrical delays to successively fired transducer elements can be used to focus the ultrasound beam.

the vertical edges of the image display) to the depth of interest, lateral resolution is improved at this level (Fig. 4.3a).

It is possible to select *multiple focal zones* (Fig. 4.3b) such that multiple pulses are transmitted along each scan line, each electronically focused to a different selected depth. As the system has to wait for each pulse to return before the next pulse is transmitted, firing multiple pulses along each scan line will normally reduce the frame rate. A number of modern systems use various focusing algorithms and digitally encoded pulses that allow the use of multiple, simultaneous transmissions. This enables manufacturers to maintain reasonable frame rates even when multiple focal zones are selected. Since the breast is a relatively static structure, a high frame rate is not essential. If, however, the frame rate drops below around 12 frames per second, it becomes difficult to assess normal tissue when surveying the breast if the transducer is moved too quickly (Stavros 2004).

Focusing of the beam can also be achieved on reception using a sequence of electronic delays similar to those used on transmission. By varying these delays with time, the beam is focused to the precise depth of each returning echo. This function is automatically controlled within the machine, the operator having no direct control, the focal depth varying constantly to correspond with the pulse–echo transit time (Hoskins et al 2003, p. 32). This *dynamic focusing on reception* is not dependent on the transmission of multiple pulses so there is no loss of frame rate.

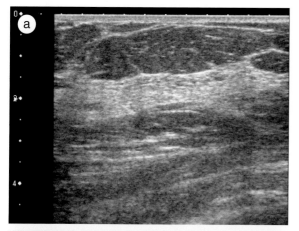

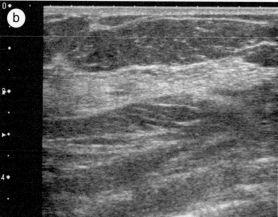

Figure 4.3   (a) The depth of a single focal zone should correspond to the depth of the parenchymal breast tissue—the focal zone is indicated by an arrowhead (at 2 cm) on the depth scale at the left hand side of the image. (b) Multiple focal zones are placed adjacent to and just below the parenchymal breast tissue—this reduces the frame rate, giving a slightly 'smoother' image.

By combining electronic focusing on transmission and dynamic focusing on reception, it is possible to maintain good, uniform lateral resolution throughout the imaged depth. The target value for lateral resolution identified by the MDA is 3 mm over the whole depth range with a limiting value of 4 mm (MDA 1998a). With recent advances in transducer technology, these targets may need to be revised.

In practice, the initial selection of multiple or single focal zones may be part of the application pre-set. It may still be necessary for the operator to adjust the transmit focus throughout the examination. This is particularly important for large breasts or very superficial lesions where use of a stand-off should also be considered (see below).

Slice thickness (short axis)

The short axis width of the beam (at 90° to the image plane) is normally significantly greater than the lateral (long axis) beam width and varies with depth. The effect of slice thickness artifact is a significant limiting factor in spatial resolution and is most significant when imaging small fluid-filled structures (see Ch. 3). The volume averaging that occurs due to slice thickness will limit the ability of the system to demonstrate small fluid-filled structures, such as ducts and tiny cysts, as completely echo free.

SHORT AXIS FOCUSING

In conventional linear array transducers, electronic focusing is not possible perpendicular to the scan plane (the short axis). The width of the ultrasound beam in this direction (the slice thickness) is determined by fixed mechanical focusing and is limited to one depth. This is set by the manufacturer and cannot be altered by the operator. General purpose high frequency linear array probes are designed to image to a depth of up to approximately 70 mm. This allows the transducer to be used for varied applications including lower limb arterial studies that require such image depth. The fixed focusing in the short axis plane is therefore set to around 30–40 mm (Stavros 2004, GE 2005a, Philips 2005a). The depth of tissue to be examined when the breast is flattened against the chest wall is typically less than 40 mm for most patients, highlighting the need for a transducer that is designed specifically for breast imaging.

Target values for slice thickness published by the MDA are 3 mm with a limiting value of 4 mm over the entire image range. A technical assessment of commercially available ultrasound systems undertaken by the MDA on behalf of the UK NHSBSP (MDA 2001) showed that the majority of systems evaluated could not meet these target values. The mean slice thickness was 4.76 mm with a maximum thickness in excess of 10 mm for over a third of the transducer combinations tested.

Again, where short axis resolution is poor, small cysts may appear as solid lesions; it is also likely that small solid lesions might be missed since they may appear isoreflective with surrounding tissue (Stavros 2004).

1.5D ARRAY TRANSDUCERS

One of the most significant advances in breast ultrasound over recent years has been the development of matrix (multiple row) or 1.5D array transducers. In a conventional array, each element occupies the full width of the transducer surface. In 1.5D arrays, each element is subdivided into between three and eight sections (Fig. 4.4).

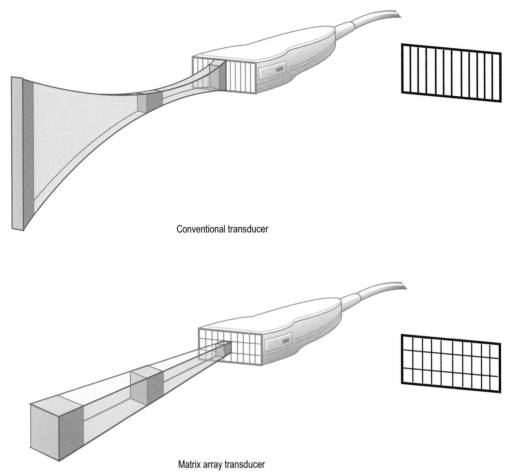

Conventional transducer

Matrix array transducer

Figure 4.4   Whilst conventional ultrasound transducers have fixed scan plane focusing, matrix array transducers allow dynamic focusing in the elevation plane.

This allows limited dynamic focusing in the elevation plane. The benefit is greater uniformity of resolution with depth and a significant reduction in slice thickness, particularly close to the transducer (Garra 2005).

CONTRAST RESOLUTION

Contrast resolution is essentially the ability of the system to detect and display differences between different types of tissue and is a function of both anatomical structure and electronic signal processing. Excellent contrast resolution is particularly important when scanning the breast, as often there is little difference between the inherent reflectivity of areas of pathology and surrounding normal tissues.

Low contrast gray-scale resolution can be defined as the ability of the system to display regions of similar reflectivity as discrete and separate structures, e.g. demonstration of a subtle lipoma within an area of normal subcutaneous fat.

High contrast gray-scale resolution can be defined as the ability of the system to differentiate structures of similar reflectivity in a mixed field of strong/weak reflectors, e.g. a small cancer within an area of dense glandular tissue. Both high and low contrast will be affected by equipment performance and set-up.

The ability to distinguish changes in echo brightness is a complex process. The degree to which a lesion appears 'conspicuous' will depend on characteristics of the lesion, the imaging system itself, the observer's visual acuity and the conditions under which the image is viewed (Hoskins et al 2003). The absolute brightness of a displayed echo within the image and the difference in brightness between adjacent structures not only are influenced by the nature of the reflector from which the echo has arisen, but are also dependent upon spatial resolution, frequency, gain, dynamic range, gray-scale allocation and the presence of artifact within the image.

OPTIMIZATION OF EQUIPMENT SETTINGS—GETTING THE BEST OUT OF THE EQUIPMENT

Excellent spatial and contrast resolution have been identified as key parameters for breast imaging. These depend not only on equipment specification, but also on the skilled use of equipment settings. All currently available systems allow the operator to select application-specific *default pre-sets* (Fig. 4.5). These provide an excellent baseline from which scanning parameters can be adjusted to meet the imaging requirements of individual patients and pathologies. Default pre-sets are usually programmed by the equipment manufacturers and include a wide range of individual parameters, most of which rarely need to be altered. However, it is possible to develop individualized department pre-sets and, given the inherent subjectivity of human visual perception, it is not unusual for individual operators to want to 'save' their own particular combination of preferred equipment settings to avoid having to make repeated adjustments at the start of every examination.

Individual equipment settings that affect image quality are now considered; the following list is not exhaustive, but includes the parameters that will need most frequent adjustment by the operator—optimization criteria for B-mode equipment controls are summarized in Table 4.3.

Equipment settings that improve spatial resolution

As outlined above, spatial resolution can be considered in three distinct planes: axial, lateral (long axis) and slice thickness (short axis).

Axial resolution is improved at high frequency. When surveying the breast, the operator should always select the highest transmit frequency that provides adequate penetration to the chest wall. Where superficial pathology is suspected or detected, the frequency should be increased to interrogate this area of interest in more detail.

Lateral resolution is improved with beam focusing. Focal zones should therefore be adjusted throughout the scan to align them at the depth of particular interest. The effective width of the beam is also affected by 'gain' settings. If the overall gain is set too high, the effective

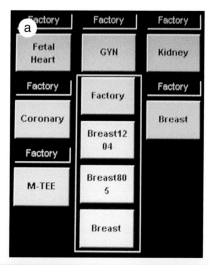
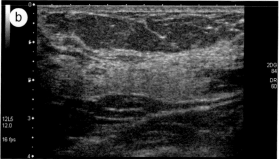
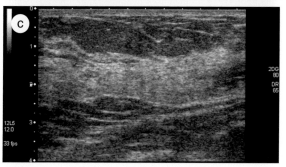

Figure 4.5 (a) Application-specific 'pre-sets' allow rapid operator selection of a default combination of baseline scan parameter settings at the beginning of each examination. (b and c) Application pre-sets can be customized to suit individual operator preferences.

beam width increases and lateral resolution is degraded (Fig. 4.6).

Slice thickness is predetermined at any specific depth and is not normally adjusted by the operator. Use of a dedicated breast transducer with or without a stand-off is essential. Where available, a 1.5D array provides better, uniform resolution in the short axis.

Table 4.3 How to optimize B-mode settings

Control	Optimization criteria	Incorrect adjustment
Frequency	For best spatial resolution, use highest frequency available that will allow penetration to the chest wall. For a large or dense attenuating breast, it may be necessary to change to a lower frequency if increased gain and increased power fail to demonstrate the chest wall.	Use of low frequency is associated with poorer spatial resolution. Use of too high a frequency will fail to demonstrate deep structures.
Gain/TGC	Adjust to visualize breast anatomy in useful density range and to avoid saturation of the image. Ensure adequate visualization of structures from skin surface to chest wall.	Too much gain reduces both spatial and contrast resolution. Incorrect adjustment can make it difficult to distinguish cysts from solid lesions—lack of increased through transmission should raise the possibility that the lesion is solid.
Power output	Limit to minimum required to ensure adequate penetration to chest wall. May need to increase for large breasts. May need to increase in Doppler mode.	If set too low, low level echoes will be lost, solid lesions may appear cystic, deeper tissues may not be visualized. Take care to keep to minimum to reduce risks of adverse biological effects.
Focusing	Adjust to depth of interest throughout examination. Select multiple focal zones (3) to improve resolution throughout depth of breast.	When surveying a large area with multiple focal zones selected—try to keep frame rate above 12 fps to reduce image blurring
Dynamic range	Increased dynamic range improves contrast resolution—but may not improve perceived image quality.	If set too high, the image appears gray and flat (low contrast) with in-filling of cystic areas. If set too low (high contrast). solid lesions may be misclassified as cysts.
Compound imaging	Reduces shadowing and increased through transmission.	If compound imaging is activated by selection of a default pre-set, it may be necessary either to reduce or to deactivate this to determine the through transmission characteristics of a focal lesion.

TGC = time gain compensation.

Equipment settings that improve contrast resolution

Current state-of-the-art equipment utilizes complex signal processing and noise reduction algorithms designed to improve contrast resolution. Breast-specific application pre-sets will be tailored to optimize these settings for the majority of patients and it is rarely necessary for the operator to adjust them. However, in the presence of subtle pathology and in the occasional 'difficult to scan' patient, an appreciation of the impact of these controls is useful since skillful operator manipula-tion of signal processing functions may sometimes improve diagnostic capability (Box 4.3).

Dynamic range adjusts the range of signal values over which the available gray-scale is utilized. In theory, increasing the dynamic range will improve contrast resolution, but will not necessarily improve the subjective image quality since the overall 'contrast' in the image is reduced, giving it a 'flat' grayer appearance (Fig. 4.7).

Noise within the image degrades contrast resolution and can be reduced through use of features such as *persistence* and *frame averaging* (Hoskins et al 2003).

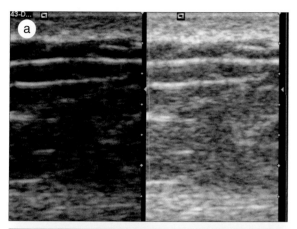

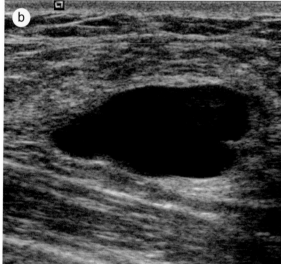

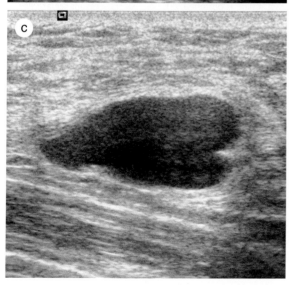

Figure 4.6 (a) Split image to show how the definition of interfaces parallel to the transducer face is improved with low overall gain. (b and c) Increasing the overall gain (c) can result in better defined edges, to this simple cyst for example, and thus improved measurement accuracy.

Box 4.3   Equipment settings that improve contrast resolution

- Focusing to improved spatial resolution
- Choose a high frequency transducer
- Choose a broad bandwidth transducer—select a higher frequency
- Good use of gain controls and focusing to suppress off-axis echoes
- Activation of tissue harmonic imaging function to suppress off-axis echoes
- Increase persistence/frame averaging to reduce noise
- Increase dynamic range
- Manipulate gray-scale processing

If persistence is set to a high level, there will be an appreciable lag in the image if the transducer is moved too quickly, as each frame is updated. Increased frame averaging will reduce the frame rate. For a static structure such as the breast, this should not be problematic if the transducer is moved slowly.

Gray-scale transfer curves are used to allocate a range of echo signal values to the available gray levels that can be displayed on the monitor. It may be useful to try different transfer curves (gray 'maps') to highlight subtle abnormalities (Fig. 4.8).

In practice, misregistered low amplitude echoes produced by off-axis beam energy degrade contrast resolution. Contrast resolution and spatial resolution are therefore inextricably linked. By optimizing basic controls such as gain settings and focusing, contrast resolution will be improved.

Choice of transducer

This is critical, as transmit frequency and transducer focusing have a significant impact on both spatial and contrast resolution. The size and shape of the transducer

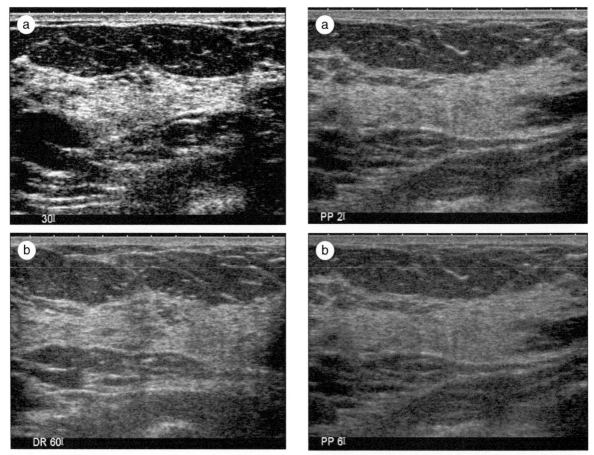

Figure 4.7 (a) High contrast images are obtained using low (30 dB) dynamic range settings. (b) Lower contrast images are obtained with higher (60 dB) dynamic range settings.

Figure 4.8 (a) The postprocessing function (PP2) alters the display characteristics of the image. (b) A 'flatter' lower contrast image is obtained with the postprocessing set at PP6.

also affect how effectively sound is transmitted into, and received back from the body.

Transmit frequencies greater than 7.5 MHz are recommended for breast ultrasound, with a range from 7.5 to 15 MHz being ideal, and achievable with broad bandwidth transducers (Madjar et al 1998, MDA 1998a, ACR 2002, AIUM 2002, RCR 2005).

The *transducer footprint* is the surface that is placed in contact with the patient's skin. The dimensions of the skin contact area need to be small enough to allow ease of access to the axilla. However, if the transducer footprint is too small, full coverage of a large breast will be time consuming as the width of the field of view is limited by the width of the transducer (Fig. 4.9). The ability to measure and demonstrate the entire perimeter of a large lesion is also limited by transducer footprint width, although the recommended width of 40 mm

(Madjar et al 1998) is adequate for most examinations. Although a curved array may give better contact in the axilla, a flat-faced linear array transducer is more suitable for the breast when it is flattened over the anterior chest wall with the patient in the standard posterior-oblique scanning position.

A number of developments in transducer design and beam forming allow the field of view to be extended beyond the width of the transducer footprint. *Extended field of view* techniques include 'trapezoid' imaging where the beam generated at the outer elements of a linear array is steered electronically (Fig. 4.10). The resultant field of view is extended laterally and is particularly useful for imaging large lesions that lie deep within the breast (GE 2005b). A number of manufacturers have developed systems that are capable of generating a static 'panorama' field of view up to 120 cm in length

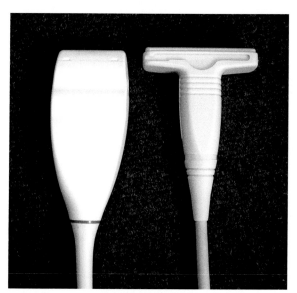

Figure 4.9   The 'footprint' width of breast ultrasound transducers varies between manufacturers.

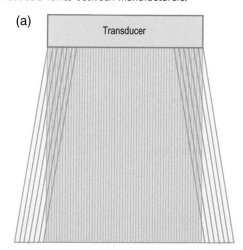

(a)

Transducer

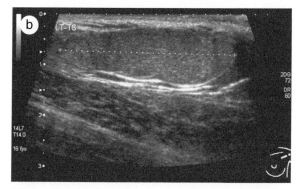

Figure 4.10   (a) Diagram to illustrate how the ultrasound beam is steered at the edges to produce a field of view wider than the transducer footprint. (b) This 'extended' field of view can be used to display the full length of a large mass.

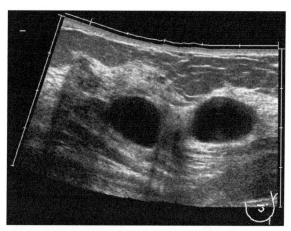

Figure 4.11   A 'panorama' extended field of view technique can be used to demonstrate the relationship of multiple large cysts within a breast.

(Fig. 4.11) (Philips 2005b, Siemens 2005). Extended field of view is a technique in which a compound image is built from multiple images obtained during a freehand translation of the transducer across a wide area of interest. The feature facilitates measurement of very large lesions, and can make it much easier to document the position of any particular lesion with reference to other lesions and/or to the nipple (Barr 2001, Stavros 2004, Ying & Sin 2005).

Use of a stand-off

Use of a thin (10 mm) acoustic stand-off pad (Fig. 4.12a) can improve visualization of very superficial lesions and the nipple–areolar complex. Since the focal depth in the elevation plane (short axis focus) of most dedicated breast transducers is around 15–20 mm (Stavros 2004, p. 21), small lesions that lie superficial to this may be missed due to volume averaging. The use of a stand-off moves a superficial lesion closer to the short axis focus where the slice thickness is narrowest (Fig. 4.12b). At this depth, volume averaging is reduced, thus spatial and contrast resolution are improved and lesion conspicuity is increased. Where a stand-off pad is not available, some operators advocate the use of a generous amount of gel to achieve a similar effect.

The routine use of a stand-off, however, is of no benefit as deep lesions may be moved out of the normal focal range of the transducer. Stavros (2004, p. 947) suggests that lesions that are both palpable and pea sized or smaller are best visualized with the use of a stand-off. Where a 1.5D array is available, use of a stand-off should not be necessary as limited short axis focusing can be achieved throughout the depth of interest.

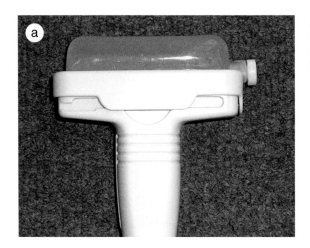

Figure 4.12   (a) A transducer with a water-path stand-off attachment. (b) Diagram to illustrate how the use of a stand-off attachment brings superficial structures into the transducer's short axis focal zone.

(b)

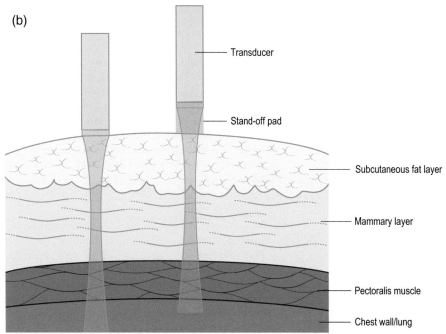

Transducer

Stand-off pad

Subcutaneous fat layer

Mammary layer

Pectoralis muscle

Chest wall/lung

DOPPLER IMAGING

Cell proliferation and tumor growth are associated with increased perfusion and the development of new blood vessels (angiogenesis). The flow velocity waveform produced in spectral Doppler mode allows an estimation of the force required to direct blood through a vessel and thus has some correlation with the density and compressibility of the tissue supplied by the vessel (Fig. 4.13). The assessment of microvascularity in breast carcinoma is known to correlate with a number of significant prognostic factors. For these reasons, considerable work has been undertaken using Doppler ultrasound to character-

ize flow within tumors in an attempt to differentiate benign and malignant disease (Chao et al 1999, Shroeder et al 1999, Moon et al 2000). Whilst Doppler may provide additional information that may raise or lower the level of suspicion for a specific lesion, Doppler criteria alone are not as useful as characteristic B-mode appearances (Stavros et al 1995, Hong et al 2005). The use of Doppler in breast imaging and the interpretation of the Doppler information are considered in more detail in Chapters 6 and 7. General aspects related to equipment specification, Doppler control settings and technique that are relevant to breast imaging are summarized in Table 4.4.

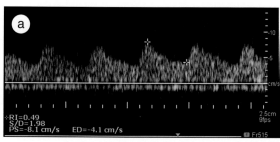 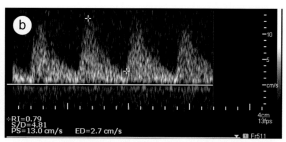

Figure 4.13 (a) Spectral Doppler display of a low resistance flow velocity waveform–typically seen in soft, compliant benign lesions. (b) A high resistance Doppler flow velocity waveform is more commonly associated with hard, dense malignant lesions.

Table 4.4 How to optimize Doppler settings

Control	Optimization criteria
Frequency	The transducer will normally default to a lower frequency (5 MHz) in Doppler mode. Manual selection of lower frequency or change of transducer may be necessary for large breasts.
Pulse repetition frequency (PRF) or scale	Low PRF (not >1 kHz) should be used to demonstrate low velocity flow.
Wall filter	Use low setting to avoid loss of low velocity flow in the breast. (50–100 Hz)
Color box	Use straight color box to maintain transducer sensitivity.
	Limit area to maintain frame rate–ensure a perimeter of 'normal' breast tissue is included for comparison when evaluating a focal lesion
Color priority	Select 'high' priority.
	In conventional color Doppler, each pixel within the color box is allocated either a color or a gray-scale level. Signals from soft tissue are of a higher intensity than the backscattered signal from red blood cells. By setting a threshold level of intensity above which a gray-scale level is allocated, the system can distinguish between blood and moving soft tissue. To image flow within the breast, a high priority level should be set to avoid overwriting flow within small vessels that may contain artifact.
Color gain	Set to minimum level just above noise–optimize this over an area of 'normal' breast (or the contralateral breast) before examining the area of interest.

The **system requirements for Doppler** imaging of the breast are similar to those for B-mode. Any Doppler system utilizes the weak backscattered signal from red blood cells. This signal normally falls below the threshold level for B-mode imaging and is close to the level of background noise. System sensitivity and signal-to-noise ratio in Doppler mode are therefore important, and both are likely to be better with a higher specification machine. The velocities of blood cells vary enormously in different vessels and, because there will be some tissue movement due to respiratory motion and transmitted cardiac pulsation, the operator needs to manipulate the Doppler controls to optimize sensitivity to blood flow, ensuring that both high and low velocities are accurately represented and that non-useful background movement information is filtered out.

In peripheral vascular applications, it is often necessary to steer the beam to achieve an adequate beam to vessel angle (Fig. 4.14). In breast imaging, this is rarely important, as the vessels are too small and tortuous to be sampled individually. Beam steering reduces transducer sensitivity and should not be used in color or power Doppler modes for breast imaging.

One of the most significant factors in the detection of flow in small vessels within the breast is the degree of pressure applied through the transducer. If even slight pressure is applied, small vessels may collapse and flow can be obliterated (Fig. 4.15). A careful scanning technique is required. It may be helpful for the operator to support their scanning arm on a pillow placed across the patient's abdomen.

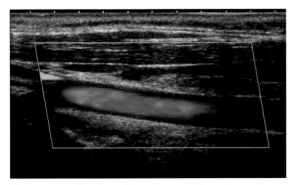

Figure 4.14   Steering of the ultrasound beam is used to optimize the Doppler angle when evaluating long straight vessels such as the carotid artery.

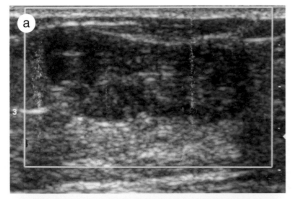

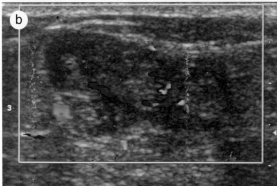

Figure 4.15   Too much transducer pressure (a) can obliterate low pressure vessels in the breast; scanning with just enough pressure to achieve good contact (b) demonstrates small caliber, low velocity, low pressure vessels, confirming that this lesion is a solid mass and not a complex fluid collection.

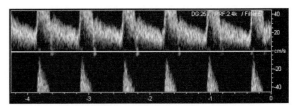

Figure 4.16   Aliasing—in spectral Doppler mode, if the pulse repetition frequency control is set too low, the Doppler signal will not be accurately represented.

The sensitivity of *power* Doppler is greater than conventional colour Doppler. The displayed colour hue within a conventional colour flow image relates to the mean Doppler shift for each pixel location. Doppler signals from small vessels that lie within each sample volume are effectively averaged for each location. As these vessels are tortuous, positive and negative directional flow will cancel out.

In power Doppler mode, the signal contribution from each small vessel is added. To achieve this, both directional and velocity information are sacrificed. However, as no velocity information is displayed, the pulse repetition frequency (PRF) is no longer limited by the need to avoid aliasing (failure to display high velocities accurately; Fig. 4.16). Use of a low PRF improves detection of low velocity flow.

One of the limitations of power Doppler is increased sensitivity to patient movement. This can result in color motion artifact. Although occasionally problematic, this effect can be utilized to evaluate the response of areas of breast tissue to deliberately induced vibration.

The assessment of response to *vocal fremitus* was first described by Sohn and Baudendistel in 1995. They noted by chance that color Doppler artifacts produced in response to thoracic vibration as the patient speaks were absent in tumor tissue, and that there might be a differential effect between benign and malignant tumors. More recently, Stavros (2004, p. 923) reported the use of power Doppler vocal fremitus, and claimed that using power Doppler made the technique more sensitive than when using color Doppler. Standard power Doppler settings are selected and the patient is asked to hum; the area of interest is interrogated and the response compared with an area of normal tissue using a split screen facility. Areas of abnormal tissue exhibit an acoustic vibratory defect, i.e. show no color artifact (Fig. 4.17). Although it is probably not possible to differentiate benign and malignant lesions reliably, the technique nevertheless seems to be useful for identifying focal lesions that have similar reflectivity to surrounding tissue.

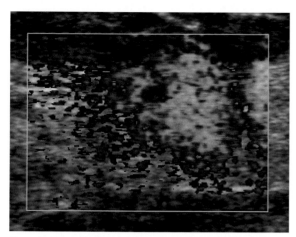

Figure 4.17 Vocal fremitus can be used to highlight breast lesions as vibratory defects.

Box 4.4   Recommended weekly user tests

- Visual inspection of transducers and cables
- Crystal drop out check
- Hard copy performance

MDA (1998a)

EQUIPMENT MAINTENANCE AND ROUTINE QUALITY ASSURANCE

Equipment manufacturers and suppliers offer a variety of equipment *maintenance contracts* that provide varying levels of service support. These should be explored at the time of purchase. A key issue for many breast units is the availability of only one ultrasound machine. It is therefore important to consider the reliability record of the equipment, as downtime can be very difficult to manage. Often the best way to check equipment reliability and the quality of support available from specific manufacturers is to speak with other users.

Medical equipment should be tested before it is first used on patients, routinely within a planned preventative maintenance program and whenever repairs or modifications are carried out. *Electrical safety testing* is a statutory requirement on delivery of any new equipment and annually thereafter (MDA 1998b). *Routine equipment testing* is recommended by the MDA (1998b) as it may provide useful information about the consistency of equipment performance; however, it is not a substitute for regular servicing. In addition to the formal 6-monthly testing regime outlined in the above document, routine weekly user tests are also recommended (Box 4.4).

The aim of a quality assurance (QA) program is to ensure that acceptance levels of performance are maintained and that performance is consistent over time. Within any QA program, there needs to be local agreement on how the information obtained during routine QA testing will be used—without a specific indication of the limits of acceptability of test results, and clear agreement on who is responsible for taking any necessary action, there is little value in such a program.

Cleaning the transducer

Numerous studies have identified the potential for the spread of infection from ultrasound transducers (Fowler & McCracken 1999, Karadeniz et al 2001). Cleaning the transducer between patients is therefore essential. Most equipment manufacturers recommend a non-alcohol-based cleaning fluid. Over time, alcohol-based solutions will damage the rubber seal on the transducer scanning surface, and their use may invalidate any manufacturer warranty.

RECENT ADVANCES IN ULTRASOUND EQUIPMENT TECHNOLOGY

In conventional B-mode imaging, each frame of information from a linear array is generated by firing groups of elements in a single sweep across the face of the transducer. Each pulse of sound is fired at 90° to the array. **Compound imaging** uses electronic beam steering to fire pulses from between three and nine separate transmit angles (Fig. 4.18) (Philips 2005c). Real time imaging is

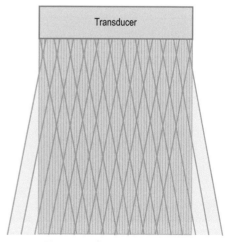

Figure 4.18 Diagram to illustrate how compound imaging uses multiple transmit angles to generate one frame of image information.

then achieved by combining the data from multiple lines of sight to generate successive frames.

By scanning from a number of different angles, artifacts such as speckle, clutter, noise and shadowing are reduced and real structures are reinforced. Benefits have been reported in breast imaging; however, the use of compound imaging is not without its limitations.

A number of authors report an improvement in delineation of capsular margins (Fig. 4.19), conspicuity of low-contrast lesions, tissue differentiation, clearer depiction of internal architecture of solid lesions, artifact reduction within cysts and clearer depiction of implants (Entrekin 1999, Huber et al 2002, Kwak et al 2004, Stavros 2004).

The key drawback of this technique is that the system is unable to distinguish between artifacts that reduce image quality and 'helpful' artifacts that may alert the operator to the presence of pathology or help to charac-terize a lesion. Compound imaging effectively removes or reduces the appearance of acoustic shadowing (Fig. 4.20). This includes a reduction in edge shadowing (typically associated with a fibroadenoma) and shadowing posterior to a malignant lesion. The appearance of increased through transmission posterior to a cyst or area of low attenuation will also be reduced.

It is not yet clear if compound imaging results in a simple improvement in the aesthetic appearance of the ultrasound image, or if it contributes to improved diagnostic capability. Whilst some operators are choosing to use compound imaging as their standard technique, and are thus incorporating it into the default pre-set, accepted sonographic criteria for lesion characterization are based on the conventional imaging format. Thus a combination of observations in conventional and compound formats is likely to yield both accurate diagnosis and optimal display.

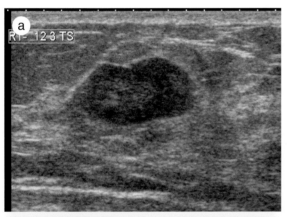

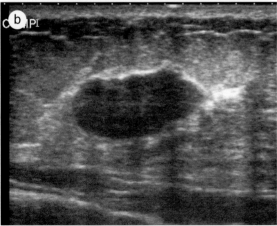

Figure 4.19   (a) A solid benign lesion (fibroadenoma) imaged using conventional B-mode imaging. (b) The same lesion imaged using the compound technique better demonstrates the lesion margins.

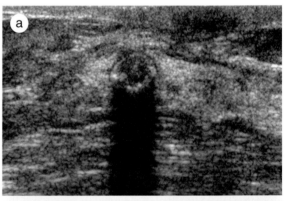

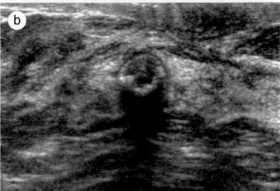

Figure 4.20   (a) A calcified cyst imaged using conventional B-mode imaging exhibits pronounced posterior shadowing. (Image courtesy of Philips Medical Systems.) (b) With the compound imaging technique, the oblique scan lines fill in some image information behind the cyst. (Image courtesy of Philips Medical Systems.)

Tissue harmonic imaging exploits the phenomenon of non-linear propagation of ultrasound through a medium. As sound propagates through tissue, it is generally assumed that the speed of propagation is a constant for a given tissue. In reality, at high amplitude, the high pressure parts of the wave (areas of compression) travel faster than the low pressure components (areas of rarefaction). This non-linear propagation of the beam results in the production of higher frequency waves. The frequency of these *harmonic* waves is a multiple of the transmitted frequency. For example, a transmitted frequency of 6 MHz would generate a second harmonic signal at 12 MHz.

Tissue harmonic imaging utilizes these higher frequency components to produce the B-mode image. Harmonics are generated by the higher amplitude central part of the transmitted beam with the weaker, off-axis part of the beam and any side lobes generating little harmonic signal. The effective beam width produced by the harmonic waves is therefore narrower than the transmitted beam, and side lobe artifacts are significantly reduced. This results in an improvement in lateral resolution, reduction of volume averaging and reduction of clutter (Hoskins et al 2003).

There are essentially two distinct ways in which harmonic imaging can be achieved. Early systems utilize a low frequency, broad bandwidth pulse on transmission. On reception, the low frequency echo components are filtered out, leaving a harmonic frequency beam with narrow bandwidth. Key disadvantages of this approach are a reduction in axial resolution associated with the reduced bandwidth and reduced penetration of the higher frequency components. Neither of these limitations is acceptable for breast imaging (Hoskins et al 2003, Stavros 2004, GE 2005a, Philips 2005d).

Pulse inversion harmonics utilizes a subtraction method of signal processing rather than filtering. By using consecutive phase-adjusted pulses, the system receiver can recognize specific return signals. Unwanted signals can therefore be subtracted regardless of any frequency overlap. It is therefore possible to maintain a broad bandwidth beam on reception without loss of axial resolution or sensitivity (Elliot 2005, GE 2005a).

Reported benefits for breast imaging include clearer differentiation of small cysts, increased conspicuity of solid lesions and better visualization of lesion capsules (Fig. 4.21) and calcifications (Kubota et al 2002, Szopinski et al 2003, Stavros 2004, Rapp & Stavros 2005).

Elastography is a developing technique that uses information from the ultrasound signal to display differences in the elastic properties of breast tissue. Occasionally, breast lesions may not be visible with conventional ultrasound and mammography techniques but are obviously palpable at clinical examination—most feeling hard

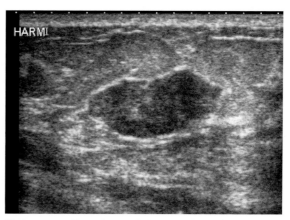

Figure 4.21 Tissue harmonic imaging further improves visualization of the margins and internal features of the fibroadenoma shown using conventional B-mode imaging in Figure 4.19a.

in comparison with surrounding breast tissue. In the same way that the clinician can feel a difference in texture, elastography detects and displays differences in tissue stiffness and thus has the potential to reveal lesions not normally visible (Bamber et al 1998, Pellot-Barakat et al 2004, Smith et al 2004). The technical requirements for elastography imaging vary between different systems, but all utilize the ability of ultrasound to detect small tissue movements in response to applied deformation, the pressure usually being applied manually through the transducer. The technique has been shown to offer improved tumor detection, grading and assessment of response to treatment (Bamber et al 1998, Hiltawsky et al 2001, Bercoff et al 2003).

3D ULTRASOUND

(with Sandra Twardun, Ultrasound Applications Specialist, GE Healthcare)

When performing a conventional two-dimensional B-mode ultrasound examination of the breast, a series of essentially two-dimensional images (of very thin slices of tissue) are viewed in rapid succession in real time. From this, the operator constructs a mental impression of the three-dimensional anatomical structure. Archived (still or video) images can be reviewed by the operator or by a third party, but it can be difficult to appreciate and understand true anatomical relationships from these 2D images, in the absence of movement or without simultaneous hand–eye correlation to help interpret the moving image.

3D ultrasound involves the rapid acquisition of image data from a volume block of breast tissue and its electronic manipulation to display multiple planes and slices of the 3D structure.

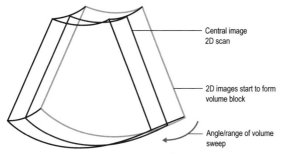

Figure 4.22   The 3D volume block. (Diagram courtesy of GE Healthcare.)

Using a specially designed transducer, the 3D data set is acquired as the ultrasound field is swept automatically through a volume of tissue (Fig. 4.22). The user holds the transducer still as the internal mechanism sweeps once, from one margin to the other margin, completing the angle selected. Volume data sets are readily stored to the ultrasound machine hard drive and then recalled for diagnostic review and manipulation, perhaps after the patient has left the examination room, and for teaching purposes. Image resolution is related to the number of slices obtained, but increased slice acquisition (and therefore improved resolution) requires longer data acquisition times.

The data set is initially viewed, similar to the 2D image slices, but in three orthogonal planes (A, B and C) centrally pivoted around a reference dot (Fig. 4.23);

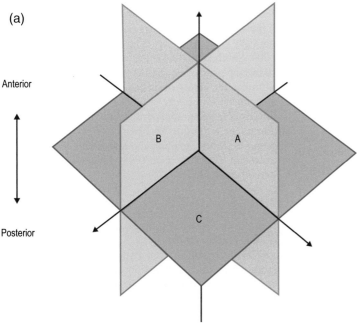

(a)

Figure 4.23   (a) The three orthogonal section planes A, B and C. (Diagram courtesy of GE Healthcare.)

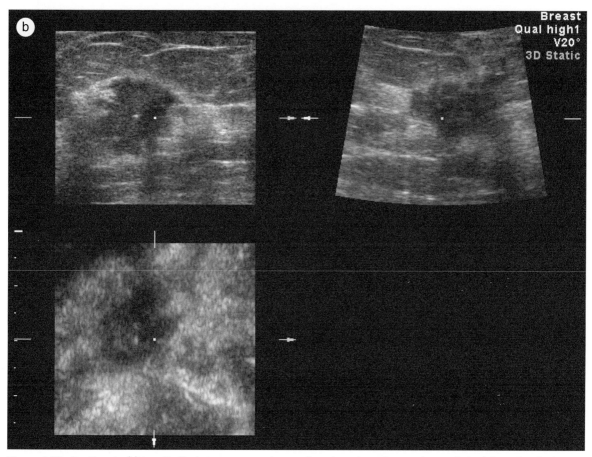

Figure 4.23, *Continued*   (b) Longitudinal, transverse and coronal sections through a carcinoma derived from the 3D data set. (Image courtesy of GE Healthcare.)

the reference dot is moved through the volume to display successive adjacent slices. The three images, with a 90° relationship to each other, can be displayed simultaneously or separately. There is also the option to display a series of contiguous anatomical slices in one particular plane—tomographic ultrasound imaging (Fig. 4.24). The information can be viewed in a variety of planes, with the ability to reconstruct in coronal planes, i.e. to demonstrate anatomical planes parallel to the skin/chest wall, proving particularly useful for evaluating the branching ductal anatomy and assessing intraduct disease extension

(Fig. 4.25). The technique can also be used in color or power Doppler mode to display vascular information.

Reported advantages of 3D breast ultrasound include clearer definition of tumor margins, improved accuracy and reproducibility of tumor volume measurement and assessment of tumor size variation over time, better appreciation of the internal structure of lesions, improved visualization of biopsy needles (Fig. 4.26) and easier visualization of breast structure as an aid to surgical planning (Chen et al 2004, Smith et al 2004, Shipley et al 2005).

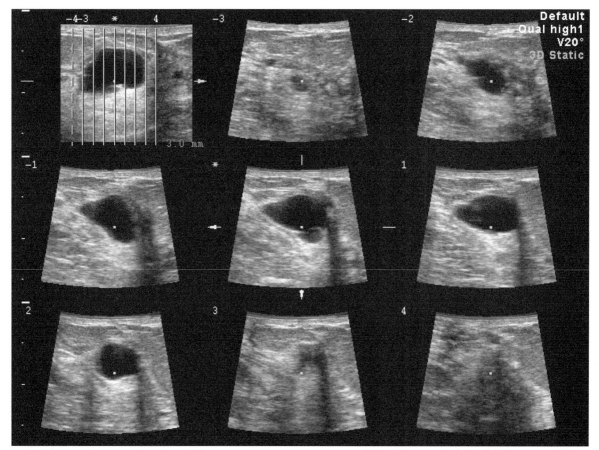

Figure 4.24   Nine contiguous 'tomographic' 3D slices through a cyst derived from the 3D data set. (Image courtesy of GE Healthcare.)

A further interesting development is the semi-automated acquisition of 3D ultrasound data with simultaneous acquisition of digital mammograms. Registration of mammogram and ultrasound image volumes seems possible, when the breast is stably compressed, and appears to offer better correlation of ultrasound and mammography findings (Kapur et al 2004, Shipley et al 2005).

SUMMARY

The amount and quality of information obtained during the ultrasound examination is fundamentally dependent upon the quality of ultrasound equipment used and on the selection and manipulation of scanning parameters by a skilled and knowledgeable operator.

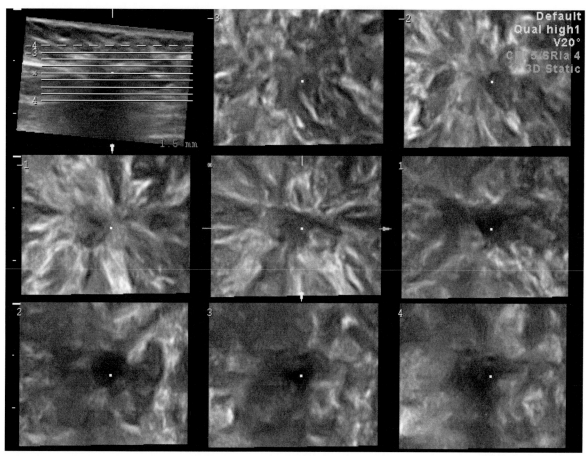

Figure 4.25 Tomographic coronal planes reconstructed from the 3D data set of a breast carcinoma readily demonstrate ductal extension. (Image courtesy of Dr Christian Weismann, Salzburg, Austria.)

As technological prototypes move from the design laboratory into the clinical environment, the quantity, type and quality of information displayed in the image continues to expand and improve. The ultrasound operator is challenged to continually keep up to date with new developments and to exploit and capitalize on each innovation in order to justify increased financial outlay in terms of enhanced diagnostic yield.

An awareness and appreciation of key system performance requirements (Table 4.5) will ensure the operator is able to choose equipment that is ergonomically safe and has high diagnostic capability, and that the equipment is used to its maximum diagnostic potential.

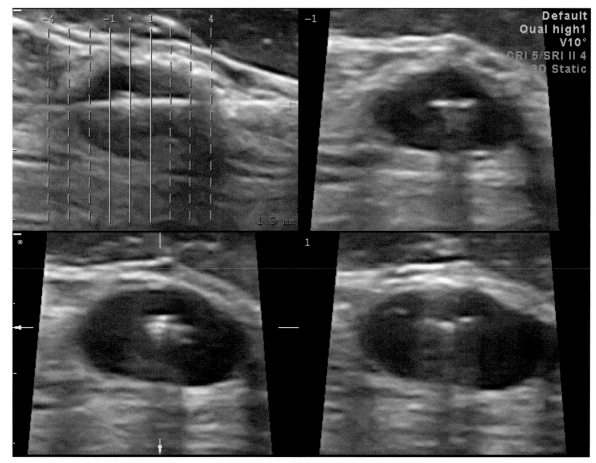

Figure 4.26 Multiple planar sections demonstrate how a biopsy sampling needle track passes centrally through a lesion. (Image courtesy of GE Healthcare.)

Table 4.5 Summary of system performance requirements for breast ultrasound

Essential	Desirable	Essential	Desirable
Imaging capability		**Transducer requirements**	
High resolution	Compound imaging	Excellent near field focusing	
High sensitivity	Tissue harmonics	(focal depth in elevation	
Excellent contrast	Extended field of view	plane 12–20 mm)	
resolution		Light weight but large enough	
Color, spectral and		for palmar grip (footprint	
power Doppler capability		width 40 mm)	
Transducer requirements		**Ergonomic features**	
High frequency (above	1.5D array	Lightweight and maneuvrable	Footswitch
7.5 MHz)		Adjustable height keyboard	Voice activation
Penetration depth to at	Stand-off facility	and monitor	software
least 40 mm			Keyboard and monitor
Broad bandwidth			tilt facility
		Additional features	
		Hard copy imaging device	Digital archiving and
			retrieval facilities

References

ACR 2002 ACR practice guideline for the performance of a breast ultrasound examination. Reston, VA: American College of Radiology.

AIUM 2002 AIUM standard for the performance of breast ultrasound examination. Laurel, MD: American Institute of Ultrasound in Medicine.

Bamber JC, Doyley M, Miller N et al 1998 Freehand elasticity imaging to improve breast tumour diagnosis. Annual Research Report. London: Institute of Cancer Research/Royal Marsden NHS Trust. 119 pp. Online. Available at: http://enjoy.underwired.com/portfolio/sites/icr/research_pdf/imaging98.pdf. Accessed on 18 March 2006.

Barr RG 2001 Breast ultrasound: a bright future. Medica Mundi 45(2):8–13. Online. Koninklijke Philips Electronics N.V. Available at: http://www.medical.philips.com/main/news/publications/medicamundi/archive/ Accessed on 18 March 2006.

Bercoff J, Chaffai S, Tanter M et al 2003 In vivo breast tumour detection using transient elastography. Ultrasound in Medicine and Biology 29(10):1387–1396.

Chao TC, Lo YF, Chen SC et al 1999 Color Doppler ultrasound in benign and malignant breast tumors. Breast Cancer Research and Treatment 57(2):193–199.

Chen DR, Chang RF, Chen CJ et al 2004 Three-dimensional ultrasound in margin evaluation for breast tumor excision using Mammotome. Ultrasound in Medicine and Biology 30(2):169–179.

Dodgeon J, Newton-Hughes A 2003 Enabling sonographers to minimise work related musculoskeletal disorders. BMUS Bulletin 11(3):16–21.

Elliot ST 2005 A user guide to tissue harmonic imaging. Ultrasound 13(4):243–248.

Entrekin RR 1999 Real time spatial compound imaging in breast ultrasound: technology and early clinical experience Medica Mundi 43(3):35–43. Online. Koninklijke Philips Electronics N.V. Available at: http://www.medical.philips.com/main/news/publications/medicamundi/archive/ Accessed on 18 March 2006.

Fowler C, McCraken D 1999 Ultrasound probes. Risk of cross infection and ways to reduce it—comparison of cleaning methods. Radiology 213(1):299–300.

Garra BS 2005 Processing, technology improves breast imaging. Higher frequencies, better transducers, and new techniques portend an era of faster speeds and greater detail. California: Diagnostic Imaging. Online. Available at: http://www.diagnosticimaging.com/AdvancedUS/breast.jhtml Accessed on 9 March 2006.

GE 2005a LOGIQ 700 transducers: LA39 boad spectrum transducer. Online. Available at: www.gehealthcare.com/usen/ultrasound/education/products/msula39.html Accessed on 18 March 2006.

GE 2005b LOGICView extended field of view imaging. Online. Available at: www.gehealthcare.com/euen/ultrasound/products/general-imaging/logiq-7/truscan-architecture.html Accessed on 18 March 2006.

Hiltawsky KM, Kruger M, Starke C et al 2001 Freehand ultrasound elastography of breast lesions: clinical results. Ultrasound in Medicine and Biology 27(11):1461–1469.

Hong AS, Rosen EL, Soo MS et al 2005 BI-RADS for sonography: positive and negative predictive values of sonographic features. American Journal of Roentgenology 184(4):1260–1265.

Hoskins PR, Thrush A, Martin K et al 2003 Diagnostic ultrasound physics and equipment. London: Greenwich Medical Media.

Huber S, Wagner M, Medl M et al 2002 Real time spatial compound imaging in breast ultrasound. Ultrasound in Medicine and Biology 28(2):155–163.

Kapur A, Carson PL, Eberhard J et al 2004 Combination of digital mammography with semi-automated 3D breast ultrasound. Technology in Cancer Research & Treatment 3(4):325–334.

Karadeniz YM, Kılıç D, Altan SK et al 2001 Evaluation of the role of ultrasound machines as a source of nosocomial and cross-infection (Technical report). Investigative Radiology 36(9):554–558.

Kubota K, Hisa N, Ogawa Y et al 2002 Evaluation of tissue harmonic imaging for breast tumors and axillary lymph nodes. Oncology Reports 9(6):1335–1338.

Kwak JY, Kim EK, You JK et al 2004 Variable breast conditions. Comparison of conventional and real-time compound ultrasonography. Journal of Ultrasound in Medicne 23(1):85–96.

Madjar H 2000 The practice of breast ultrasound. Stuttgart: Thieme.

Madjar H, Rickard M, Jellins J et al (eds) 1998 IBUS guidelines for the ultrasonic examination of the breast. European Journal of Ultrasound 9:99–102.

MDA 1998a Further revisions to guidance notes for ultrasound scanners used in the examination of the breast, with protocol for quality testing. Evaluation Report MDA/98/52. London: Medical Devices Agency, Department of Health.

MDA 1998b Medical device and equipment management for hospital and community based organisations. Device Bulletin 9801. London: Medical Devices Agency, Department of Health.

MDA 2001 A comparative evaluation of eleven ultrasound scanners for examination of the breast. MDA 01024. London: Medical Devices Agency, Department of Health.

Miles J 2005 Work related upper limb disorders in sonographers. Synergy. London: Society of Radiographers. October, pp. 6–11.

Moon WK, Im J-G, Noh D-Y et al 2000 Nonpalpable breast lesions: evaluation with power doppler US and a microbubble contrast agent—initial experience. Radiology 217(1):240–246.

NHS PASA 2005 Ultrasound: radiology. Online. Reading: NHS Purchasing and Supply Agency. Available at: http://www.pasa.nhs.uk/dme/radiology/ultra.stm Accessed on 8 March 2006.

Pellot-Barakat C, Frouin F, Insana MF et al 2004 Ultrasound elastography based on multiscale estimations of regularized displacement fields. IEEE Transactions on Medical Imaging 23(2):153–163.

Philips 2005a Transducers. Online. Available at: www.medical.philips.com/main/products/ultrasound/transducers/ Accessed on 18 March 2006.

Philips 2005b HDI 5000 Panoramic imaging. Online. Available at: http://www.medical.philips.com/main/products/ultrasound/general/hdi5000/features/panoramic.html Accessed on 18 March 2006.

Philips 2005c SonoCT Real time compound imaging. Online. Available at: http://www.medical.philips.com/us/products/ultrasound/general/hdi5000/upgrades/sonoct/index.html Accessed on 18 March 2006.

Philips 2005d HDI 5000 Pulse inversion harmonics. Online. Available at: http://www.medical.philips.com/main/products/ultrasound/general/hdi5000/features/pulse_inversion.html Accessed on 18 March 2006.

Rapp CL, Stavros AT 2005 Coded harmonics in breast ultrasound: does it make a difference? Online. Available at: http://www.gehealthcare.com/inen/rad/us/education/edu_rapparticle.html Accessed on 18 March 2006.

RCR 2003 Guidance on screening and symptomatic breast imaging. 2nd edn. BFCR(03)2. London: Royal College of Radiologists.

RCR 2005 Standards for ultrasound equipment. BFCR(05)01. London: Royal College of Radiologists.

SDMS 2003 Industry standards for the prevention of work-related musculoskeletal disorders in sonography. Plano, TX: Society of Diagnostic Medical Sonography.

Shipley JA, Duck FA, Goddard DA et al 2005 Automated quantitative volumetric breast ultrasound data-acquisition system. Ultrasound in Medicine and Biology 31(7):905–917.

Shroeder RJ, Maeurer J, Vogl TJ et al 1999 D-Galactose-based signal-enhanced color Doppler sonography of breast tumors and tumorlike lesions. Investigative Radiology 34(2):109–115.

Siemens 2005 Siescape panoramic imaging. Online. Available at: http://www.medical.siemens.com/webapp/wcs/stores/servlet/ProductDisplay?productId=13712&storeId=10001&langId=-11&catalogId=-11&catTree=100001,12805,12823*483748584&level=0 Accessed on 18 March 2006.

Smith AP, Hall PA, Marcello DM 2004 Emerging technologies in breast cancer detection. Radiological Management 26(4):16–24.

Sohn C, Baudendistel A 1995 Differential diagnosis of mammary tumors with vocal fremitus in sonography: preliminary report. Ultrasound in Obstetrics & Gynecology 6(3):205–207.

Stavros AT 2004 Breast ultrasound. Philadelphia: Lippincott Williams & Wilkins.

Stavros AT 2005 Potential future developments for breast imaging. Online. Proceedings of the 5th Scientific Meeting of the Australasian Society for Breast Disease, Queensland, Australia 24 September 2005. pp. 81–83. Available at: http://www.asbd.org.au/handbook.pdf Accessed on 23 March 2006.

Stavros AT, Thickman D, Rapp CL et al 1995 Solid breast nodules: use of sonography to distinguish between benign and malignant lesions. Radiology 196(1):123–134.

Szopinski KT, Pajk AM, Wysocki M et al 2003 Tissue harmonic imaging. Utility in breast sonography. Journal of Ultrasound in Medicine 22(5):479–487.

UKAS 2001 Guidelines for professional working practice. London: United Kingdom Association of Sonographers.

Ying M, Sin MH 2005 Comparison of extended field of view and dual image ultrasound techniques: accuracy and reliability of distance measurements in phantom study. Ultrasound in Medicine and Biology 31(1):79–83.

Chapter **5**

Breast anatomy and normal ultrasound appearances

Mike Stocksley and Anne-Marie Dixon

BREAST DEVELOPMENT

The female breasts or mammary glands are accessory organs of the female reproductive system. Originating as ectodermal modified sweat glands at birth, the mammary glands in males and females are undeveloped and appear as minimal elevations on the chest wall. In the female, thelarche (commencement of breast development) starts between 10 and 12 years of age during puberty, a developmental phase that marks the change from childhood to physical maturity. Prior to the onset of thelarche, approximately at the age of 8 or 9 years, biochemical changes, predominantly in the adrenal gland, take place. The ovaries develop multiple small follicles in response to nocturnal luteinizing hormone surges and this coincides with the first noticeable development of the breast; the breast bud. Breast development has been classified by Tanner (Fig. 5.1).

Endocrine malfunction may cause breast development at an early age.

Precocious puberty describes the development of secondary sexual characteristics before the age of 8 years. It is identical to normal puberty but occurs early owing to premature activation of the hypothalamic–pituitary–gonadal axis. Associated gynecological ultrasound signs include enlarged ovaries containing multiple follicles and a 'large for age' uterus with signs of estrogen-responsive endometrial proliferation.

Pseudoprecocious puberty describes the condition where secondary sexual characteristics are present, e.g. isolated pubic hair, as a result of excess androgen production. This condition may result from an ovarian or adrenal neoplasm. Ultrasound may demonstrate large ovarian follicles, and although the child does not ovulate regularly since the ovaries are prematurely functional transient breast development occurs.

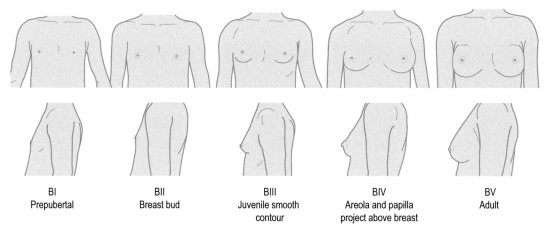

BI	BII	BIII	BIV	BV
Prepubertal	Breast bud	Juvenile smooth contour	Areola and papilla project above breast	Adult

Figure 5.1   Tanner breast development classification. (After Tanner, 1962.)

Isolated premature thelarche, defined as isolated breast development without progression through puberty, can occur in infants between 6 months and 2 years of age. Breast development is often asymmetrical. Unlike precocious puberty, there is no associated axillary or pubic hair development or growth spurt, and developed ovarian follicles are fewer but larger.

In the breasts of prepubescent children, both males and females have a rudimentary glandular system consisting mainly of lactiferous ducts with a small number of alveoli, the internal structures being the same in males and females.

At puberty, breasts in the female start to develop after the release of the female sex hormones, estrogen and progesterone, by the ovaries. Ovarian secretion is ultimately controlled by follicle-stimulating hormone (FSH) which is secreted in response to gonadotropin-releasing factor (GnRF) by the hypothalamus. Estrogen stimulates the formation of additional ducts and the elongation of existing ducts and development of the milk-secreting glands, with progesterone stimulating lobule formation. Breast enlargement is usually the first sign of normal puberty, with menarche (onset of menstruation) occurring after breast development (Tanner stage IV). With the onset of ovulation and the formation of the corpus luteum, there is further mammary development. The ductule system matures, fat deposits are laid down, the glands increase in size, and the areola and nipple become pigmented. Their primary role being lactation, the breasts are normally in a resting state and only reach full functional development during the latter stages of pregnancy.

After puberty, during childbearing years and during pregnancy, continued estrogen and progesterone stimulation cause increased breast tissue development; after the menopause when estrogen production is reduced, the breast tissue will undergo atrophy.

It is typical for one breast to be slightly larger than the other (typically the left is the larger), but sometimes development is markedly asymmetrical. Sudden onset or progressive asymmetry requires investigation as it is usually associated with underlying pathological change. Breast development is very rarely unilaterally absent; Poland's syndrome describes the condition in association with underlying muscular, cartilaginous and bony anomalies.

In men, the breasts are functionless and normally remain undeveloped. Gynecomastia (enlargement of the male breast) may however occur and is particularly associated with treatment for cancer of the prostate, excess estrogen, obesity, Cushing's syndrome, cirrhosis of the liver, hyperthyroidism, and with some testicular and adrenocortical neoplasms (see Ch. 12).

GROSS ANATOMY OF THE BREAST

Most females have two breasts; the adult female breast is normally hemispherical in shape and protrudes from the anterior chest wall overlying the second to sixth ribs bilaterally (Fig. 5.2). The breasts are usually sited between the lateral borders of the sternum and the anterior axillary line. In the erect position, the superior aspect of each breast gradually rises from the infraclavicular fossa while the lateral, medial and inferior borders are relatively more well defined.

There is significant biological and physiological variation in actual breast size, shape and composition, with orientation and mobility also varying naturally with age, functional status and anatomical arrangement of stromal and parenchymal elements. The predominantly 'fatty' breast has a soft consistency with parenchymal tissue, which is often more prevalent in the lateral and upper

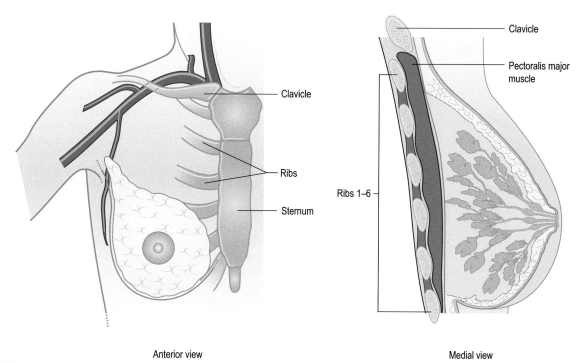

Anterior view   Medial view

Figure 5.2   Position of the adult female breast on the anterior chest wall. (Adapted from www.siefmedgraphics.com)

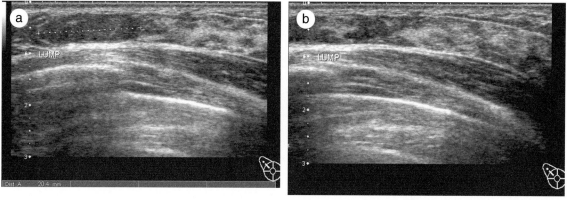

Figure 5.3   (a) Accessory breast tissue in the axilla. Clinically this presented as a palpable lump; on ultrasound the appearances suggested a slightly hyporeflective focal mass. (b) By rotating the transducer, it was possible to demonstrate that the accessory tissue is continuous with, and of similar architecture to, normal breast tissue in the upper outer quadrant of the breast.

outer parts of the breast, feeling much firmer. Breast consistency will vary throughout the menstrual cycle as the lobules swell and regress in response to hormonal stimulation. Multiparous women tend to have larger and more pendulous breasts.

The skin covering the breast, especially over the upper quadrants, is often thinner than the skin over the axilla and adjacent chest wall, with veins readily visible under the skin surface. In the supine position, the breast is relaxed over the chest wall and can extend into the axilla and over the upper chest wall if large. A triangular portion of breast tissue—the axillary tail (tail of Spence), extends towards the axilla. The axilla is the underarm fossa containing regional lymph nodes, and is traversed by lymphatic drainage channels, blood vessels and nerves.

Accessory breast tissue, either isolated from or contiguous with the main parenchyma, is most commonly found in the axilla (Fig. 5.3), but may occur anywhere

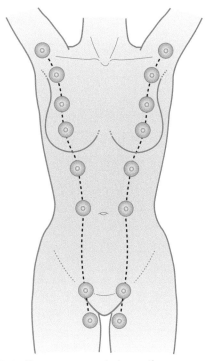

Figure 5.4 Supernumerary nipples and/or accessory breast tissue may occur anywhere along the 'milk lines'. (Redrawn from *Gray's Anatomy Online*, 39th edn, Churchill Livingstone.)

between the axilla and groin along the 'milk line' (Fig. 5.4). Up to 5% of the female population have supernumerary nipples, and these may be present with or without associated parenchymal (functional) tissue.

BREAST STRUCTURE

The adult female breast consists of parenchymal elements, the lobes with lobules of glandular tissue and ducts, adipose tissue and stromal elements of fibrous connective tissue that hold the lobes together (Fig. 5.5). It is essentially the amount of adipose tissue that gives the breast its form and determines its size. The normal adult female breast consists of approximately 80–85% fat.

Each breast consists of a surface covering of skin and variable thickness layers of subcutaneous fat and retromammary fat. Between the fat layers lies the parenchymal tissue enveloped in the superficial fascia of the anterior chest wall. The parenchymal tissue consists of approximately 15–20 breast lobes surrounded and separated by adipose and fibrous tissue. The lobes are positioned with the base nearest to the ribs and the apex close to the areola and nipple (Fig. 5.6). Each lobe contains a group

of lobules, the lobules measuring between 1 and 8 mm in diameter in the non-pregnant state—most measure between 1 and 2 mm. There can be hundreds, even thousands of lobules within each breast.

In the mature breast, the lobules consist of clusters of grape-like, potentially milk-secreting, rounded alveoli or acini (ductule-like terminal secretory units) opening into a terminal lactiferous ductule, there being 30–50 ductules in each lobule. Ductules are the smallest, blind-ending tubular epithelial structures that make up the resting mammary gland (Fig. 5.7). The terminal duct—the most distal terminal branch of the mammary duct system—and alveolus is termed the terminal ductal lobular unit (TDLU) (Fig. 5.8). The ductule is lined with epithelium and it is here that the majority of breast pathologies are considered to originate. The alveoli radiate around the small extralobular terminal ducts, this arrangement allowing for expansion of the TDLU in all directions during pregnancy and lactation.

The ductules unite to form larger tributaries of the terminal lactiferous ducts, each of which drains one lobe. Each lactiferous duct widens to form a lactiferous sinus or ampulla (acting as a reservoir for milk during lactation) then narrows again as it runs towards the areola, opening on the surface of the nipple (Fig. 5.9). An increase in size, tenderness and firmness in pregnancy is caused by the number of lobules multiplying.

Each breast has an areola and nipple situated anteriorly, and these are covered with pigmented squamous epithelium (Fig. 5.10). The areola is a circular area 2–6 cm in diameter whose pigment varies in color between pale pink to deep brown depending on a woman's age, skin color and parity. During a first pregnancy, the areola darkens and never regains its original light color. The areola has several small, raised bumps and beneath these are the sebaceous glands responsible for lubrication of the nipple; this helps prevent nipple and areolar cracking and fissure formation especially during breastfeeding. These 'Montgomery's' glands enlarge markedly during the third trimester of pregnancy.

The nipple is a raised mound of tissue in the middle of the areola, usually found at the level of the 4th intercostal space but varying in position according to how much the suspensory ligaments have been stretched. The base of the nipple is surrounded by a circular band of smooth muscle, Sappey's plexus (after Marie-Philibert-Constant Sappey, the nineteenth century French anatomist). Longitudinal smooth muscle fibers (Meyerholtz's muscle, after the nineteenth century German anatomist), branch out radially from the circular band to encircle the major lactiferous ducts that converge towards the nipple. Occasionally the nipple is congenitally inverted, sudden nipple inversion requiring investigation to rule out underlying inflammation or malignancy.

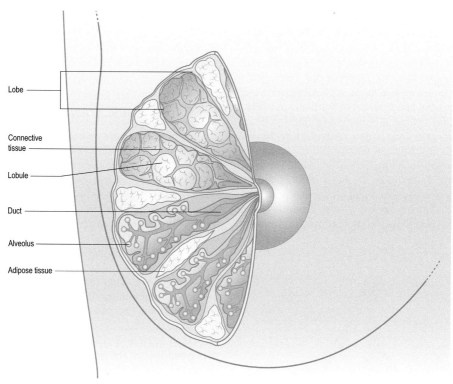

Figure 5.5   Cut-away diagram to show the macroscopic structure of the breast. (Adapted from www.breastdiagnostics.com)

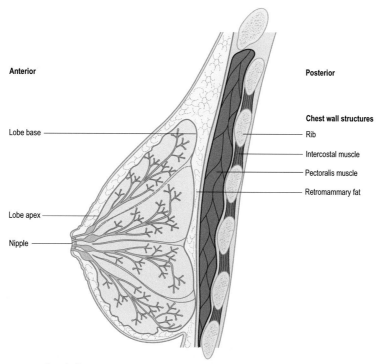

Figure 5.6   Sagittal cross-sectional diagram to show the orientation of the breast lobes in relation to the chest wall and nipple. (Adapted from Fig. 3.1 Madjar 2000.)

The lobules are held in place by fatty tissue and a net of loose connective tissue which supports blood vessels and ducts. The amount of fatty tissue increases towards the apex of each lobule, giving the breast its volume and characteristic shape. Most of the breast disk lies superficial to the pectoralis muscle fascia, with some overlying the anterior serratus and external oblique muscles (Fig. 5.11). The fascial stroma, a derivation of the superficial stroma of the chest wall, forms multiple fine bands, running radially from the breast into the subcutaneous tissues and the skin overlying the breast. These bands of fascia, or Cooper's suspensory ligaments (after Sir Astley Paston Cooper, the English surgeon who first described them in 1845), support and anchor the glandular structures of the breast between the skin and against the deep layer of the superficial fascia. Stretching of the suspensory ligaments (as occurs in pregnancy), or when the ligaments become loose with advancing age or illness, causes 'sagging' of the breast inferiorly onto the chest wall and in extreme cases onto the upper abdomen.

VASCULAR SUPPLY AND DRAINAGE

The breast is supplied with blood by several arteries (Fig. 5.12). The medial half of the breast and the pectoralis major and minor muscles are supplied by perforating branches of the internal thoracic artery which traverse the second, third and fourth intercostal spaces passing through the intercostal muscles and anterior intercostal membrane. These arteries enlarge during pregnancy and in advanced breast disease. The medial half of the breast is also supplied by small branches from the anterior intercostal arteries.

Laterally, the outer half of the breast is supplied by the pectoral branch of the thoraco-acromial branch of the axillary artery and the lateral mammary branches of the lateral thoracic artery. The medial and lateral arteries branch generally in the supra-areolar region such that the upper half of the breast has approximately double the arterial supply of the lower half.

The venous drainage pattern of the breast generally follows that of the arterial supply (Fig. 5.13). Blood is returned to the superior vena cava via the axillary, internal thoracic and internal jugular veins, and via the vertebral venous plexuses that are fed from the intercostal and azygos vein. An anastamotic plexus of superficial breast veins is found below the areola—this can often be

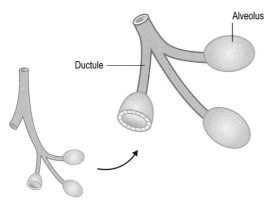

Figure 5.7 Diagrammatic representation of a breast ductule. (Adapted from www.kellyman.com)

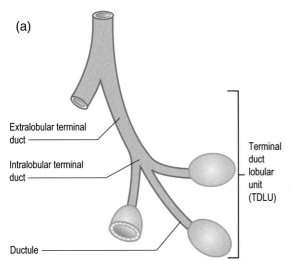

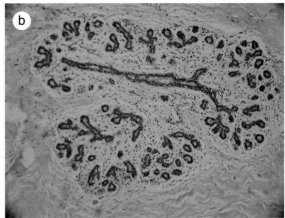

Figure 5.8 (a) Diagrammatic representation of a terminal duct lobular unit (TDLU). (b) Histological appearance of a TDLU. (Image courtesy of Dr J. Lowe, University Hospital of North Tees, UK.)

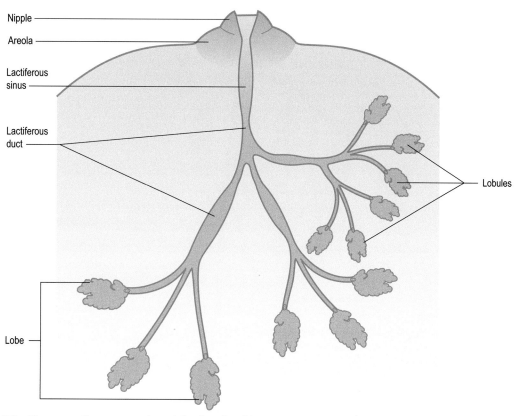

Nipple

Areola

Lactiferous sinus

Lactiferous duct

Lobules

Lobe

Figure 5.9   Diagrammatic representation of the ductal architecture of the breast. (Adapted from www.breastsource.com)

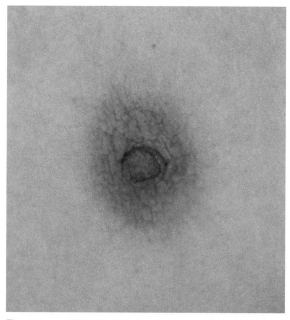

Figure 5.10   The nipple areola complex—the nipple rises centrally from the pigmented areola.

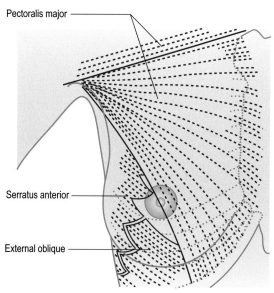

Pectoralis major

Serratus anterior

External oblique

Figure 5.11   The underlying muscular anatomy of the chest wall. (Adapted from Fig. 4.14 in Lumley 2002.)

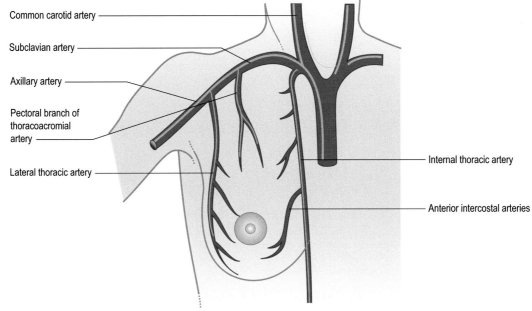

Figure 5.12   The arterial supply to the breast. (After www.breastcancersource.com)

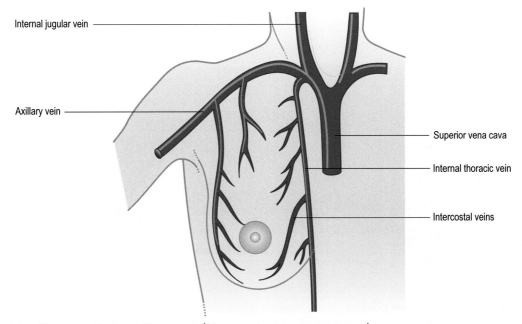

Figure 5.13   The venous drainage of the breast. (After www.breastcancersource.com)

seen in women with lighter, thinner skin and is obvious during pregnancy. Venous flow in the upper half of the breast is greater than in the lower half.

Hematogenous metastatic spread from breast tumors is often through the migration of malignant cells along branches of the axillary, intercostal and internal thoracic veins, promoting disease dissemination to the capilliary bed of the lungs, and via the vertebral plexus to the axial skeleton.

INNERVATION OF THE BREAST

Sensory nerves arising from the 2nd to 6th intercostal nerves that give rise to pain and pressure sensation in the breast extend upwards from the muscle layer through the breast to terminate in the skin layers, and are highly sensitive especially around the nipple and areola. It is for this reason that biopsy around the nipple and areola region is avoided whenever possible and why an intra-dermal technique is used for prebiopsy local anesthetic administration.

The thoraco-dorsal nerve, a branch of the posterior cord of the brachial plexus, innervates the superior half of the latissimus dorsi muscle. The long thoracic nerve supplies filaments to the serratus anterior muscle. Three minor cutaneous nerves—the intercostal brachial

nerves—supply the skin of the medial surface of the upper arm after passing from the lateral chest wall across the base of the axilla. Medial and lateral pectoral nerves pass from the axilla to the lateral chest wall to the two pectoral muscles (Fig. 5.14).

LYMPHATIC DRAINAGE OF THE BREAST

The lymphatic drainage pathways of the breast are important when assessing loco-regional spread of malignant disease. The lymphatic drainage of the breast follows either the superficial and cutaneous route or the deep parenchymal drainage system (Fig. 5.15).

The nipple, cutaneous and subcutaneous areas around the areola are drained by a large superficial lymphatic plexus lying just beneath the areola. This plexus also drains the deep central parenchymal region of the breast, the lymph rising from the deeper tissues to pool in the superficial plexus.

The deep parenchymal lymph channels drain most of the breast. Ductal and acinal lymph channels collect parenchymal lymph and deliver it to the large interlobar lymphatics. Cutaneous and periareolar lymph drains either directly into the subareolar plexus or deeply into the parenchymal lymph channels and then to the sub-areolar plexus.

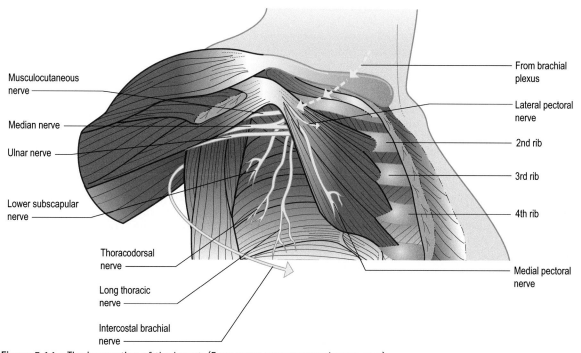

Figure 5.14   The innervation of the breast. (From www.cancersupportivecare.com)

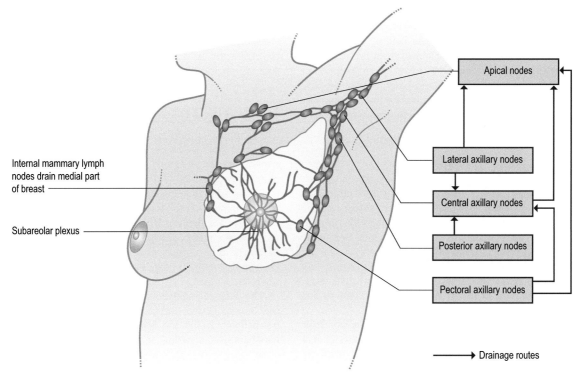

Figure 5.15   The lymphatic drainage of the breast. (Adapted from connection.lww.com)

Lymph from the retroareolar plexus and deep inter-lobar lymphatics passes via two major trunks to the axillary group of nodes. One lymphatic trunk drains the half of the breast above the areola and the other drains lymph from below the areola. Most breast lymph drains to the anterior axillary or subpectoral group of nodes that lie just deep to the lateral border of pectoralis major, near the lateral thoracic artery. From here, lymph usually passes superiorly via the axillary chain of lymph vessels and nodes to nodes positioned beside the upper half of the axillary vein. The lymph eventually reaches the highest nodes of the axilla (see below).

This is the main path of flow, although there are others (Fig. 5.16). Sentinel node mapping (see Ch. 13) has been particularly useful in mapping lymphatic drainage pathways, and therefore routes of early tumor spread. Lymph may drain directly from the breast to the highest axillary nodes (often found with tumors in the upper half of the breast), the midaxillary nodes lying deep to pectoralis minor tendon, the subscapular axillary nodes or via lymphatics adjacent to the axillary vein, and to the most inferior group of supraclavicular cervical nodes. With tumors in the medial half of the breast, lymphatic drainage has been noted across the midline to the lymphatics of the contralateral breast, directly to contralat-

eral axillary lymph nodes and to the internal mammary nodes in the parasternal region.

GROSS ANATOMY OF THE AXILLA

Although the axilla usually contains no functional breast tissue, it is important in breast imaging since it contains the lymph nodes likely to receive the majority of the lymphatic drainage of the breast, and as such it is often the site of reactive lymphadenopathy and early metastatic spread. Postmastectomy and axillary clearance, hematomas or seromas may form in the axilla and this may result in blood vessel compression; postoperative venous thrombosis may occur in the axillary vessels.

The axilla is situated between the supero-lateral chest wall and the upper arm. It consists of four walls, an apex and a base, is a repository for lymph nodes, is traversed by blood vessels, nerves and lymphatic channels, and contains variable amounts of fatty tissue.

The anterior axillary wall has two layers of muscle (Fig. 5.17). The superficial layer consists of pectoralis major and its fascia, and the deep layer comprises pectoralis minor, subclavius and fascia and the clavipectoral fascia that runs from the clavicle to the base of the axilla.

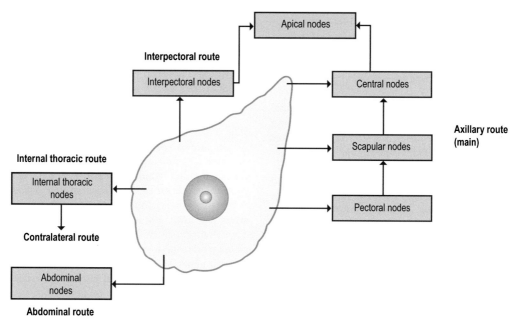

Figure 5.16   Common lymphatic drainage pathways from the breast. (Adapted from Fig. 2.11 in Winchester et al 2006.)

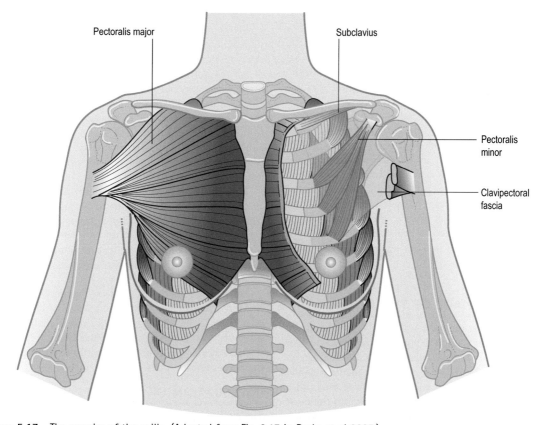

Figure 5.17   The muscles of the axilla. (Adapted from Fig. 3.17 in Drake et al 2005.)

The posterior or scapular wall is formed mainly by the subscapularis muscle and inferiorly by teres major and latissimus dorsi muscles.

The medial or thoracic wall is formed by the second to sixth ribs and intercostal muscles, and partly by the serratus anterior muscle.

The lateral or humeral wall is formed by the bicipital groove of the humerus containing the tendon of the long head of biceps. The two lips of the groove are the sites for attachment of the muscles forming most of the anterior and posterior axillary walls.

The apex stops at the outer border of the first rib and is limited by the clavicle anteriorly, the superior margin of the scapula posteriorly and medially by the first rib. Adipose tissue of the apex is continuous with the postero-inferior region of the neck.

The base of the axilla is composed of skin, subcutaneous tissue and the axillary fascia, and extends from the lateral border of the pectoralis major muscle to the anterior border of the latissimus dorsi muscle.

BLOOD SUPPLY TO THE AXILLA

The axillary artery is the major artery supplying the axilla—it runs deep to pectoralis minor. It is a continuation of the subclavian artery at the first rib and, after crossing the axilla, becomes the brachial artery at the lower border of teres major. The axillary artery has three parts, the first part lies close to the anterior aspect of the shoulder joint. Its single branch, the highest thoracic artery, runs to the superior and lateral chest wall where it anastamoses with the internal thoracic and anterior intercostal arteries. The second part has two branches, the thoracoacromial trunk and the lateral thoracic (external mammary) artery. This gives off lateral mammary and chest wall branches. The mammary branch runs to the lateral border of the pectoralis major muscle before turning medially to supply the lateral quadrants of the breast. The third part lies close to the surgical neck of the shaft of the humerus. Its major branch is the subscapular artery which supplies the posterior axillary wall.

VENOUS DRAINAGE OF THE AXILLA

The axillary vein is the most superficial structure in the axilla. It begins at the lower border of teres minor with the confluence of veins accompanying the brachial artery. It then joins the basilic vein, continuing medially as the axillary vein becoming the subclavian vein at the border of the first rib. Much venous blood drains into the most superior part of the axillary vein via the cephalic vein just below the first rib.

LYMPHATIC DRAINAGE OF THE AXILLA

The axilla contains between 15 and 40 relatively large (2–8 mm) lymph nodes and many lymphatic channels interspersed between fatty areolar tissue. The lymphatic channels and nodes lie in close proximity to venous structures, particularly the axillary vein.

The axillary nodes are divided into five groups (Fig. 5.18).

The **lateral (or axillary vein) group** of nodes (3–8 in number) drain most of the upper extremity and in turn drain into the **apical (or subclavicular) nodes**. The **pectoral (anterior or external mammary) nodes**, again 3–8 in number, lie along the course of the lateral thoracic artery and lower border of the pectoralis major muscle. They drain much of the chest wall, receive most of the primary drainage from the breast and drain the abdominal wall above the level of the umbilicus. The pectoral nodes drain into the central and apical axillary nodes. The **subscapular (scapular or posterior) nodes** (3–6 in number) drain lymph from the skin and muscular areas of the posterior chest wall and the back of the neck. In addition, they drain some lymph directly from the lateral area of the breast. Subscapular nodes drain into the central axillary nodes.

The **central axillary nodes** (4–6 in number) are usually the largest of the axillary nodes and are relatively superficial and easy to palpate. They receive lymph from the lateral, pectoral and subscapular nodes and also directly from the breast and upper extremity. The central nodes drain into the apical nodes.

The **apical nodes** of the axilla (6–10 in number) are the most superior nodes in the axilla, receiving lymph from all other axillary lymph areas. They also receive lymph from the lymphatic channels associated with the cephalic vein and from the lymphatics draining the upper inner quadrant of the breast.

The lowest axillary lymph nodes, lateral and inferior to pectoralis minor, are referred to as Level I nodes (subscapular, lateral and pectoral groups). Level II nodes are located deep to pectoralis minor (central and possibly some apical) and Level III nodes are found medial and superior to pectoralis minor in the mid-clavicular line (apical).

Efferent lymphatic vessels from the apical nodes join to form a narrow lymphatic trunk—the subclavian lymphatic trunk which drains lymph into the junction of the subclavian and internal jugular veins, the right lymphatic or thoracic duct; occasionally, lymphatic drainage is via the deep cervical nodes.

INNERVATION OF THE AXILLA

Medial, lateral and posterior cords of the brachial plexus are arranged around the first and second parts of the

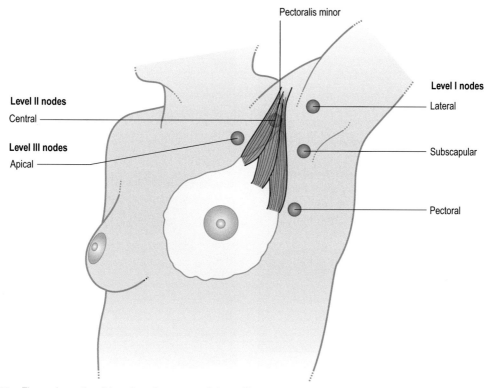

Pectoralis minor

Level II nodes

Central

Level III nodes

Apical

Level I nodes

Lateral

Subscapular

Pectoral

Figure 5.18   The main regional lymph node groups of the axilla.

axillary artery, the terminal branches of the cords being arranged around the third part. The presence of the cords of the brachial plexus and their branches in the axilla renders them susceptible to surgical damage with associated loss of sensation and muscle wastage.

NORMAL ULTRASOUND APPEARANCES OF THE BREAST

The female breast varies considerably in its ultrasound appearance according to age, hormonal status and in pregnancy. The density of the breasts is reduced after the menopause as the breast involutes, with the fat components becoming more prominent and the mammary ducts undergoing atrophy. Breast density also varies with ethnic origin, increased density being more prominent in Asian and Japanese women.

The normal breast contains glandular breast tissue, fat and vessels in varying proportions. On ultrasound images, the breast tissue has a stratified appearance with three distinct layers (Fig. 5.19).

The **anterior subcutaneous** or **premammary layer** contains the skin, nipple, areola, distal extensions of the anterior connective tissue (suspensory ligaments) and subcutaneous fat.

The **parenchymal layer** or **middle mammary** layer contains the functional breast parenchyma—the glandular tissue, lactiferous ducts and interconnecting tissues.

The deepest, posterior layer—the **retromammary layer**—contains retromammary fat lobules and the deep connective tissues, and lies immediately anterior to the pectoralis major fascia.

In the premammary layer, nearest to the transducer and therefore uppermost on the ultrasound image, the **skin** is demonstrated as two thin parallel hyper-reflective lines normally measuring no more than 3 mm in antero-posterior (vertical) thickness (Fig. 5.20). The skin of the lower half of the breast is often slightly thicker. The thickness of the skin layer also depends upon skin type and will vary with force of transducer compression.

The **nipple and areola** attenuate ultrasound slightly more than the rest of the breast due to their denser connective tissue composition, and therefore look slightly darker. The nipple is of intermediate level reflectivity (mid-gray) and exhibits strong posterior acoustic shadowing if scanned with the transducer directly over that

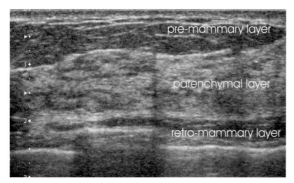

Figure 5.19   Normal ultrasound appearances of the superficial premammary, central parenchymal and deep retromammary layers of the breast.

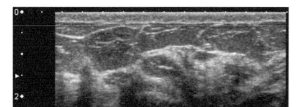

Figure 5.20   The skin is seen uppermost in the ultrasound image as two horizontal hyper-reflective lines separated by a thin layer of homogeneous tissue of mid-reflectivity. The total skin thickness should be no more than 3 mm.

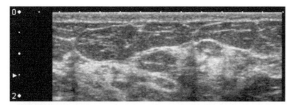

Figure 5.21   The superficial fat lies between the skin and the parenchymal breast tissue—it has a dark-gray speckled lobulated appearance.

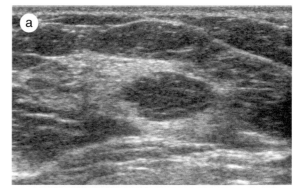

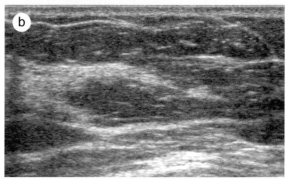

Figure 5.22   (a) Using a transverse scan plane—a fat lobule mimics a focal lesion. (b) By rotating the transducer into a longitudinal scan plane, it can be shown that the 'pseudolesion' is in fact a continuation of the superficial fatty tissue.

area, the shadowing obscuring the deeper subareolar tissues. Loss of contact, and therefore image voids also occur due to the steep angle at which the edges of the nipple rise from the areolar surface. The area behind the nipple is also difficult to evaluate because of dense attenuating fibrotic connective tissue around the lactiferous ducts; a combination of scanning approaches is required to overcome these limitations (see Ch. 6).

Subcutaneous fat lies immediately deep to the skin layer, and the amount (thickness or depth in the image) varies with body habitus, age, parity and hormonal status. Ultrasound appearances are similar in all women—homogeneous, but slightly speckled, dark-gray fat lobules interspersed with thin hyper-reflective suspensory ligament fibers (Fig. 5.21). Fat lobules in the breast are of lower reflectivity, and are thus displayed darker than the parenchymal glandular tissue. The 'fatty breast', having a predominance of hyporeflective fat lobules and very little parenchymal tissue, might be considered better suited to mammographic evaluation rather than ultrasound imaging owing to its relatively poor sound transmission characteristics.

Breast **fat lobules** are relatively well defined by their connective tissue envelopes. Seen best in longitudinal section, fat lobules have smooth margins and their shape tapers at the extremes of their long axis. Seen transversely, fat lobules appear ovoid and are easily compressed.

Since the fatty tissue invests and surrounds the fibroglandular tissue, sometimes 'fat islands' appear and can mimic hyporeflective focal lesions. By rotating the transducer and scanning from different angles, it can be demonstrated that these pseudolesions are not isolated masses and are in fact contiguous with the superficial or retromammary fat layer (Fig. 5.22).

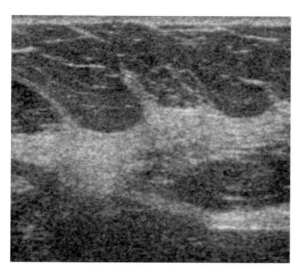

Figure 5.23   Cooper's ligaments anchor the breast parenchyma to the superficial fascia—they are hyper-reflective and traverse the superficial fat layer between the fat lobules.

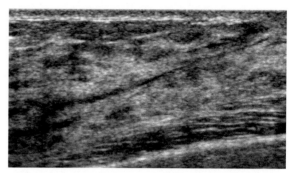

Figure 5.24   In a radial scan plane, breast ducts are well-defined echo-free channels with hyper-reflective smooth walls that taper peripherally.

Cooper's suspensory ligaments are seen as highly reflective curvilinear structures separating the fat lobules. They invariably cause some acoustic shadowing, sometimes making it difficult to image deeper structures; compound imaging reduces this effect (Fig. 5.23).

The middle parenchymal layer contains the **fibroglandular breast tissue**, and this layer shows the greatest sonographic variability. The parenchymal layer is separated from the subcutaneous layer by the premammary fascia—demonstrated as a horizontal (often discontinuous) hyper-reflective (white) line superficially (towards the top) in the image. Almost all the main ducts and TDLUs are in this layer, along with a variable amount of stromal, fatty and fibrous tissue. Normal parenchymal glandular tissue is hyper-reflective—towards the white end of the gray-scale spectrum, with the ductal structures visible as linear echo-free channels (Fig. 5.24). The glandular tissue may be heterogeneous in reflectivity, depending upon the amount of interspersed fatty tissue and the prominence of the ductal architecture; localized patches of reduced reflectivity may be associated with areas of benign breast change such as fibroadenosis.

The varying amount of fat within the normal breast results in a range of ultrasound appearances, from the entirely adipose hyporeflective (dark gray) breast, to an almost completely hyper-reflective (bright) glandular breast (Fig. 5.25). This variation broadly correlates with mammographic appearances.

Lactiferous (milk) ducts are normally visualized particularly when minimally distended in the late stage of the menstrual cycle. They are seen as hyporeflective or echo-free tubular structures, 2–4 mm diameter at a radial orientation to the nipple. Their caliber increases centrally towards the lactiferous sinuses.

The retromammary layer is separated from the middle mammary (parenchymal) layer by the retromammary fascia. The deep retromammary layer is usually thin on ultrasound images since the patient is normally scanned in the supine or supine oblique position and the breast is compressed gravitationally against the chest wall. The retromammary layer may be further obliterated by firm transducer pressure. This deep layer contains variable amounts of retromammary fat and some suspensory ligaments, and is bounded posteriorly (at the bottom of the ultrasound image) by the anterior chest wall structures.

The **pectoral muscles** (pectoralis major and minor) lie deep to the breast tissues and are demarcated by the hyper-reflective fascia. Since their orientation is parallel to the skin, on ultrasound images they are readily seen deep in the image as a striated layer of varying thickness that has a laminated hyper- and hypo-reflective appearance (Fig. 5.26). The muscles are particularly well visualized in the transverse plane in the upper outer quadrant towards the axillary tail of the breast (Fig. 5.27). The pectoralis muscles are more prominent in small breasts and can be quite large in athletic types.

The pectoralis muscles lie immediately anterior to the **ribs, intercostal muscles and costal cartilages**. When scanning over the lateral part of the breast in longitudinal section, the anterior surfaces of the bony ribs are seen as hyper-reflective anteriorly convex structures that exhibit strong posterior acoustic shadowing; more medially,

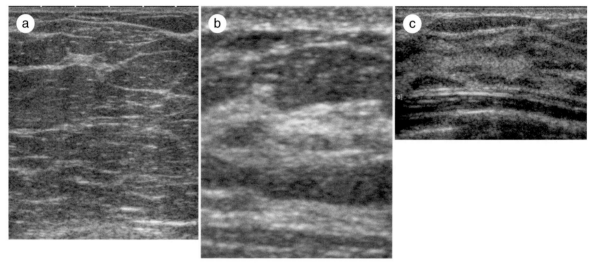

Figure 5.25 (a) A predominantly 'fatty' breast is uniformly dark gray apart from the linear connective tissue strands. (b) A mixed 'fatty/glandular' breast has a hyper-reflective central layer of parenchymal tissue between the darker gray superficial and deep fatty layers. (c) A predominantly 'glandular' breast is uniformly hyper-reflective and has minimal or no darker fat layers above or below.

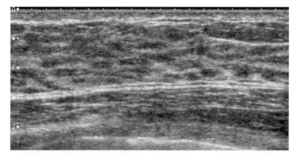

Figure 5.26 The striated muscles of the chest wall should be included across the bottom of the image.

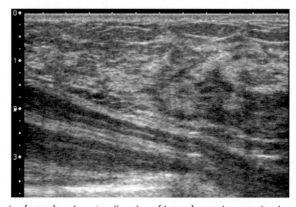

Figure 5.27 The pectoralis major (upper) and pectoralis minor (deeper) muscles are clearly seen when scanning the upper outer quadrant/axillary tail of the breast.

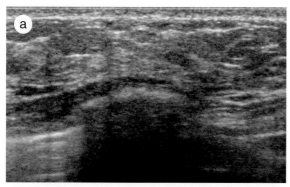

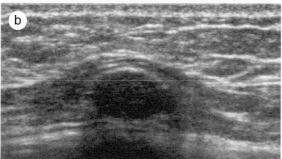

Figure 5.28 (a) The anterior surface of the rib produces a distinct acoustic shadow. (b) The costal cartilages attenuate the ultrasound beam and cause some shadowing, but the entire circumference is usually seen unless the cartilage is heavily calcified.

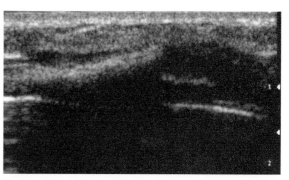

Figure 5.29 The costo-chondral junction can be demonstrated by scanning parallel to the rib long axis—sometimes the costo-chondral junction is responsible for the perception of a palpable mass.

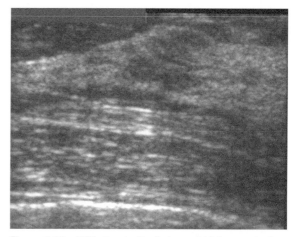

Figure 5.30 With the depth of view set high enough, the pleural membrane can be seen as a white horizontal line across the bottom of the image—in real time this can be observed moving with respiration.

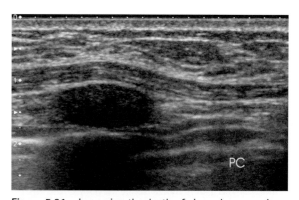

Figure 5.31 Increasing the depth of view when scanning the left breast will demonstrate the pulsatile anterior pericardium (PC) deep to the chest wall.

cross-sections of the costal cartilages are seen as hyporeflective oval masses (Fig. 5.28). Scanning in transverse section, along the long axis of the rib, the change in reflectivity is readily apparent at the costo-chondral junction (Fig. 5.29). Between the ribs lie the intercostal muscles, and deep to the thoracic cage the pleura–lung interface can be observed as a thin hyper-reflective line that moves in phase with respiration (Fig. 5.30). With sufficient image depth, the anterior surface of pericardium might also be demonstrated deep to the left anterior chest wall (Fig. 5.31). The proximity of the pleura and pericardium (often within 3–4 cm of the skin surface) should alert the observer to the potential risks of needle interventional procedures in the breast.

Normal **blood vessels** may occasionally be seen in two-dimensional B-mode images of the breast, most often coursing a straight or gently curved path, parallel to and just below the skin surface or along the surface of the glandular tissue. Superficial blood vessels are anechoic tubular structures that are easily compressed with too much transducer pressure; blood vessels can be discriminated from dilated lymphatic channels using color Doppler (Fig. 5.32).

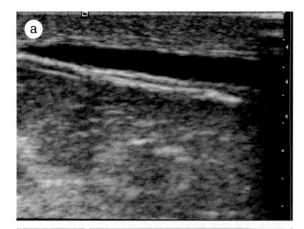

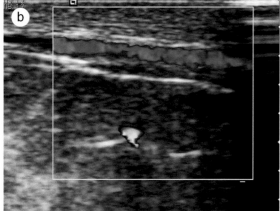

Figure 5.32 (a) Superficial echo-free channels may represent veins or dilated lymphatics. (b) Color flow Doppler can be used to differentiate blood vessels from lymphatics, lymphatic flow being too slow to detect.

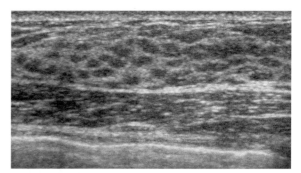

Figure 5.33 The adolescent breast has a 'honeycomb' appearance.

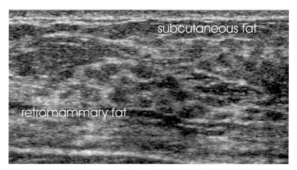

Figure 5.34 There is usually very little subcutaneous or retromammary fat in the adolescent breast.

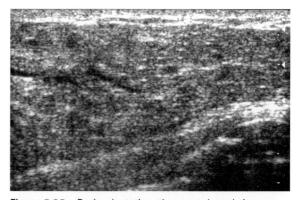

Figure 5.35 During lactation, the parenchymal tissue becomes thickened with the milk content, giving rise to a hyper-reflective and 'speckled' appearance in the ultrasound image.

Deeper parenchymal vascularity is readily demonstrated using an appropriately sensitive Doppler technique (see Chs 6 and 7), with breast vascularity being more pronounced in pregnancy, during lactation and with inflammatory and malignant disease.

AGE- AND HORMONE-RELATED PHYSIOLOGICAL CHANGE IN THE BREAST

The **teenage breast** often contains little or no subcutaneous and retromammary fat. In early puberty, the ultrasound appearance is of an initial hypo-reflective nodule which should not be confused with a hypo-reflective tumor; as the parenchymal tissue develops, the breast becomes more hyper-reflective—often having a honeycomb appearance (Fig. 5.33). Generally there is little or no interspersed intramammary fat, and the subcutaneous

and retromammary fat layers are thin and barely discernible (Fig.5.34).

In the **lactating breast**, the general reflectivity of the parenchymal tissue is increased and it tends to have a 'speckled' appearance (Fig. 5.35). Whilst the breast

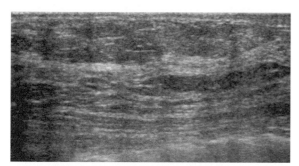

Figure 5.36 Around the menopause, the breast becomes hyper-reflective and the parenchymal layer becomes thinner.

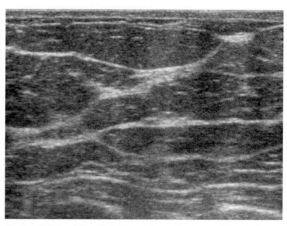

Figure 5.37 After the menopause, the parenchymal tissue involutes and the breast has a hyporeflective 'fatty' appearance.

ducts are collapsed in the non-lactating breast, during lactation they may measure up to 8 mm diameter in the subareolar region and between 2 and 4 mm peripherally. Breast milk in the ducts sometimes appears as diffuse low-level echoes or has a particulate hyper-reflective 'speckled' appearance. The galactocele, an area of focal cystic duct dilatation, appears as a well-circumscribed fluid mass containing 'speckled' fluid. Blood flow to the breast is also increased during pregnancy and lactation, resulting in an increased color Doppler signal.

With advancing age as ovarian function decreases, the breast undergoes fibrotic change and the parenchyma becomes more hyper-reflective. The **perimenopausal breast**, however, has thicker subcutaneous and retromammary fat layers and the relative amount of fibroglandular tissue reduces with advancing age and is replaced by connective tissue (Fig. 5.36). Both breasts, if normal, should be similar in appearance.

In the **postmenopausal breast**, the overall density, and therefore ultrasound reflectivity, is much reduced if women do not take hormone replacement therapy (HRT). HRT modifies the density of the breast, with a year's estrogen and progesterone therapy doubling breast density—giving the breast a much 'younger' appearance on mammography and ultrasound images. Without hormone supplement, the fat components of the aging breast become more prominent, and the ducts, lobules and glandular tissues begin to atrophy. Glandular tissue slowly involutes, the involuting parenchymal tissue being homogeneous in appearance with mid to low reflectivity (mid to dark gray), eventually resulting in a predominantly adipose (fatty) breast (Fig. 5.37). Since most malignant tumors are similarly hypo-reflective, they appear less conspicuous.

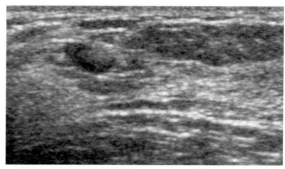

Figure 5.38 Intramammary lymph nodes are occasionally seen within the breast tissues. Normal lymph nodes are well-defined oval structures with a dark gray outer rim and an a characteristic lighter hilum towards one side.

NORMAL ULTRASOUND APPEARANCES OF THE AXILLA

When scanning the axilla, blood vessels, lymph nodes and the proximal pectoralis muscle should be readily identified. Occasionally, normal lymph nodes are seen in the breast (intramammary lymph nodes) usually in the upper outer quadrant (Fig. 5.38), but lymph nodes are most often only demonstrated in the axilla, parasternal nodes not being visible unless enlarged. Normally ovoid in shape, the symmetrical circumferential lymphoid tissue is hypo-reflective and the central, fatty hilar tissue is hyper-reflective (Fig. 5.39). A thin hyper-reflective surrounding capsule delineates the lymph node margins making size and margin regularity easy to assess, normal lymph nodes having a maximum short-axis diameter of

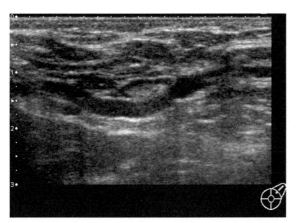

Figure 5.39 Lymph nodes can often be seen adjacent to the axillary vessels.

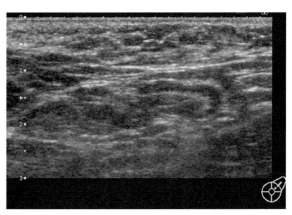

Figure 5.41 Normal axillary lymph nodes are often isoechoic with surrounding tissue and can be difficult to delineate.

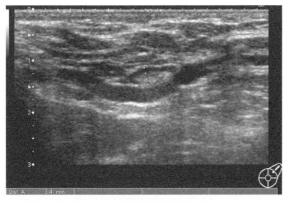

Figure 5.40 Lymph node size should be assessed using a short axis diameter—this should normally be no more than 10 mm.

no more than 10 mm (Fig. 5.40). In practice, identifying normal lymph nodes can be difficult as they invariably have a similar appearance to the normal fatty tissue of the axilla—with careful technique and experience, however, it should be possible to demonstrate representative normal lymph nodes during most examinations (Fig. 5.41).

Careful examination of the axilla for accessory breast tissue is important as this may contain pathology similar to that found in the main breast parenchyma.

Bibliography and suggested further reading

Bock K, Hadji P, Schultz KD, Wagner U, Duda VF 2004 Differential diagnosis of Poland syndrome versus unilateral accentuated thelarche. Ultraschall in der Medizin 25(5):377–382.

De Bruyn R 2004 Paediatric ultrasound, How, why and when. Edinburgh: Churchill Livingstone.

Drake R, Vogl W, Mitchell A 2005 Gray's anatomy for students. Churchill Livingstone.

Gray H, Williams PL 1995 Gray's anatomy: the anatomical basis of medicine and surgery. 38th edn. British. Edinburgh: Churchill Livingstone.

Heywang-Kobrunner SH, Dershaw DD, Screer I 2001 The normal breast. In Diagnostic breast imaging. Stuttgart: Thieme, pp. 162–180.

Krontiras H, Bland KI 2006 Anatomy of the breast, axilla and thoracic wall. In Winchester DJ, Winchester DP, Hudis CA et al (eds) Breast cancer. 2nd edn. Hamilton, Ontario: Decker, pp. 15–30.

Lumley JSP 2002 Surface anatomy: the anatomical basis of clinical examination. 3rd edn. Edinburgh: Churchill Livingstone.

Madjar H 2000 Sonographic anatomy of the breast and axilla. In The practice of breast ultrasound. New York: Thieme, pp. 47–55.

Proposed classification of pathology of human mammary gland. Online. Available at: http://mammary.nih.gov/reviews/comp_path/wellings

Rutter CM, Mandelson MT, Laya MB, et al 2001 Changes in breast density associated with initiation, discontinuation and continuing use of hormone replacement therapy. Journal of the American Medical Association 285:171–176.

Stavros AT 2004 Breast anatomy—the basis for understanding sonography. In Breast ultrasound. Philadelphia: Lippincott Williams and Wilkins, pp. 56–108.

Structure of the terminal ductal lobular unit (TDLU). Online. Available at: http://ccm.ucdavis.edu/bcancercd/21/TDLU1.html

Tanner JM 1962 Growth at adolescence. 2nd edn. Oxford: Blackwell Scientific.

Winchester DP, Winchester DJ, Hudis CA, Norton L 2006 Breast cancer. 2nd edn. Elsevier.

Chapter **6**

Ultrasound examination technique

Anne-Marie Dixon

INTRODUCTION

The ability to perform breast ultrasound examinations accurately and to a high standard is not the exclusive domain of any particular healthcare profession; breast ultrasound may be undertaken by surgeons, radiologists, ultrasound or mammography radiographers and breast care nurses. The performance of accurate high quality breast ultrasound examinations is a complex process and requires thorough initial training, regular practical experience and ongoing professional development.

Ultrasound is widely acknowledged to be the most operator-dependent diagnostic imaging technique, but the use of a standardized Scheme of Work and a protocol-driven systematic approach to breast ultrasound examinations helps to ensure that the scanning process, the images produced and the examination reports generated are of high quality and are reproducible between operators and facilities.

Several professional organizations have produced guidelines to help standardize provision and promote high standards of practice in breast ultrasound, and most of these include guidance on equipment to be used, technique for performing the ultrasound examination, criteria for interpreting the ultrasound appearances and minimum standards of reporting (Madjar et al 1999, UKAS 2001, AIUM 2002, Merritt & Rumack 2003, RCR 2003).

There is little material discrepancy in the recommendations made by the various organizations, and individual departments offering a breast ultrasound service should devise a local Scheme of Work that aligns with the professional guidance documents appropriate for the geographical and clinical context of the services they are providing.

CLINICAL INDICATIONS

At the outset of any breast ultrasound examination, it is important for the person performing the scan, *the operator*, to be clear as to the clinical context and intended purpose of the examination.

In the UK, breast imaging services are provided within the context of either the National Health Service Breast Screening Programme (NHSBSP) or as part of a symptomatic breast referral service. Within either of these contexts, the ultrasound examination forms part of the 'triple assessment' process, sometimes in conjunction with X-ray mammography, as the imaging assessment, after a clinical assessment and before any invasive pathology assessment (RCR 2003).

For the majority of referrals, ultrasound is performed as a targeted examination localized to a particular area of concern; however, whole breast ultrasound examinations may be appropriate in some cases. The most common clinical indications for undertaking breast ultrasound examinations are given in Box 6.1.

Prior to the patient's attendance for an ultrasound examination, previous imaging investigation reports and/or images should have been retrieved and reviewed, and they should remain available for comparison during subsequent image interpretation and reporting (Merritt & Rumack 2003).

COMMUNICATION

Despite the availability of a large body of information and the increasingly favorable outlook for the majority of breast referrals, patients attending for breast imaging will often be anxious and sometimes fearful or distressed; they are invariably keen to get the results of the examination at the earliest opportunity. Since ultrasound is not associated with any biological hazard, departments should allow the patient to be accompanied by a supporting relative or friend, particularly when undergoing interventional procedures—this provides reassurance and enhances the patient's ability to cope with their experience (Ehrlich et al 2004, p. 87).

The need to give information to patients gives the healthcare professional an opportunity to provide emotional support, and the act of giving information can in itself be therapeutic when patients are afraid and uncertain (De Zeeuw 2001, pp. 137, 141). It is important that the ultrasound practitioner can communicate sensitively and give clear explanations to both patient and their supporters to gain their understanding and cooperation and so that examinations can proceed without unnecessary interruptions to explain or reassure in response to multiple questions.

> **Box 6.1 Clinical indications for breast ultrasound**
>
> First-line breast imaging investigation in
>
> - Women under 35 years of age
> - Women with breast implant(s) in situ
> - Pregnant and lactating women
> - Men
> - Suspected abscess, open infection
> - When clinical examination suggests benign disease, e.g. simple cyst
> - Symptoms restricted to axilla
>
> Performed in conjunction with mammography for
>
> - Focal palpable mass
> - Further evaluation of mammography-detected focal lesion
> - Technically inadequate mammography due to lesion location
>
> Guidance of interventional procedures if abnormality visible at ultrasound
>
> Breast ultrasound is NOT routinely indicated when patients present with
>
> - Pain
> - Diffuse nodularity
> - No clinical abnormality and negative mammography screening
>
> Whole breast ultrasound MAY be appropriate for
> Suspected silicone implant leakage
> Defining the presence of metastatic/mutlifocal disease
> High risk women with suboptimal mammographic imaging, e.g. due to breast density or scarring from previous surgery

The person performing the scan remains in close proximity to the patient and their supporters throughout the examination, and this creates an opportunity for the operator to build up a close rapport with the patient and their supporters and allows immediate reassurance when all is well, but it can also generate a very tense and difficult atmosphere when pathology is detected, particularly if the appearances are those of malignant disease.

The willingness of the practitioner to answer the patient's technical and clinical questions can promote the patient's confidence in the operator and in the diagnostic service as it demonstrates an open, transparent and patient-centered philosophy. Patients may appreciate the opportunity to view the ultrasound images at the end of their scan, the demonstration of ultrasound findings, whether clinically negative or positive, being reassuring. When an abnormality is detected, the patient is often relieved that 'something' has been found, the find justifying their attendance at the clinic irrespective of what the lesion actually is. Demonstration of normal appearances can also be reassuring, particularly when patients can confirm that the transducer is indeed placed over the area of concern; in such circumstances, phrases such as *nothing abnormal is showing up on ultrasound* more accurately reflect the capability and limitations of the technique and are less likely to reduce confidence in both the technique and the operator if sonographically occult pathology is subsequently diagnosed.

PATIENT PREPARATION

Whenever a healthcare professional encounters a new patient for the first time, it is important they introduce themself by name and profession before informing the patient of the purpose of the encounter (RCR 1998a). This information can easily be imparted as the patient is called from the waiting area; further communication is best reserved until inside the examination room when the patient's privacy and dignity can be maintained. Breast ultrasound is considered to be a particularly intrusive intimate diagnostic examination, and the patient is likely to feel stressed and vulnerable; in the absence of an accompanying supporter, patients should be offered the opportunity to have a chaperone present throughout the examination—this is particularly important for female patients if the ultrasound operator is male (RCR 1998b).

Initially the patient must be positively and unequivocally identified. A three-point identification check is recommended whereby the patient is invited to give their name, date of birth and address—not only does this reduce the risk that the 'wrong' patient is being examined but it is not unusual for discrepancies in computerized departmental records to be identified following this procedure.

After checking patient identification, the clinical information and pertinent past medical and family history should be verified (Table 6.1). Sometimes this information has already been obtained, perhaps prior to mammography, and it is useful in these instances to explain to the patient why the information is being re-checked—primarily to help in interpretation of the ultrasound

appearances; simply asking them to confirm what has already been recorded rather than to expect them to repeat it all again is useful in this situation.

Once the ultrasound practitioner has ascertained all the information they need, it is necessary for them to give a careful explanation of how the examination will be conducted and what is expected of the patient. It is useful to do this even when patients state that they have been scanned before; some will not remember specific details and others find it reassuring to have confirmation of what they think is going to happen; the provision of written information at the time of referral allows the patient to consider what is likely to happen beforehand. The patient should be given the opportunity to ask questions or seek clarification, and then, once clear informed verbal consent has been obtained, the examination may proceed (RCR 1998b). At the outset of the examination, the patient's identifying information should be entered into the ultrasound machine and the appropriate baseline scanning parameter pre-set selected (see Ch. 4).

The patient will need to undress above the waist and should be provided with private, warm, comfortable and secure facilities for this (RCR 1998b). It is important that the patient's privacy and dignity is maintained in the ultrasound examination room with the door locked and the patient reassured that no one else can enter during the examination; alternatively, facilities might be provided for a curtain to be drawn between the scanning area and the room's entrance door. The use of blouse-style front-opening hospital gowns, with Velcro or press-stud fastenings, facilitates repeated undressing for successive clinical and imaging examinations when patients are attending symptomatic one-stop or screening assessment clinics. A supply of such gowns in a variety of sizes, with functioning fastenings, will be required, and additional attention must be paid to ensure privacy in waiting areas used by patients not fully dressed in their own clothes.

Women attending for mammography are usually asked to refrain from using underarm deodorant as this can mimic microcalcification on the images. There is no such complication with ultrasound image appearances; however, acoustic coupling gel does combine with underarm deodorant to form a rather uncomfortable gritty compound. This is unpleasant for both the patient and the operator, and it is prudent to allow the patient to remove deodorant prior to the start of the scan if the axilla is to be examined.

MAMMOGRAPHIC CORRELATION

When the ultrasound examination has been requested to provide further information about an abnormality visible on mammograms, it is important to be able to correlate

Table 6.1 Information to check with patient prior to examination

Information type	Components	Reason
Identification	Full name Date of birth Address	Ensure correct patient examined
Clinical history Signs and symptoms	Breast: size, shape and symmetry Skin: reddening, edema, dimpling, thickening Nipple: inversion, discharge, Paget's Pain: location, nature, duration Lumps: location, duration, mobility	Establish reason for seeking investigation Ensure correct area examined

Family and lifestyle
   history
	Known risk factors for breast cancer
	   Age
	   Affected relatives
	      Breast and gynaecology
	   Obstetric history
	   Menstrual history
		Informs image interpretation and differential
		   diagnosis

Past diagnostic
   investigations
	Ultrasound
	Mammography
		Ascertain how much explanation of procedure
		   is required
		Compare previous/complementary imaging
		   appearances

Past medical and
   surgical history
	Breast
	   Document scars
	   Ascertain histology
	Systemic
	
	Heart valve replacements
		Aids interpretation/diagnosis
		Informs style and tone of communication
		May aid image interpretation
		Co-existing conditions may have impact on
		   patient care and management
		May aid image interpretation
		May need antibiotic cover for interventional
		   procedures

Current medication/
   health conditions
	Anticoagulants
	
	Hormones
		May influence subsequent investigations—
		   particularly interventional procedures
		Refines level of suspicion during image
		   interpretation

two-dimensional mammographic lesion display with a three-dimensional anatomical location in the breast. The operator must know how to place the ultrasound transducer at an appropriate location on the breast surface to obtain sonographic images of the correct area (UKAS 2001, p. 42).

Ideally, the breast ultrasound practitioner will have an awareness of mammographic positioning and image orientation. When the breast ultrasound practitioner is occupationally competent in mammographic technique and/or mammographic image interpretation, the tasks of viewing mammograms correctly, identifying each breast quadrant and localizing a focal abnormality are readily performed (Fig. 6.1).

If the ultrasound operator does not have these competencies, careful consultation and effective communication between the respective mammographic and ultrasound healthcare professionals is required to correlate the two components of the diagnostic imaging investigation; over time, this will lead to informal development of competency and a mutual awareness of the relative contributions of each examination to the overall image-based diagnostic process.

PATIENT POSITIONING

Choice of patient position depends on many factors (Box 6.2). Where possible, breast ultrasound is performed in

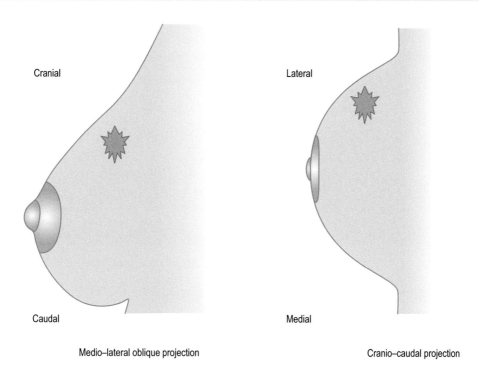

Cranial

Lateral

Caudal

Medial

Medio–lateral oblique projection

Cranio–caudal projection

N.B. Lesion (✳) lies in upper outer quadrant

Figure 6.1 Mammograms should be viewed prior to the ultrasound examination to localize an abnormality. Lesions that appear towards the top of a medio-lateral projection are in the upper half of the breast; lesions appearing near the top of a cranio-caudal projection are in the outer half of the breast.

Box 6.2 Factors influencing patient positioning

- Correlation with position used for breast surgery
- Easy and comfortable for patients to achieve and maintain
- Facilitates clinical examination of palpable masses
- Allows use of technical features that optimize spatial and contrast resolution
- Facilitates reproducible technique and lesion location

a similar position to that in which breast surgery is performed to facilitate correlation of ultrasound and surgical localization of any abnormality. In addition to this clinical consideration, the position should be easy and comfortable for patients to achieve and maintain, it should

facilitate the clinical localization of palpable masses and it should allow the use of ultrasound equipment features that give the best spatial and contrast resolution. A supine or supine oblique position meets these requirements (Fig. 6.2).

The patient should initially be asked to lie on their back on the examination couch; this supine position gives good access to the medial half of each breast. If the lateral aspect of the breast is to be examined, the patient should be asked to raise the affected side and a foam pad used to support them in this supine, contralateral posterior oblique position (Heywang-Kobrunner et al 2001, p. 92). With the patient in the left posterior oblique position, the right breast becomes flattened and assumes a more even thickness on the anterior chest wall with the nipple in a central position (Fig. 6.3). The degree of obliquity will need to be varied according to each individual patient's breast size, larger breasts requiring a steeper angle to prevent the breast tissue slipping laterally.

Raising the patient's ipsilateral (side under examination) arm onto the pillow above their head further reduces breast tissue thickness and additionally stretches

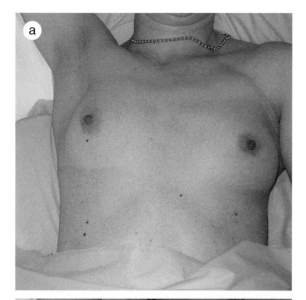

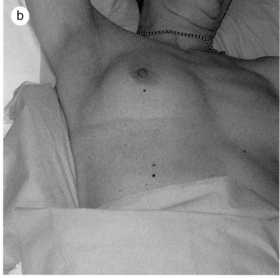

Figure 6.2 (a) The 'supine' position is appropriate for scanning the inner half of the breast. (b) The 'supine oblique' position can be achieved by raising the side under examination and supporting the patient on a foam wedge-shaped pad.

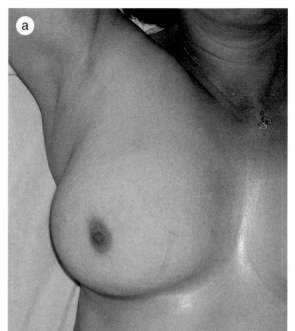

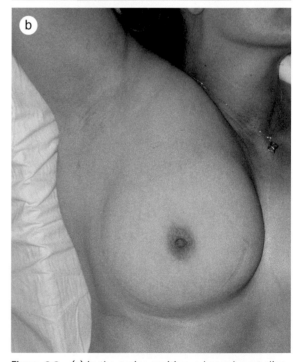

Figure 6.3 (a) In the supine position, a larger breast slips laterally. (b) Using the contralateral posterior oblique position will centralize the breast tissue over the chest wall—it becomes flattened, of uniform thickness and is better immobilized.

the underlying pectoralis muscle, helping to immobilize the breast and facilitate examination of the axilla.

Reducing breast thickness reduces the volume of tissue to be insonnated and thus the amount of ultrasound penetration required; this means higher transducer frequencies can be used optimizing spatial resolution.

Whilst this is the standard and universally recommended position in which breast ultrasound examinations should be performed, the technique is versatile enough to enable limited examinations to be performed in other positions. This makes ultrasound particularly useful when a patient's physical or cognitive impairment precludes diagnostic mammography, but it must be remembered that a systematic and comprehensive whole breast examination is unlikely to be possible with an adapted technique.

CLINICAL EXAMINATION

Before the ultrasound examination begins, the operator should perform a limited clinical examination of the patient's breast to localize a palpable lesion or feel the area that the patient reports to be abnormal or unusual (UKAS 2001, p. 42). The physical confirmation of such an abnormality by the healthcare professional is both reassuring for the patient and helps the operator correlate ultrasound transducer position and image appearance with the area of concern. In practice, it is possible to keep a finger on the abnormality, or to immobilize it between two fingers, to aid positioning of the ultrasound transducer directly over the area for a localized examination of a 'target' area.

When abnormalities are difficult to palpate, perhaps due to their small size or deep location, it is useful if the examining surgical clinician referring the patient annotates the area of concern on the patient's skin surface using a non-permanent marker. In the absence of such identifying information, it may be necessary, and should be operationally feasible, to call the clinician into the ultrasound examination to identify the specific area of interest directly—this is particularly useful when no definite ultrasound abnormality can be identified.

In some cases, the ability to palpate a lesion is positional, and the patient or clinician may only be able to locate the lesion with the patient seated or standing. In such cases, it is possible to locate the lesion with the patient erect and then apply the transducer to the breast and perform an initial limited exploratory examination in this position. Once a lesion is identified, however, it should still be examined and documented with reference to the standard examination position.

OPERATOR AND EQUIPMENT POSITION

Performance of ultrasound examinations is associated with increased risk of work-related musculoskeletal disorders, particularly in the spine and upper limb; it is important that the operator takes care to minimize the need to twist and over-reach during examinations by placing themselves, the ultrasound machine and the area

to be scanned as close together as possible (Dodgeon & Newton-Hughes 2003).

The selection of the relative position of operator, patient, examination couch and the ultrasound scanning machine, and selection of the technique for performing the examinations, requires careful balancing of technical and clinical factors and health and safety considerations to achieve high quality diagnostic accuracy and minimize the risk of occupational injury.

Dodgeon and Newton-Hughes (2003) suggest that the ultrasound machine should be positioned parallel to the examination couch (Fig. 6.4), with the control panel directly in front of the operator and the image display monitor at a height that allows the operator when seated or standing, with a straight spine, to see over the top if looking directly ahead (Fig. 6.5).

Madjar suggests that operators should adopt a relaxed position sitting level with the patient (Fig. 6.6) and using the wrist, rather than the arm, to move the transducer over the breast (Madjar 2000, p. 34). The adoption of a standing position, however, still enables wrist-guided transducer movement but keeps the shoulder position within a biomechanically safe zone of operation (Fig. 6.7). Most techniques will allow the operator to rest their arm lightly on the patient's anterior chest wall during scanning.

SCANNING PROTOCOLS

The performance of breast ultrasound scans should be comprehensive, systematic and reproducible to ensure that all relevant normal and pathological structures in the area of interest are visualized (Madjar et al 1999). The examination may involve a combination of B-mode and Doppler techniques to demonstrate anatomy and vascular supply and perfusion, and should be comprehensive and extended to include the 'whole breast' and axilla, or localized to a specific 'targeted' area, depending on a particular patient's individual clinical presentation (UKAS 2001, p. 42).

It is recommended that departments have evidence-based Schemes of Work that describe a standard technique for performing the examination and the structures to be demonstrated (Box 6.3). Quality assurance and audit systems should be in place to reduce interoperator variability by ensuring that Schemes of Work are adhered to by all members of staff.

For descriptive purposes, each breast is considered to consist of four anatomical areas, the upper and lower outer and medial quadrants, and to have a central nipple/areolar section (Fig. 6.8) (Tot et al 2000, p. 32). In addition, segmental location is described with reference to an analog clock face (Fig. 6.9).

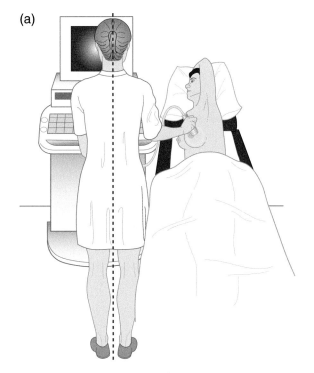

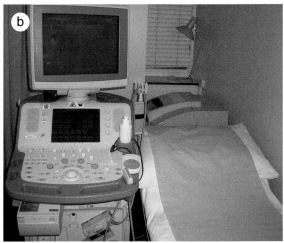

Figure 6.4 (a) The operator should be able to maintain a straight spine whilst scanning. (b) The ultrasound machine should be positioned parallel to the patient couch.

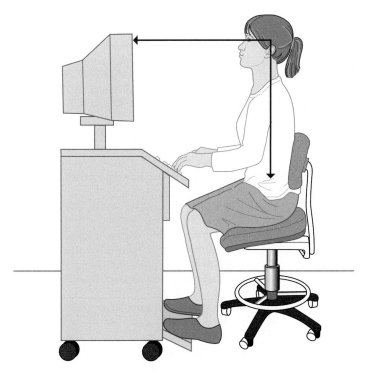

Figure 6.5 To reduce the risk of work-related musculoskeletal disorder, the ultrasound machine keyboard should be positioned so that the operator's forearms are parallel to the floor; the viewing monitor height should allow the operator just to see over the top.

SCANNING TECHNIQUE

A liberal amount of acoustic coupling gel is applied to the skin surface over the area to be examined so that the transducer can be moved smoothly without dragging the patient's skin or disturbing the underlying spatial relationships of breast anatomy.

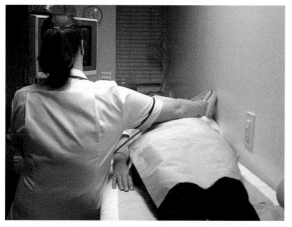

Figure 6.6 When sitting level with the patient, the operator's forearm can be supported on the patient's abdomen and wrist movements used to guide the transducer over the breast.

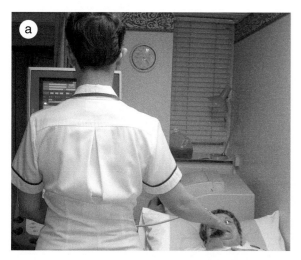

Figure 6.7 (a) With the operator standing, shoulder abduction remains within the biomechanically safe zone. (b) To reduce the risk of WRULD (work-related upper limb disorder), shoulder abduction should remain within the biomechanically 'safe' zone. Prolonged positions within the 'danger' zone should be kept to a minimum. (Diagram courtesy of Ms J. Dodgeon, University of Salford, UK.)

Careful attention must be paid to how the transducer is held to reduce the risk of carpal tunnel syndrome. A dynamic grip (Fig. 6.10) combines features of both power and precision grips, with the transducer held against the palm of the hand and distal phalanges used to brace it against the heel of the hand (Dodgeon 2005). This minimizes fatigue and nerve pressure whilst maintaining the ability for fine control when required (Dodgeon & Newton-Hughes 2003).

If the transducer is held near to the scanning contact area, the medial aspect of the operator's hand and little finger are in contact with the patient and glide over the skin of the breast during the examination (Fig. 6.11). This technique allows tactile feedback to improve the operator's spatial awareness of the position of the transducer on the breast and combines with visual feedback from the ultrasound image to improve hand–eye coordination. This contact of the operator's hand with the patient's skin is particularly useful when investigating palpable lesions; when the operator feels their finger slide over the 'lump', they are alerted to its impending, or immediately preceding (depending on the direction of scan movement) appearance of the area of abnormality on the viewing monitor.

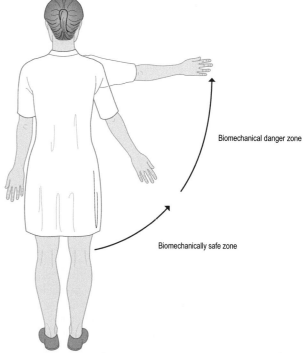

Biomechanical danger zone

Biomechanically safe zone

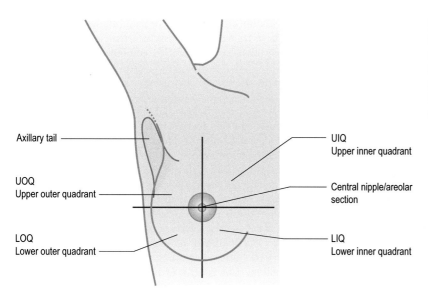

Figure 6.8 Quadrant annotation for describing anatomical locations within a breast. (After Smeltzer and Bare (2001), Brunner and Sudarth's Textbook of Medical-Surgical Nursing, 10th edn, with permission of Lippincolt Williams and Wilkins.)

Box 6.3 Structures to be demonstrated at breast ultrasound (After UKAS (2001), with permission of United Kingdom Association of Sonographes, London)

Breast

- Skin, nipple and areola
- Subcutaneous fat
- Superficial and deep layers of the superficial fascia
- Lactiferous ducts and sinuses
- Fibroglandular breast and interspersed fatty tissues
- Cooper's ligaments
- Retromammary space
- Pectoralis major, pectoralis minor and serratus anterior muscles

Axilla

- Lymph nodes
- Muscles and fatty tissue
- Axillary vessels

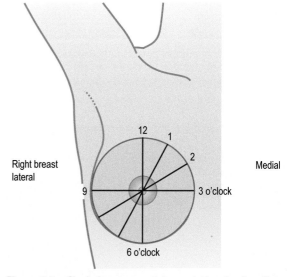

Figure 6.9 Clock-face segmental annotation for describing anatomical locations within the breast.

During all transducer movement across the breast, the transducer face should be maintained at a perpendicular orientation to the skin surface to maintain efficient sound transmission across the transducer–skin boundary and to optimize penetration of sound deep into the breast. The amount of pressure with which the transducer is applied to the skin should be the minimum required to maintain adequate transducer–skin contact; this maximizes patient comfort, minimizes occupational risk to the operator and reduces the risk of compressing and thus obliterating some superficial abnormalities. Additional pressure can be applied intermittently as a diagnostic maneuver to

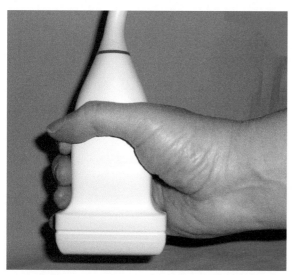

Figure 6.10   The ideal way to hold the transducer is in a 'dynamic' grip—the body of the transducer is held against the palm of the hand and the distal phalanges are used to brace it against the heel of the hand. If you are not used to this grip, it may take a while to become comfortable with it—persevere to reduce your risk of WRULD!

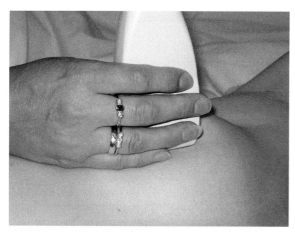

Figure 6.11   By keeping the medial aspect of the little finger and palm in contact with the patient's skin surface, the operator has better spatial awareness of the position of the transducer on the breast and can relate observed image appearances to the location of the nipple and any palpable mass.

assess normal tissue and focal lesion compressibility and mobility, or to reduce the acoustic shadowing associated with refraction and scattering of the ultrasound beam by oblique anatomical interfaces such as those formed by Cooper's ligaments (Fig. 6.12).

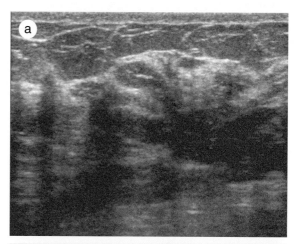

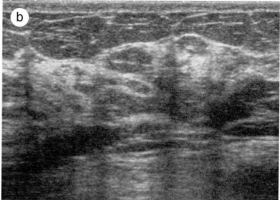

Figure 6.12   (a) The oblique orientation of Cooper's ligaments often gives rise to posterior acoustic shadowing which obscures deeper structures. (b) This artifact can be reduced by the application of gentle transducer pressure to flatten out the interfaces.

Scanning should initially always be performed in two perpendicular planes (Fig. 6.13), and operators may choose to interrogate systematically either a localized area or the whole breast, using contiguous and overlapping longitudinal and transverse scan planes or radial and antiradial planes.

If an abnormality is suspected, it must be remembered that ultrasound is a dynamic real-time imaging technique; the transducer can be angled, rotated and tilted to achieve additional customized scan planes that fully demonstrate the spatial extent and sonographic characteristics of the abnormality. The dynamic and versatile nature of the technique is particularly useful for delineating the complex interconnecting fibroglandular and fatty tissue; this overcomes the limitation of the

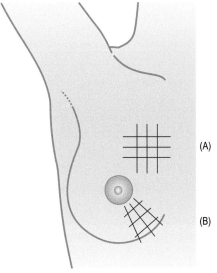

Figure 6.13 Scan plane orientation—orthogonal scan planes can be achieved in either (A) longitudinal and transverse sections or (B) radial and antiradial (tangential) planes.

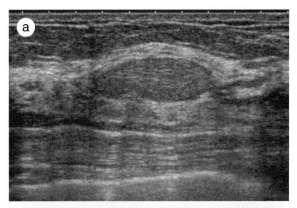

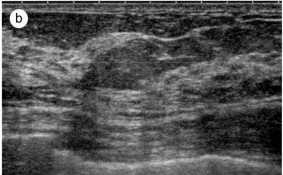

Figure 6.14 (a) The pseudolesion: scanning this area of the breast in a transverse plane revealed a possible focal lesion—it may represent a fibroadenoma. (b) By rotating the transducer through 90° into a longitudinal section, it was possible to demonstrate that the hyporeflective area was continuous with, and an extension of, the superficial fatty tissue.

ultrasound image being a two-dimensional representation of three-dimensional anatomical relationships and helps differentiate artifacts and 'pseudolesions' from real tumors (Fig. 6.14).

OPTIMIZATION OF IMAGE DISPLAY

Once the image is displayed on the monitor, the operator must adjust the scanning controls from the baseline pre-set values to optimize visualization and display of the sonographic features for each individual patient (Fig. 6.15).

Initially the field of view should be adjusted using the 'depth' control to ensure the anterior chest wall is included just above the lower border of the image. The focal zone(s) should be placed at depth in the image, or corresponding to the depth of a particular area of interest, and then the overall gain and time gain compensation controls altered to ensure that the received echo signals are displayed at appropriate gray-scale levels throughout the whole depth of the image.

Throughout the examination, the depth control should be adjusted to ensure the area of interest is magnified to occupy the majority of the display area (Fig. 6.16) and the overall and time gain controls adjusted to compensate for tissue attenuation differences as the scan plane traverses successive anatomical cross-sections (Fig. 6.17).

LONGITUDINAL AND TRANSVERSE SCAN PLANES

The use of longitudinal and transverse scan planes aligns with most other medical ultrasound practice and therefore is familiar to breast imaging practitioners with an ultrasound background. The use of longitudinal and transverse scan planes is recommended as an initial starting point in the breast ultrasound examination as it allows a relatively easy and rapid survey of either the whole breast or a particular area of interest. If focal abnormalities are present, scan planes can be aligned with the axis of a specific lesion in order to assess its size and differentiating acoustic features; radial/antiradial scan planes can be employed specifically to assess the ductal architecture.

To perform a targeted scan of a localized area or a specific focal lesion using the longitudinal section and transverse section technique, the transducer is initially

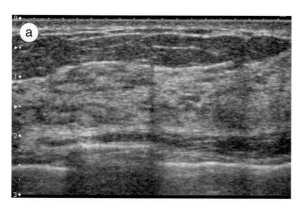

Figure 6.15 (a) Initially the field of view should be set to include the whole depth of the breast and anterior chest wall from the skin surface at the top of the image to the ribs and pleural membrane at the bottom of the image—a depth of 3 cm is usually adequate. The overall gain and time gain compensation should be adjusted so that the whole range of echo signals throughout the image is displayed at appropriate gray-scale levels. The focal zones should be placed at the depth of interest—usually at the depth of the parenchymal tissue. (b) Diagrammatic representation of the sectional anatomy that should be identifiable in the breast ultrasound image.

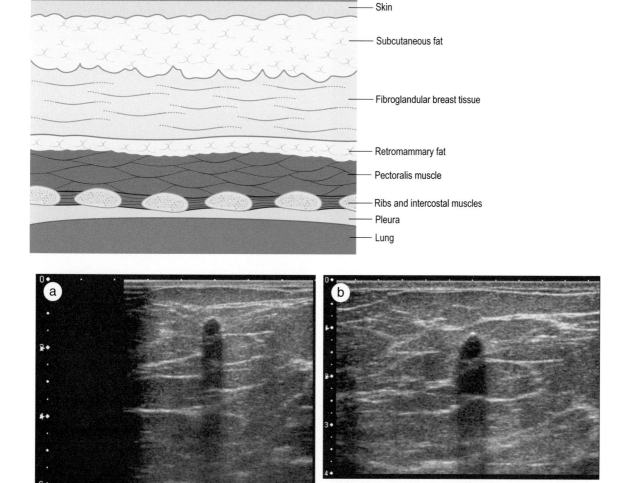

Figure 6.16 (a and b) When focal abnormalities are identified on an initial survey using a full depth of view (a), small superficial lesions should be examined in more detail by reducing the depth of view and magnifying areas of particular interest (b).

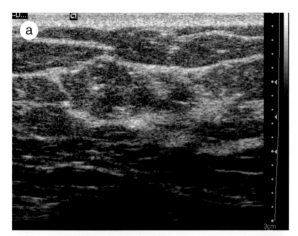

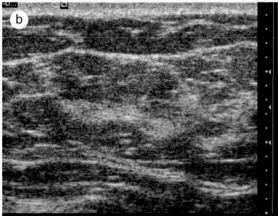

Figure 6.17 (a and b) Deeper structures in the image will not be adequately demonstrated (a) if the time gain compensation control is not correctly adjusted. By increasing the TGC at depth (b), echo signals from the retromammary layer and anterior chest wall are now displayed at useful gray-scale levels.

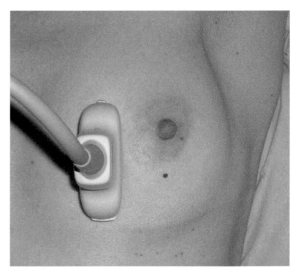

Figure 6.18 To obtain images in longitudinal section, the long axis of the transducer is positioned parallel to the patient's medial sagittal plane.

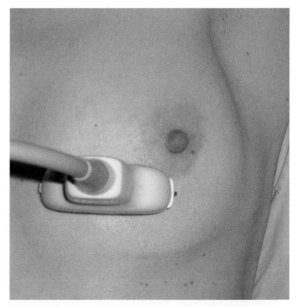

Figure 6.19 To obtain images in transverse section, the long axis of the transducer is positioned perpendicular to the patient's medial sagittal plane.

placed in a parasagittal orientation and moved over the area of interest (Fig. 6.18). The transducer is then rotated through 90° (Fig. 6.19) and swept over the area of interest from its superior to inferior aspect. This technique requires movement mainly at the operator's shoulder for the transverse scans and at the elbow for the longitudinal scans with minimum movement at the wrist.

When whole breast ultrasound (WBUS) is performed, a systematic evaluation of each of the four quadrants of the breast using contiguous and overlapping scan planes is required. Each breast can be examined by moving the transducer across and down the breast in a systematic and comprehensive sequence.

The breast is first examined in parasagittal sections with the transducer face aligned parallel to the median sagittal plane. Starting at the parasternal edge, medially

in the upper inner quadrant (Fig. 6.20: position 1), the transducer is moved laterally across the upper half of the breast to the lateral aspect of the upper outer quadrant in the axilla (position 2). The transducer is then *translated* inferiorly to a position overlapping by approximately 10 mm (position 3), and a second sweep of the transducer is made across the breast in a lateral to medial direction towards the sternum. At the sternum (position

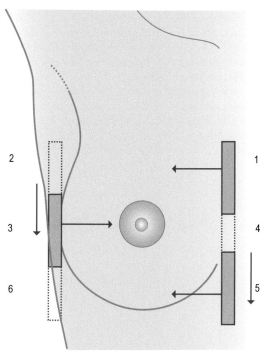

Figure 6.20 To undertake a longitudinal survey of the whole breast, the transducer is passed across and down the breast in continuous right-to-left and left-to right sweeps (positions 1–6) ensuring overlap.

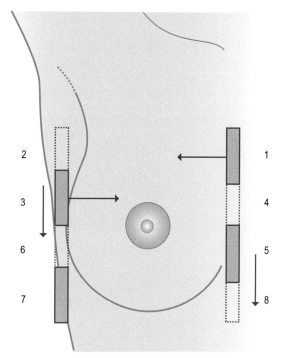

Figure 6.21 With large breasts, or smaller footprint transducers, additional sweeps (1–8) are required to ensure full coverage and complete visualization of the whole breast.

4), the transducer is moved inferiorly again (position 5), and a further overlapping sweep of the transducer, from medial to lateral across the lower half of the breast, is made (position 6). These three *passes* should be sufficient to give complete breast coverage with most transducers; however, the number of passes required depends on relative image field of view size (determined by the area of the transducer face) and the size of the breast; with smaller transducers and larger breasts, additional passes are required to ensure comprehensive coverage (Fig. 6.21).

Examination of the breast in transverse section is achieved by *rotating* the transducer through 90° and systematically scanning in contiguous and overlapping axial sections. Returning to the parasternal edge, with the transducer perpendicular to the long axis of the sternum, the transducer is moved caudally over the breast from the superior extent of the upper inner quadrant to the inferior aspect of the lower inner quadrant. The transducer is then moved laterally a distance just less than its own width (to ensure scan plane overlap) and the central section of the breast is examined from inferior to superior extent. A third, downward sweep of the transducer through the upper outer and lower outer quadrants will ensure comprehensive visualization of the entire breast for the majority of patients with most trans-

ducers; small transducers and large breasts requiring additional passes as before.

RADIAL AND ANTIRADIAL (TANGENTIAL) SCAN PLANES

Radial and antiradial planes align more with the natural architecture of the breast and therefore are considered by some to demonstrate ductal abnormalities more readily (Madjar et al 1999). Although some would argue that this alignment with the natural anatomy of the breast makes radial/antiradial scanning appropriate for surveying the whole breast, in practice it is difficult to achieve a systematic technique that gives complete coverage, particularly around the nipple and breast periphery, and that is not prohibitively time consuming (Madjar 2000, p. 42).

Radial/antiradial scanning is perhaps appropriate to investigate localized duct ectasia as the resultant scan plane orientation allows tracking along and visualizing the length of dilated ducts. Radial scan plane orientation is also useful when evaluating focal lesions to look for extension of the tumor along the ducts. In such cases, however, rather than adopting a systematic radial technique, the operator should align the scan plane with reference to the anatomical appearances demonstrated as opposed to with reference to the relative position of the transducer to the 'whole breast'.

Radial scanning requires the operator to keep one end of the transducer near to the nipple of the breast under examination whilst rotating the other end around the periphery of the breast in a clockwise sweeping motion. This maneuver requires a twisting action at the operator's elbow and wrist, and requires careful changing of transducer grip as it is performed to reduce pressure in the carpal tunnel (Dodgeon & Newton-Hughes 2003). If this technique is used to perform a whole breast survey, and each quadrant is examined in turn, care should be taken to ensure overlap of coverage at the 12, 3, 6 and 9 o'clock positions. Alternatively, a continuous *spiral* pathway can be employed, starting at the nipple/areolar area and gradually moving outwards towards the chest wall (Hagen-Ansert 2004).

On the ultrasound monitor, the relative positions of the nipple and breast periphery remain constant, but this means that medial and lateral orientation and superior and inferior orientation are reversed at the 3 and 9, and 12 and 6 o'clock positions, respectively (Fig. 6.22).

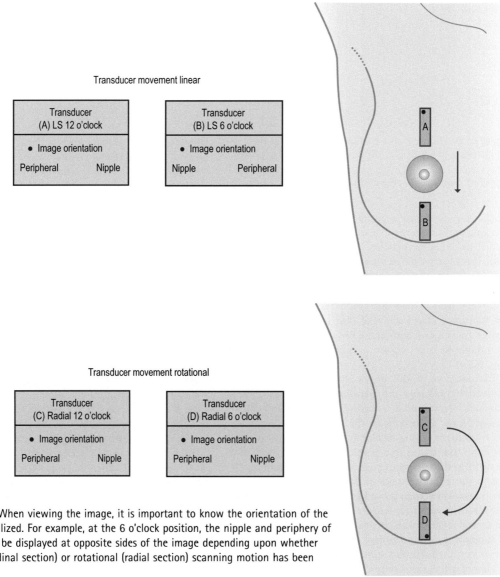

Transducer movement linear

Transducer (A) LS 12 o'clock
• Image orientation

Peripheral	Nipple

Transducer (B) LS 6 o'clock
• Image orientation

Nipple	Peripheral

Transducer movement rotational

Transducer (C) Radial 12 o'clock
• Image orientation

Peripheral	Nipple

Transducer (D) Radial 6 o'clock
• Image orientation

Peripheral	Nipple

Figure 6.22 When viewing the image, it is important to know the orientation of the scan planes utilized. For example, at the 6 o'clock position, the nipple and periphery of the breast will be displayed at opposite sides of the image depending upon whether linear (longitudinal section) or rotational (radial section) scanning motion has been used.

From the radial orientation (Fig. 6.23), the transducer is rotated through 90° until it is perpendicular to the architectural pattern of the ducts for the antiradial, or tangential scans (Fig. 6.24). It is then moved in centripetal and centrifugal sweeps towards and away from the nipple. The whole breast can be examined by sequentially circling around the breast in clockwise fashion and, although this will naturally give considerable overlap of scan planes towards the central nipple/areolar region, care must be taken to ensure overlap at the periphery where adjacent scan planes diverge (Madjar 2000, p. 43).

The nipple and areola

Examination of the areola and nipple is technically challenging for several reasons. Since the nipple is raised from the surface of the breast, it is difficult to maintain transducer contact and this creates voids in the image where transducer-skin contact is lost (Fig. 6.25). Additionally, the nipple, along with the skin and subcutaneous tissue layers, lies superficial in the image, making it difficult to include in the focal zone where resolution is best. Finally, the nipple and periareolar regions contain a lot of dense, sound-attenuating connective tissue that reduces sound penetration to the deeper tissues (Fig. 6.26). The prob-

lems of contact, proximity to the transducer face and sound attenuation can be overcome in several ways.

A *stand-off* device can be interposed between the transducer face and the breast skin surface. This is most commonly achieved by connecting a customized transducer attachment (Fig. 6.27 and Fig. 6.28). The stand-

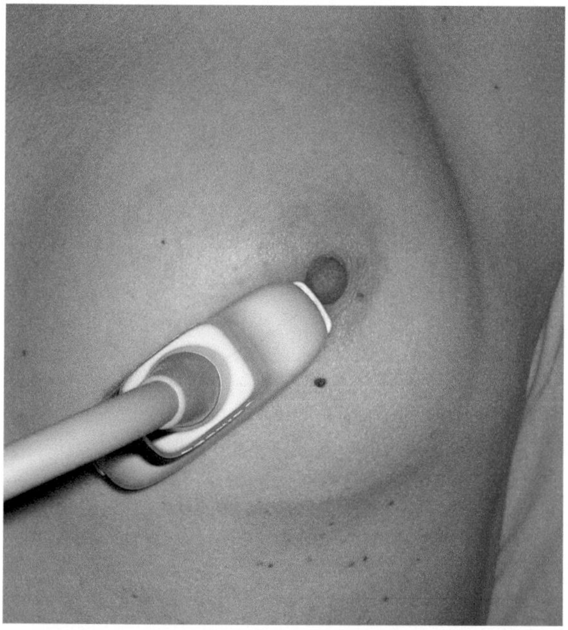

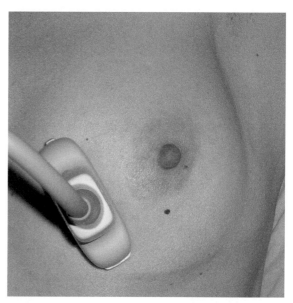

Figure 6.24   To obtain images in a plane at 90° to the radial planes the transducer long axis is placed tangentially on the breast and moved towards and way from the nipple—again circling around in a similar motion to clock face hands.

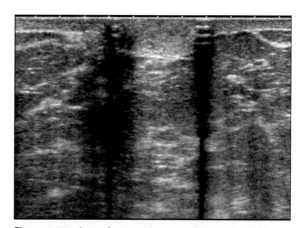

Figure 6.23   To obtain images in radial sections, the long axis of the transducer is positioned with one end close to the nipple and the other end towards the periphery of the breast, and is rotated around the breast in a similar motion to clock face hands.

Figure 6.25   Loss of contact between the transducer face and the areola surface adjacent to the nipple results in image voids—sometimes this can be avoided by placing copious amounts of coupling gel around the nipple (see Fig. 6.26).

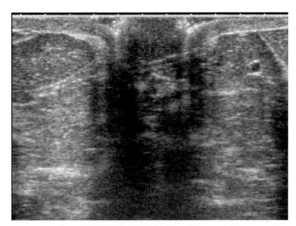

Figure 6.26   High attenuation in the dense nipple–areola complex tissues reduces the amplitude of echo signals from the subareolar region.

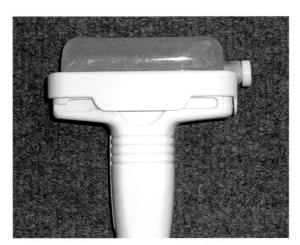

Figure 6.27   A proprietary water-filled transducer stand-off attachment.

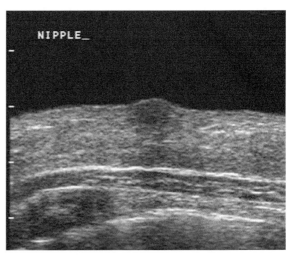

Figure 6.28   Ultrasound appearances over the nipple when a stand-off attachment has been utilized. There are no 'loss of contact' image voids and the nipple lies deeper within the image and is therefore more likely to be at the short axis focus. (Image courtesy of Mrs A. Hampshaw, Calderdale & Huddersfield NHST, UK.)

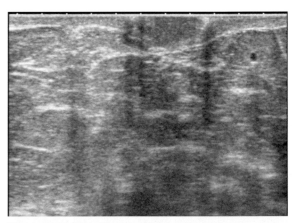

Figure 6.29   The effect of nipple/areola shadowing can be reduced by applying gentle but firm transducer pressure and increasing the overall gain.

off material surface is soft and molds to the skin contour ensuring good contact and thus efficient transmission of ultrasound across the skin boundary. An improvised stand-off can be achieved by applying copious amounts of additional coupling gel around the nipple and taking care to apply minimal transducer pressure to maintain this in the scan plane.

The nipple and subareolar tissues can sometimes be demonstrated by applying additional transducer pressure to compress the nipple's convex contour to give a flat-tened contact area; the overall gain will need to be increased (Fig. 6.29) although this may still not elimi-nate acoustic shadowing enough to get a clear view of the retroareolar anatomy.

Visualization can be improved by moving the trans-ducer slightly away from the nipple and areola and angling the sound beam obliquely into the retroareolar region.

In the absence of a stand-off attachment, however, the most effective technique to visualize the subareolar tissue is to use a coronal scanning approach. This is achieved by placing the transducer contact surface against the medial or lateral aspect of the breast so that the transducer, and therefore the scan plane, is parallel to the chest wall (Fig. 6.30). The operator's non-scanning hand can be used to push the opposite side of the breast up against the transducer as it is slowly moved away from the chest wall to examine the tissue behind the nipple and areola. Alternatively, single-handed coronal scanning can be performed by turning the patient onto the ipsilateral side and placing a towel roll under the lateral aspect of the breast (Fig. 6.31); the breast is thus supported and stabilized, allowing imaging of the nipple and subareolar region from the medial surface (Fig. 6.32) (Philips 2003). This approach is particularly useful for demonstrating subareolar ductal anatomy using a radial scanning technique (Fig. 6.33), with anatomical appearances correlating to the medio-lateral oblique mammogram projection.

The axilla

Palpable masses in the axilla are readily demonstrated using ultrasound and will usually be lymph nodes made prominent as a result of non-specific reactive

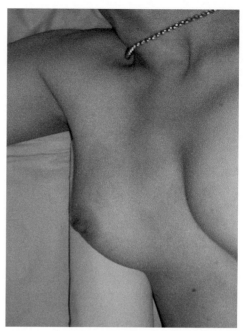

Figure 6.31   Coronal scanning can also be performed using lateral decubitus patient positioning with the lateral aspect of the breast rested on a paper roll.

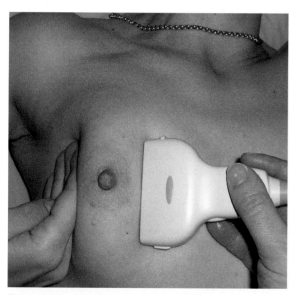

Figure 6.30   In order to avoid nipple/areola artifacts, the subareolar tissue can be visualized using coronal planes. With the patient in the supine/supine oblique position, the transducer is positioned parallel and against the chest wall. The breast is stabilized between the transducer footprint and the operators non-scanning hand as the transducer is lifted away from the chest wall towards the nipple. 'Two-handed' scanning techniques such as this necessitate an assistant, footswitch, cine-loop or video recording facilities!

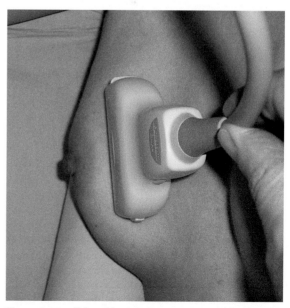

Figure 6.32   Using this technique enables one-handed coronal scanning.

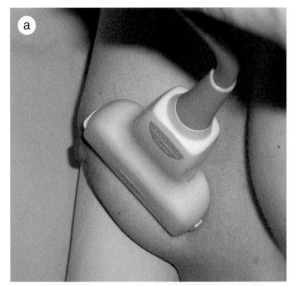

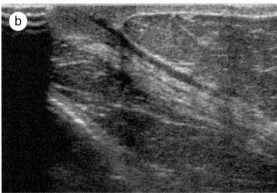

Figure 6.33 (a and b) In the lateral decubitus position, radial scan planes (a) give ultrasound images that correlate with medio-lateral oblique mammography projections. This technique is particularly useful for examining the subareolar ducts (b).

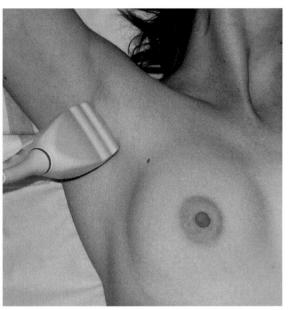

Figure 6.34 To image the axilla in longitudinal section, the transducer is placed obliquely and swept from anterior to posterior gradually working up (or down) the axillary fossa.

enlargement or enlargement due to tumor infiltration in locally metastatic disease. A breast ultrasound examination should be extended to include the axilla as a matter of routine whenever a lesion suspected to be malignant is detected. Assessment of ipsilateral axillary lymph nodes can also help refine the level of suspicion of a focal lesion that has equivocal ultrasound appearances.

The axilla is examined using longitudinal and transverse scan planes that run parallel and perpendicular to the edge of the pectoralis major muscle and the axillary blood vessels. A systematic meandering pattern of contiguous overlapping transducer passes, similar to that used over the breast, is used to ensure thorough

visualization of the lymphatic drainage pathways in the axilla. Care should be taken to adjust the depth of view, far gain and transducer frequency controls, to ensure that the deep axilliary vessels are included and visualized posteriorly on the image and thus to ensure that the full extent of the axillary fossa has been interrogated.

The transducer is initially placed obliquely on the upper outer quadrant of the breast over the axillary tail of the breast disk and aligned parallel with the underlying pectoralis major muscle fibers (Fig. 6.34). The transducer is then swept from a postero-lateral to antero-medial position (and vice versa) maintaining the longitudinal orientation. A series of overlapping side-to-side passes of the transducer are made, gradually moving upwards away from the chest and through the axilla towards the patient's upper arm. To ensure good transducer contact with the skin, it is important that the axilla is stretched and taut and presents a slightly convex, and not a concave scanning surface (Fig. 6.35).

To examine the axilla in transverse section, the transducer is rotated through 90°. From an initial position over the lateral aspect of the upper outer quadrant of the breast, the transducer is swept upwards through the axilla until the head of the humerus is visualized. The transducer is then moved horizontally across the arm to a position that overlaps the first by approximately 10 mm,

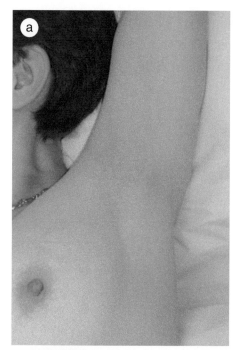

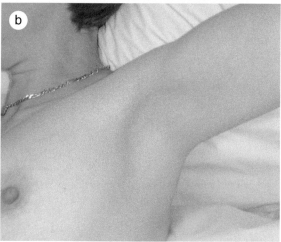

Figure 6.35 (a) Ideally the patient is positioned so that the axilla presents a taut convex skin surface to ensure good transducer footprint contact. (b) A concave axillary fossa skin surface will result in poor contact (and thus image void) and reduced transducer maneuvrability (incomplete visualization).

and is swept downwards towards the chest again. Similar meandering up and down passes are made until the whole width of the axilla has been interrogated in transverse section.

Internal mammary lymph nodes lie in close proximity to the internal thoracic arteries deep to the intercostal

muscles in the parasternal region (Heywang-Kobrunner et al 2001, p. 313). Normally they are small and not visualized during ultrasound examinations. When abnormally enlarged with metastatic disease, they may be demonstrated as hyporeflective round extrapleural masses in the intercostal spaces adjacent to the upper sternum (Madjar 2000, p. 53).

MEASUREMENTS

The maximum diameter of any focal lesion should be ascertained by measuring it in at least two planes and images recorded both with and without the on-screen measurement callipers in position (Merritt & Rumack 2003); extensions of stellate (malignant) lesions should not be included (Tot et al 2002, p. 128). Complex hemorrhagic, serous or inflammatory fluid collections, and diffuse abnormalities, should be measured in three planes to demonstrate their two-dimensional area (length and width in longitudinal and transverse planes) and their antero-posterior depth (Fig. 6.36). This defines the overall extent of the abnormality, allows estimation of fluid volume and facilitates serial monitoring of progression, resolution or response to treatment.

DOPPLER ULTRASOUND

Doppler ultrasound is used to provide additional information to that displayed at 2D B-mode imaging for both focal lesions and diffuse areas within the breast. The perfusion characteristics around and within focal lesions can be assessed and the vascularity of non-specific areas of diffuse or subtle abnormality can be compared using 'normal' areas of the ipsilateral or contralateral breast as a 'control'.

Although the most useful diagnostic ultrasound criteria are those demonstrated using black and white 2D B-mode imaging, additional evaluation of tissue vascularity may be useful for refining the level of suspicion attributed to abnormalities that have equivocal or non-specific B-mode features.

Doppler examination of the breast requires a sensitive technique to detect and display low amplitude ultrasound echo signals from low velocity blood flow in normal breast tissue; increased pulse repetition frequency may be needed to prevent aliasing when evaluating hypervascular tumors.

As with conventional B-mode imaging, Doppler ultrasound is very operator, and indeed also equipment, dependent in performance and interpretation. The use of locally customized manufacture pre-set scanning parameters (Table 6.2) helps to optimize the image and standardize the technique between operators and over serial attendances.

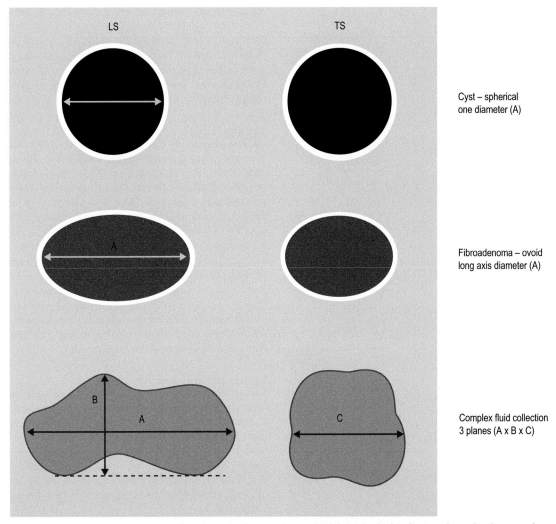

Figure 6.36 Measuring focal abnormalities. A single diameter is required for spherical lesions such as simple cysts. A single, long axis measurement of oval lesions should be recorded. Complex lesions and fluid collections should be measured in three planes.

Color flow mapping (CFM) and power Doppler (PD) are used to display flow in the blood vessels of the breast, with CFM additionally showing direction of flow. Spectral Doppler displays the relative velocities of blood flow over the cardiac cycle, the *flow velocity waveform*, and allows quantitative analysis; dense malignant lesions tend to have high velocity, high resistance spectral waveform patterns.

Once a decision is made to investigate an area with Doppler, the CFM function is activated to display the 'color box' on the image monitor; this is then adjusted in size and position to include the lesion or area of interest (Fig. 6.37). Detection of flow requires minimal transducer pressure so as not to compress small caliber vessels and occlude flow (Fig. 6.38), and very slow movement of the transducer over the area of interest. The operator will need to manipulate the transducer orientation carefully to overcome the inherent limitation that signals from vessels running at acute angles to the transducer face will be very weak; a variety of insonation angles must be tried to optimize the scanning angle and maximize the Doppler signals. When evaluating Doppler characteristics of a specific vessel, the transducer should be held quite still, to demonstrate the spontaneous phys-

Table 6.2   Optimization of Doppler scanning parameters

Parameter	Optimal setting
Frequency	High 5–10 MHz
	≥5 MHz
Wall filter	Minimum 50–100 Hz
PRF	Low 500–1000 Hz CFM
	1000–3000 Hz PWD
Power	Minimum to achieve adequate penetration
Color receiver gain	Just below background noise level
Sample volume size	2 mm
Angle correction	≤60°
Transducer scanning pressure	Minimum to achieve adequate contact

CFM = color fow mapping; PRF = pulse repetition frequency; PWD = pulsed wave Doppler.
UKAS (2001, p. 43).

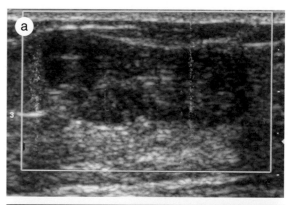

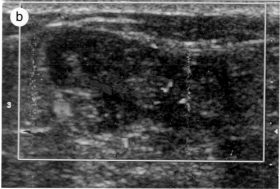

Figure 6.38   (a and b) If too much transducer pressure is applied when scanning the breast in color flow Doppler mode, small low pressure blood vessels will be compressed and their flow obliterated (a). By using minimal transducer pressure, slow velocity flow in lesions (b) and normal breast tissue is more likely to be demonstrated.

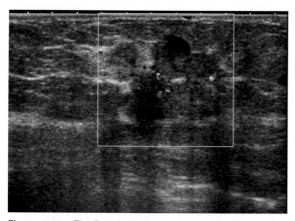

Figure 6.37   The Doppler 'color box' should be placed over the area of interest and adjusted in size to include a small margin of the surrounding 'normal' tissue.

iological movement within the scan plane; if the transducer itself is moved, spurious Doppler signals will be generated.

The color box should be kept relatively small to optimize temporal resolution, but when investigating the Doppler characteristics of a focal mass the Doppler color box should include a margin of surrounding normal breast tissue as a comparative 'control' and to enable evaluation of the orientation of any feeding vessels (Fig. 6.39). When evaluating the vascular characteristics of a more diffuse area, the Doppler scanning parameters can be set up over an area of 'normal' breast in the same or contralateral breast as a reference standard.

PD displays Doppler signal intensity and is not angle dependent, but is more susceptible to image degradation due to motion artifact, particularly from chest wall movements during normal breathing. When using PD to display vascularity, extra care must be taken to reduce the motion of both the transducer and the patient, sometimes employing arrested respiration, during scanning.

If spectral Doppler is to be performed, the vessel of interest is first identified using CFM mode and the 'sample volume' cursor displayed and placed in position over the vessel before activating the spectral function (Fig. 6.40). At this point, the image display usually splits into a small 2D image and a larger real-time spectral tracing (Fig. 6.41). In Duplex mode, the spectral trace is periodically suspended momentarily to refresh the 2D

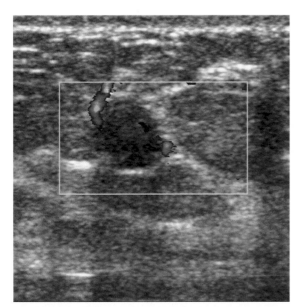

Figure 6.39 Including a margin of surrounding tissue in the color box enables the vascularity of adjacent tissue and the direction of lesion feeding vessels to be evaluated.

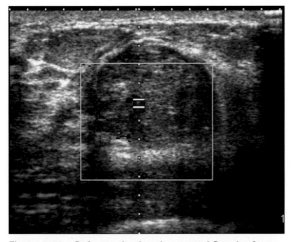

Figure 6.40 Before activating the spectral Doppler function, the sample volume 'gate' should be positioned over the vessel to be interrogated in color flow mapping mode.

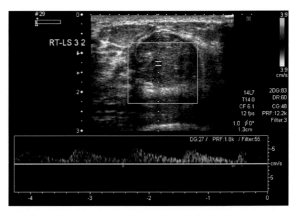

Figure 6.41 Once the spectral Doppler function is activated, the image usually splits to show both the B-mode image with color box and Doppler gate position, and the spectral Doppler flow velocity waveform.

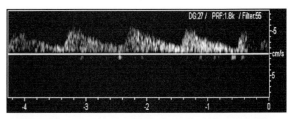

Figure 6.42 The spectral Doppler flow velocity waveform displays changes in blood velocity over time—ideally the waveform should be assessed over at least three cardiac cycles.

image. Small adjustments to sample volume position can be made by listening to the audible Doppler signal and adjusting insonnation angle and position to maximize the signal, but if the signal disappears completely the operator will need to revert to 2D CFM function and reposition the sample volume, before activating the spectral trace again.

The scale, time base and spectral gain parameters must be adjusted to show a clear trace of the flow velocity waveform over at least three cardiac cycles (Fig. 6.42). Doppler assessment using flow velocity waveforms should be undertaken over a range of vessels within a lesion or abnormal area of the breast, as tumors in particular show flow variability. Assessment of the flow velocity waveform can be undertaken both qualitatively and quantitatively; however, great care must be exercised in the latter since this is fraught with both technical and performance error.

Measurement of flow velocity is difficult to perform since a reasonable length of vessel must be displayed and its relative orientation to the ultrasound sound beam displayed using the 'angle correction' control. Doppler ratio measurements, resistance index (RI) and pulsatility index (PI), are not angle dependent and are considered to be more reliable discriminating parameters (Schelling et al 1997).

PATIENT AFTERCARE

At the end of the ultrasound examination, the patient should be informed that their ultrasound scan is complete and that they may wipe away all the acoustic coupling gel, and they should then be allowed to dress in privacy.

Breast ultrasound is most likely to be performed in a woman who has presented with symptoms or has been recalled after a positive screening mammogram—in both situations, the patient is likely to have raised anxiety and be particularly worried about the potential outcome of the examination and the effect this will have on themselves and their family (Evans & Wilson 2003). Wherever possible, the operator should give the patient (and any accompanying supporters) a brief indication as to the success of the examination and a summary of the relevance of the findings in the overall diagnostic pathway.

The way that information is given to patients can have a significant effect on the amount of anxiety and stress they feel, their perception of the standard of care they are receiving, their response to any treatment offered and their clinical outcome (Lloyd & Bor 2004, p. 45). Although a full discussion of the results and their clinical significance may sometimes be within the remit and capability of the operator, the ultrasound room is not a suitable environment for this and such a practice invariably causes operational difficulties.

The processes and facilities for 'breaking bad news' in particular require careful planning and preparation. It is not unusual for patients with malignant disease to have an idea that all is not well; despite this, hearing the news confirmed is still a shock (Leeming 2005 personal communication). Breaking bad news is not a single event, and similar to their part-contribution in ascertaining a diagnosis, the ultrasound operator only has a part role to play in giving results. Ideally, the ultrasound operator will have ascertained what the patient already understands and knows about their condition and should be guided by clues from the patient as to how much additional information they would like and when, responding to their questions and reactions on an individual basis (Penson & Slevin 2002 cited in Dias et al 2003). The presence of a clinical nurse specialist at the time of a malignant diagnosis has a positive psychological impact on most patients, as they will continue to use them as a point of contact and source of support on their 'cancer journey' (Higgins 2002, McCulloch 2004).

Departmental Schemes of Work should contain guidance about the scope and amount of information that

---

Box 6.4 Suggestions for routine phrases to be used by the non-medical sonographer when communicating ultrasound findings

When no abnormality is detected:

- Nothing abnormal is showing up with this test
- The breast tissues all look normal with this test
- There is nothing in the breast that shouldn't be there
- I can feel the lump but it is just caused by normal breast structures
- If the doctor is still worried, (s)he may request some different tests

When a focal lesion is detected:

- The lump is a simple fluid-filled cyst/normal lymph node and is nothing to worry about
- I can see the lump and
  - I agree with the doctor that it seems to be a . . . . .
  - I have taken some pictures of the lump and will let the doctor/surgeon know what it looks like and how big it is
  - It is not possible to be sure what it is with this test alone, the doctor will probably want to take get a sample of tissue from it to look at under the microscope

---

ultrasound operators can divulge to patients. The guidance needs to take into account the context of the timing of the ultrasound examination in the patient's care pathway, the location of the scanning facilities and the professional background of the ultrasound operator, and how all of these are integrated in a framework of multidisciplinary team delivery of the service. Unless additional information is requested, information given routinely immediately after the ultrasound examination might specifically pertain to the ultrasound findings and be somewhat generic and non-specific (Box 6.4).

Continuity of care must be ensured, and therefore it is important to establish that the patient knows what will happen next. If patients are sent directly home after their ultrasound examination they must be advised when and where they will get their examination results. Patients

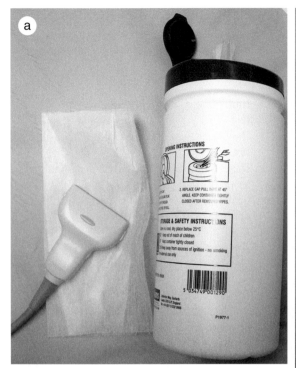 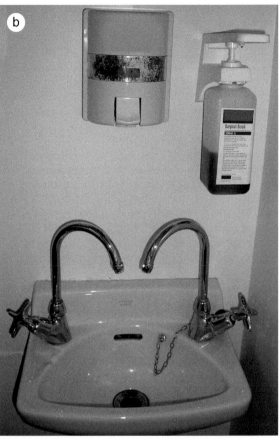

Figure 6.43 (a) At the end of the examination, the transducer and scanning machine must be cleaned according to the manufacturer's instructions and local policy in order to minimize the risk of cross-infection. (b) Hand-washing facilities should be available in the scanning room to ensure staff can comply with local infection control policies.

progressing through an investigation pathway within a symptomatic one-stop or screening assessment clinic must be shown where to wait and told what will happen next; the ultrasound operator must take responsibility for ensuring that the patient progresses to the next stage of their care pathway.

As the person performing the ultrasound examination, it is the operator's responsibility to ensure that the examination is formally reported and that the report is communicated to the clinician responsible for the care of the patient—examination reporting is discussed further in Chapter 7.

At the end of the examination, patient identification should be cleared from the scanning machine, effective infection control measures employed for hand washing and equipment cleaning (Fig. 6.43), and the scanning room restored and prepared ready for the next patient.

SUMMARY

In order to perform breast ultrasound to a high standard, and one that meets patient and service needs, the operator needs thorough knowledge of breast anatomy, ultrasound principles and equipment operation. Well-developed psychomotor skills are required to apply this knowledge to optimize demonstration and facilitate recognition of normal anatomy and pathological change. The use of standardized Schemes of Work helps to ensure that examinations are comprehensive, systematic and reproducible between operators and over successive attendances. The performance of breast ultrasound also requires the operator to apply sophisticated interpersonal skills in order to minimize the anxiety and distress of patients and their supporters and to foster effective professional relationships with colleagues in the multidisciplinary breast care team to provide an accurate, coherent and integrated diagnostic breast service.

References

AIUM 2002 Standard for the performance of breast ultrasound examination. Laurel, MD: American Institute of Ultrasound in Medicine.

De Zeeuw N 2001 Informational support. In Burnet KL (ed.) Holistic breast care. London: Balliere Tindall, pp. 137–151.

Dias L, Chabner BA, Lynch TJ et al 2003 Breaking bad news: a patient's perspective. The Oncologist 8:587–596.

Dodgeon J, Newton-Hughes A 2003 Are you sitting comfortably? Enabling sonographers to minimise work related musculo-skeletal disorders. BMUS Bulletin 11(3):16–21.

Ehrlich RA, McCloskey ED, Daly JA 2004 Patient care in radiography. St Louis, MO: Mosby.

Evans A, Wilson ARM 2003 Psychological issues and communication. In Lee L, Stickland V, Wilson R et al (eds) Fundamentals of mammography. 2nd edn. Edinburgh: Churchill Livingstone.

Hagen-Ansert S 2004 Sonographic evaluation of the breast. Online. General Medical Systems, Ultrasound Online CME Courses. Available at: http://gemedical-systems.com/rad/us/education/msucmebr.html Accessed 19 January 2004.

Heywang-Kobrunner SH, Deershaw DD, Schreer I 2001 Diagnostic breast imaging. 2nd edn. Stuttgart: Thieme.

Higgins D 2002 Breaking bad news in cancer care. Part 2: practical skills. Professional Nurse 17(11):670.

Lloyd M, Bor R 2004 Giving information. In Lloyd M, Bor R (eds). Communication skills for medicine. 2nd edn. Edinburgh: Churchill Livingstone. pp. 45–55.

Madjar H 2000 The practice of breast ultrasound. New York: Thieme.

Madjar H, Rickard M, Jellins J, Otto R (eds) 1999 IBUS guidelines for the ultrasonic examination of the breast. European Journal of Ultrasound 9:99–102.

McCulloch P 2004 The patient experience of receiving bad news from health professionals. Professional Nurse 19(5):276.

Merritt CRB, Rumack CM 2003 ACR practice guideline for the performance of a breast ultrasound examination. Reston, VA: American College of Radiology.

Philips Medical Systems 2003 Guide to sonography of the breast. Eindhoven, The Netherlands: Philips Medical Systems.

RCR 1998a Interprofessional roles and responsibilities in a radiology service. BFCR(98)6. London: Royal College of Radiologists.

RCR 1998b Intimate examinations. BFCR(98)5. London, Royal College of Radiologists.

RCR 2003 Guidance on screening and symptomatic breast imaging. BFCR(03)2. London: Royal College of Radiologists.

Schelling M, Gnirs J, Braun M et al 1997 Optimized differential diagnosis of breast lesions by combined B-mode and color Doppler sonography. Ultrasound in Obstetrics and Gynecology 10:48–53.

Tot T, Tabar L, Dean PB 2002 Practical breast pathology. New York: Thieme.

UKAS 2001 Guidelines for professional working standards: ultrasound practice. London: United Kingdom Association of Sonographers.

Chapter 7

Ultrasound image interpretation, recording and reporting

Anne-Marie Dixon

INTRODUCTION

Interpretation of the breast ultrasound image is a dynamic process that takes place during the examination itself. Images may be recorded to provide a visual representation of the findings, with the written ultrasound report in the patient's medical notes being the permanent and legal record of the examination (DH 1999, RCR 1999).

The process of breast ultrasound image interpretation involves interrogation of the image to identify normal anatomy and to recognize any architectural distortion or alteration of normal physical interaction of ultrasound with tissue that could represent disease. Where appropriate, ultrasound practitioners need to extend the scope of their examination on the basis of abnormal findings, to include other relevant anatomy (UKAS 2001, p. 43).

One of the primary goals of image interpretation when abnormality is detected is the reliable identification of malignancy and its discrimination from normal or benign appearances. Several *sonographic criteria* have been described to aid this differentiation (Table 7.1). The ultrasound examination provides a significant amount of useful information when the patient has malignant disease that helps to inform patient management and prognosis. To maximize this potential, the ultrasound practitioner must be able to communicate their findings to other healthcare colleagues in an accurate, understandable and unambiguous way (RCR 1999).

IMAGE INTERPRETATION

As with performance of the technique itself, ultrasound *image interpretation* is highly operator dependent.

Table 7.1 Differentiating sonographic criteria: B mode

Sonographic criterion	Typically benign	Typically malignant
Shape/contour	Round/spherical Oval, ellipsoid	Irregular
Margin (border) contour	Smooth, lobulated Encapsulated	Irregular, extending, infiltrating or spiculated
Margin definition	Well defined Well circumscribed	Ill-defined
Internal reflectivity (echodensity)	Anechoic (echo free) Slightly hyporeflective Hyper/isoreflective	Hyporeflective
Reflectivity pattern (echo pattern)	Homogeneous Uniform	Heterogeneous (inhomogeneous) Varied
Through transmission (posterior acoustic properties)	Increased (enhancement) Edge shadowing	Reduced (central shadowing) Varied
Mobility	Mobile	Fixed Immobile
Compressibility	Compressible	Rigid
Depth–width ratio (lesion axis)	<1 Wider than deep Horizontal or round (cyst) Parallel to chest wall Aligned with tissue planes	≥1 Deeper than wide Vertical or round (solid) Perpendicular to chest wall Cross tissue planes
Adjacent tissue plane architecture	Unaltered Raised or displaced	Discontinuity Destruction

Accurate image interpretation requires a detailed knowledge of breast anatomy, physiology and pathology, and the ability to correlate current ultrasound appearances with the results of mammography, other breast imaging studies and any previous ultrasound examination findings (Madjar et al 1999, AIUM 2002). Appearances must also be interpreted in the context of each patient's individual referral information taking into consideration patient risk factors, the findings of a current clinical examination and any other diagnostic tests that have been performed (Merritt & Rumack 2003, CoR 2005).

Individual ultrasound practitioners must recognize and work within their own level of competence, acknowledge their limitations and know when to seek further opinion or advice (CoR 2005). Experienced ultrasound practitioners can be expected to achieve a more accurate and informed interpretation of an examination since they are more reliable and consistent in the application of the semi-objective sonographic criteria to observed appearances (Chen et al 1999).

A variety of lexicons for describing sonographic appearances and focal lesion characteristics exists, but, in spite of slight differences in terminology, there is reasonable consensus on which features are the most reliable discriminators between benign and malignant disease. It is nevertheless desirable that standardization of terminology exists between operators within an individual breast ultrasound service.

Observations

Interpretation of the breast ultrasound image can only be performed if the entire area of interest is included in the field of view and scanning parameters are optimized to demonstrate normal anatomy and highlight pathological change. Throughout the ultrasound examination, the image should be systematically interrogated in real time to identify and assess the relevant anatomical appearances of the breast, axilla and chest wall (Box 7.1) as pertinent to the clinical referral information.

In the first instance, the identification of normal sonographic anatomical appearances, as described in Chapter 5, is reassuring and, after a thorough and competent examination of an appropriately referred patient, greatly reduces the risk that significant pathology is present.

When a specific focal abnormality has been identified, careful consideration must be paid to its precise position, size, shape, sonographic and Doppler characteristics (Tables 7.1 and 7.2). Two-dimensional B-mode (2DBM) sonographic characteristics are used to describe ultrasound appearances and they form the primary basis of lesion classification and differential diagnosis. Colour flow mapping (CFM) and power Doppler (PD) show anatomical vascularity, allowing the number, distribution, caliber and course of blood vessels to be assessed. Pulsed wave spectral Doppler (PWSD) gives some information about tissue metabolism, with the graphical display of the flow velocity waveform allowing quantification of blood flow characteristics.

The most useful differentiating criteria are the 2DBM characteristics: lesion shape, margin definition and depth–width ratio (Stavros et al 1995, Rahbar et al

Box 7.1   Breast anatomy to be evaluated during image interpretation

- Skin, nipple and areola
- Subcutaneous tissue
- Cooper's ligaments
- Superficial and deep mammary fascia
- Ductal and lobular glandular tissue
- Interlobular fibro-fatty tissue
- Retromammary fat
- Anterior chest wall structures
  - Pectoralis major, pectoralis minor, serratus anterior muscles
  - Ribs and intercostal muscles and spaces
  - Pleural membrane
- Breast, axillary and internal thoracic vasculature
- Subdermal, axillary, internal thoracic and cervical lymphatic drainage pathways

Table 7.2   Differentiating sonographic criteria: Doppler mode

Doppler criterion	Typically benign	Typically malignant
Overall vascularity	Low–hypovascular	High–hypervascular
Perfusion	Increased with:	Increased
	Proliferative disease	
	Pregnancy	
	Lactation	
	Inflammation	
Vessel number	Absent or singular	Increased (>3)
	Increased with inflammation	
Vascular density	Low–few vessels compared with lesion size	High–lots of vessels in comparison with lesion size
Vessel distribution	Peripheral	Peripheral and central
		Necrotic lesions have more peripheral vessels
	Single radial/segmental	Intratumoral
Vessel course/caliber	Straight and tapering	Chaotic and branching
		Ramifying pattern
Vessel orientation	Capsular	Penetrating, radial and converging
	Adjacent vessels displaced around mass	
Flow velocity	Low (<0.15 ms^{-1})	High (>0.15 ms^{-1})
Flow resistance	(inflammation–high)	
RI		
PI	Moderate (<0.7)	High (>0.7)
	Less than 1.0	More than 1.0

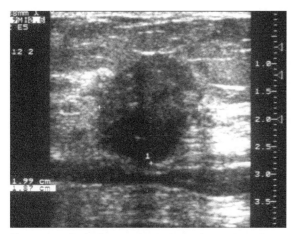

Figure 7.1 Typically a malignant lesion has an irregular margin and is deeper than it is wide.

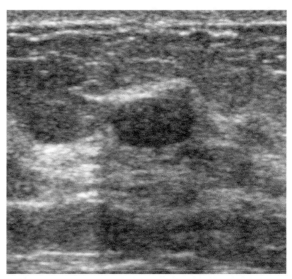

Figure 7.2 Benign lesions typically have a well-defined smooth margin and are oval in shape with a horizontal long axis (wider than deep).

1999, Hong et al 2005). Malignant lesions tend to have an irregular shape and ill-defined spiculate margins, and to be deeper than they are wide (Fig. 7.1); lesions that are round or oval, well circumscribed and that lie parallel to the chest wall are more likely to be benign (Fig. 7.2).

Doppler characteristics in themselves are not reliable discriminating parameters, but can increase sensitivity and specificity when used in conjunction with 2DBM appearances. When 2DBM ultrasound appearances are equivocal or atypical, Doppler findings may be used to substantiate a clinically suspicious diagnosis and/or raise the level of suspicion above the threshold for histological evaluation (Fig. 7.3).

This chapter provides an explanation of how to categorize and describe observed appearances, but the pathological and clinical correlates of these observations are explained in more detail in Chapters 8 and 9.

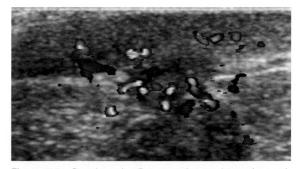

Figure 7.3 Doppler color flow mapping mode can be used to demonstrate hypervascularity in an area or lesion that has an 'equivocal' or otherwise non-specific gray-scale appearance. Hyperemia may raise the suspicion of infection or malignancy.

Sonographic characteristics—2DBM features

Number of lesions

Whilst benign disease is likely to give rise to multiple focal abnormalities, it must also be remembered that up to 40% of breast cancers are multifocal (multiple tumor foci confined to one breast quadrant) or multicentric (multiple centers of tumor development in one or both breasts) (Madjar 2000, p. 203). In practice, the number of lesions present is not a useful discriminating feature, and where multiple abnormalities are present each lesion should be evaluated independently.

Size

Maximum lesion diameter is often significant in clinical management and is also a useful monitoring parameter if lesions are managed medically or conservatively. When evaluating the size of a focal lesion, a single 'maximum' diameter in millimeter units (Fig. 7.4) should be considered and subsequently reported. The progress of diffuse abnormalities and complex fluid collections is more accurately monitored if all three-dimensional (length, width and depth) diameters are considered (Fig. 7.5).

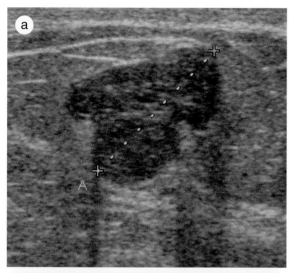

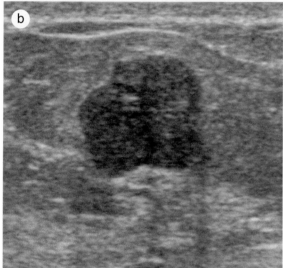

Figure 7.4 (a) Measurement callipers may be placed in any plane to measure the maximum diameter of a lesion. In this example—a lobulated fibroadenoma—the maximum dimension is demonstrated in longitudinal section with the maximum diameter lying obliquely across the lesion. (b) The transverse section area and diameters are smaller than the longitudinal section and need not be measured.

It is important to consider any interval change of an abnormality. The patient may report that it is increasing or decreasing in size since detection or measurements from previous imaging studies may have been documented. Size stability or reduction is reassuring; however, lesion progression raises the index of suspicion and may be enough to prompt consideration of diagnostic or therapeutic intervention.

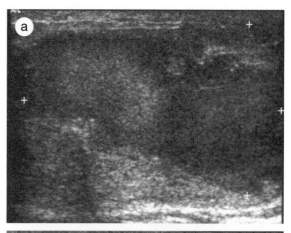

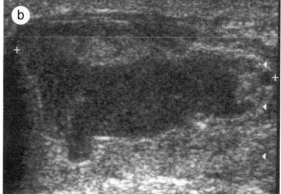

Figure 7.5 (a) With irregular and complex fluid collections, measurements in three orthogonal planes are required to obtain an estimate of the overall size of the abnormality and for serial monitoring. The long axis and vertical depth measurements of an abscess are shown. (b) The abscess short axis diameter measured on a transverse section allows estimation of overall volume.

Large benign focal lesions (>30 mm) are more likely to be aspirated (cysts) or excised (fibroadenomas), and the size of a malignant tumor is an important parameter factored into prognostic calculations (see Ch. 2).

Shape

Well-defined abnormalities can be categorized as either round, oval (elliptical) or irregular (Fig. 7.6); their three-dimensional nature can be recognized by use of the terms 'spherical' and 'ovoid' or 'ellipsoid'.

Margin/border definition

This can be classified as either sharp and well defined, or as ill defined, the former being further classified as either smooth, lobulated or irregular (Fig. 7.7). A well-defined

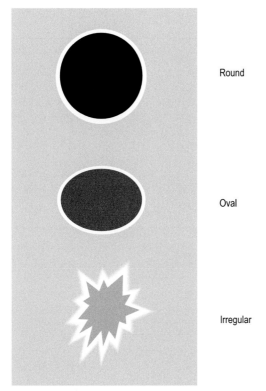

Figure 7.6 Lesions may be described as being round, oval or irregular in shape.

lesion might also be noted to appear encapsulated. Irregular lesions might also be described as spiculated or infiltrating in nature.

Depth–width ratio

This measurement is used to describe further the shape of a lesion and its orientation with reference to normal tissue planes and the chest wall (Fig. 7.8). A round, spherical lesion has a uniform diameter, is equally wide, deep and long and its depth–width ratio is 1. Lesions that are wider than deep have their longest diameter parallel to the chest wall and appear to align with the normal tissue planes; they have a horizontal axis and thus a depth–width ratio of less than 1. Lesions that are deeper than wide appear to cross normal tissue planes and have their longest diameter perpendicular to the chest wall; these lesions have a vertical axis and thus have a depth–width ratio greater than 1.

Internal appearances

The internal ultrasound appearance of a lesion depends upon both the spatial pattern and the monochromatic shading of the echo reflections within it. Descriptions of the internal structure of lesions incorporate judgments

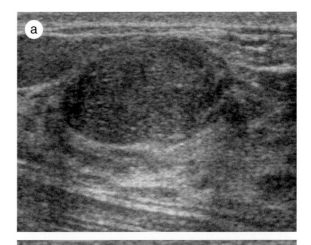

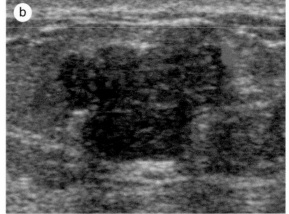

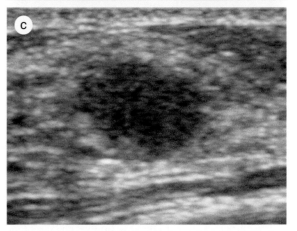

Figure 7.7 (a) Well-defined lesions, such as this fibroadenoma, may be described as having a smooth margin. (b) Some fibroadenomas have a well-defined *lobulated* lesion margin. (c) Lesions that have a reasonably well-defined but slightly irregular margin, i.e. there is no sharp distinct capsule around them, are more likely to be malignant.

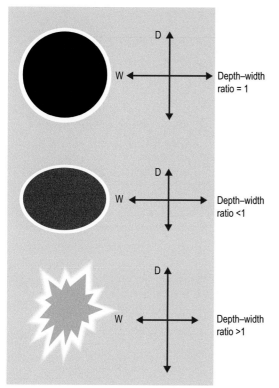

Figure 7.8   The depth–width ratio of a round lesion is 1. Lesions with a horizontal long axis have a depth–width ratio less than 1 and are more likely to be benign. Lesions with a vertical long axis have a depth–width ratio greater than 1 and are more likely to be malignant.

about both the graininess (relative location of echoes to each other) and the reflectivity (gray-scale allocation) of the echo pattern.

Homogeneous is the term used to describe appearances that are even and uniform in either texture or reflectivity, with an uneven or irregular pattern being described as inhomogeneous or heterogeneous (Fig. 7.9).

When the abnormality appears darker than adjacent tissue (Fig. 7.10), the term *hyporeflective* is used (in preference to the less technically accurate terms of hypodense or hypoechoic). Areas and lesions that have been allocated lighter shades of gray than adjacent surrounding tissue (Fig. 7.11) are termed *hyper-reflective* (as opposed to hyperdense or hyperechoic). Lesions that are similar in gray-scale shade to surrounding tissue (Fig. 7.12) are described a *isoreflective* (again in preference to the terms isodense and isoechoic).

Echo texture is separately described as being either fine or coarse grained, and again may be described as homogeneous when similar throughout the lesion/area of abnormality, or inhomogeneous if it is non-uniform (Fig. 7.13).

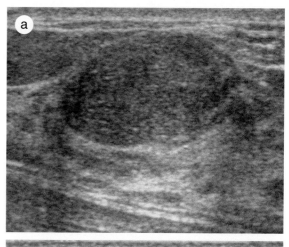

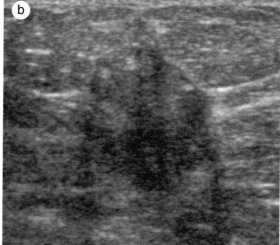

Figure 7.9   (a) The reflectivity of a lesion such as this fibroadenoma is described as being homogeneous because the gray-scale value is relatively uniform throughout the lesion. (b) Malignant lesions such as this are more likely to have heterogeneous reflectivity—the gray-scale value varies throughout the lesion with some hyper-reflective (whiter) elements and some echo-poor (darker gray) elements.

Simple fluid confined within a cyst membrane, free or collected within the breast presents a uniform transmission path to the incident ultrasound beam and as such generates no echo information. Fluid thus is demonstrated as a black area on the image (Fig. 7.14) and is described as being either echo-free or *anechoic*.

Occasionally, a fluid collection or fluid within a cyst may be complex due to the presence of cellular debris, infective exudate or hemorrhage. Such fluid often contains low-level echo signals that make it difficult to differentiate it from a solid lesion (Fig. 7.15). Clarification

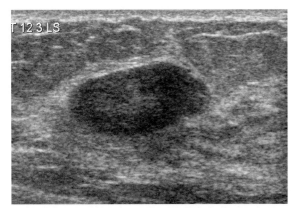

Figure 7.10 This fibroadenoma is described as a hyporeflective lesion since it is darker (produces fewer/lower amplitude sound reflections) than the surrounding tissue.

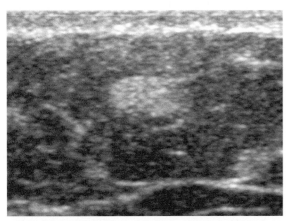

Figure 7.11 Lipomas are typically described as hyperreflective lesions since they are displayed lighter than surrounding tissue.

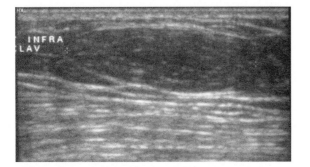

Figure 7.12 Some lesions, such as this lipoma, are described as being isoreflective since they have similar gray-scale values to the surrounding tissue. Isoreflective lesions may be very subtle in the image, making them difficult to identify and demonstrate—palpating focal lesions can help to correlate ultrasound appearances with clinical findings and improve detection of isoreflective anomalies.

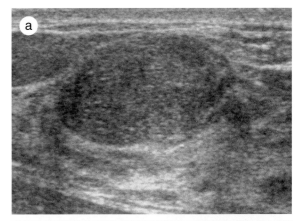

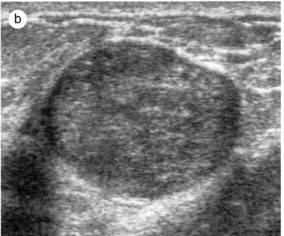

Figure 7.13 (a and b) The internal pattern of echoes within a lesion, its echotexture, may be described as fine and homogeneous (a) if it is even, or coarse and heterogeneous (b) if it is patchy.

may be achieved by observation of free-floating particles or fluid streaming if the fluid can be set in motion. Low viscosity fluid is readily set in motion either by the application of gentle oscillatory transducer pressure or by moving the patient into a different position. More viscous fluid may be seen to move using higher acoustic power; this can happen on activation of the color Doppler function and additionally allows interrogation of the lesion for internal vascularity, the presence of which defines it as unequivocally solid.

Calcification

It is possible to demonstrate calcification greater than 1 mm sonographically although sensitivity and specificity

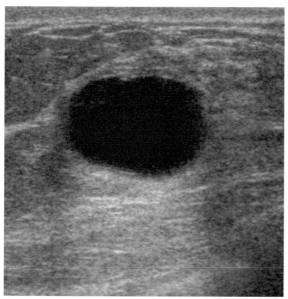

Figure 7.14   Simple fluid, as in this cyst, is echo free and is characteristically displayed black in the ultrasound image.

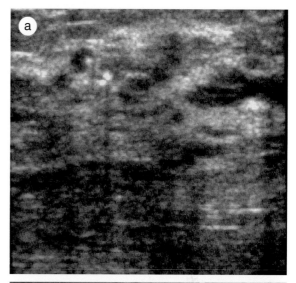

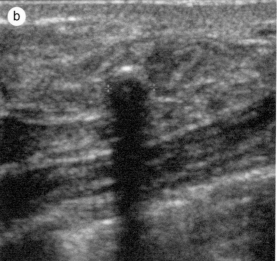

Figure 7.16   (a) With modern ultrasound equipment, it is often possible to resolve small isolated breast calcifications. (b) Calcifications, such as this calcified oil cyst, produce a characteristic acoustic shadow.

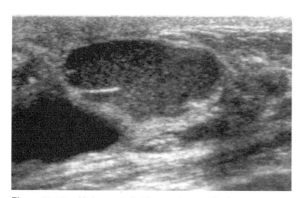

Figure 7.15   If the cyst fluid contains particulate matter, such as cellular debris or altered blood, it will not be displayed as echo free. Complicated cysts may require aspiration to confirm that they are not solid lesions.

are limited. On mammographic imaging, certain features of calcification are pathognomonic for malignancy, but no such patterns exist for ultrasound appearances.

When visualized, calcification appears as a focus of hyper-reflectivity. The calcium–soft tissue interface reflects a large proportion of the sound beam, giving a high amplitude sound echo that is represented at the white end of the gray-scale spectrum. If the ultrasound beam width is smaller than the diameter of the calcifica-

tion, no sound reaches the tissues directly behind the calcification's reflecting interface and there is a black stripe, with no image information, deep to it (see below—posterior acoustic shadowing). Small calcifications 1–2 mm in diameter are demonstrated as small white dots, with larger calcifications often presenting a white convex curved surface (Fig. 7.16). Calcification may be interspersed in the breast parenchyma or contained within a focal lesion (Fig. 7.17).

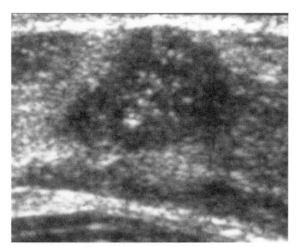

Figure 7.17   Small calcifications within a solid breast lesion raise the suspicion of malignancy.

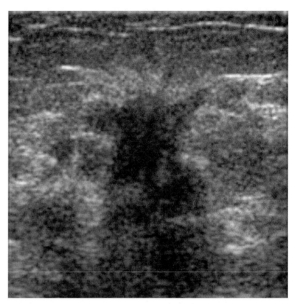

Figure 7.18   Posterior acoustic shadowing is often seen deep to malignant lesions since they absorb the sound more than adjacent tissues.

Through transmission characteristics/posterior acoustic properties

The ultrasound appearances deep to an area of abnormality or a focal lesion result from a variety of interactions between sound and body tissue that result in both reflection and absorption of the incident ultrasound beam—the physical explanations for these are described in Chapter 3.

The term *posterior acoustic shadowing* is used to describe a reduction in gray-scale level deep to a lesion. This effect may be pronounced, effectively a vertical black stripe, or more subtle, i.e. the area looks 'darker' or *hyporeflective* (Fig. 7.18).

Acoustic shadowing may be either central or an 'edge' phenomenon (see below). It is important to ensure that a posterior 'shadow' is a real effect of reflection or absorption, and not an artifact caused by refraction of the ultrasound beam as it strikes an oblique tissue interface (see Ch. 3). When shadowing is encountered, the application of increased transducer pressure will flatten oblique interfaces and improve sound transmission, reducing the artifact (Fig. 7.19). True sound-absorbing tumors or strongly reflecting (calcified) surfaces will still be associated with a posterior shadow on compression.

A lesion is said to exhibit *increased through transmission* when the area deep to it is allocated brightness levels nearer the white end of the gray-scale spectrum, i.e. it appears *hyper-reflective*. This phenomenon is most obviously seen deep to fluid-filled structures (Fig. 7.20). The traditionally used terminology 'acoustic enhancement' is increasingly avoided in this context as it more accurately describes the appearances associated with contrast agent uptake.

Edge characteristics

The phenomenon of *edge shadowing* mentioned above results from refraction of the ultrasound beam at smooth interfaces lying almost parallel to the ultrasound beam, and is a feature associated with well-defined encapsulated lesions such as fibroadenomas (Fig. 7.21). The margins of lesions with irregular, and in particular spiculated, borders may have a hyper-reflective (brighter) *halo* appearance on ultrasound images due to the complex way that the ultrasound beam undergoes multiple reflections between the lesion spiculations (Fig. 7.22).

Compressibility

Transducer pressure ca n be used to assess the compressibility of a lesion in a vertical dimension. A reduction in vertical diameter can be demonstrated in normal breast tissue and lesions that are soft, less dense and/or have an elastic tissue matrix (Fig. 7.23). The more dense, solid and inelastic tumors are firmer and show no reduction in vertical dimension but are simply displaced vertically in the breast as transducer pressure is applied (Fig. 7.24).

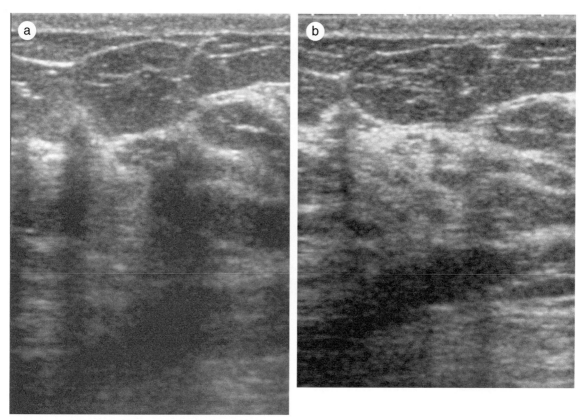

Figure 7.19 (a and b) Refraction artifact shadowing, such as that associated with Cooper's ligaments (a) can be reduced (b) by applying gentle transducer pressure; pathological shadowing will persist despite this maneuver.

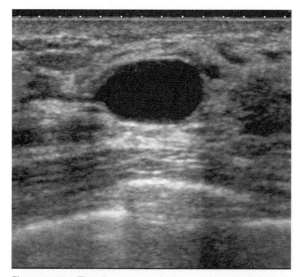

Figure 7.20 The phenomenon known as *increased through transmission* occurs deep to fluid-filled structures because sound is attenuated less as it travels through fluid than through solid soft tissue. Since the time gain compensation control operates uniformly across the transducer footprint, echo signals from behind the cyst are overamplified and displayed brighter in the image.

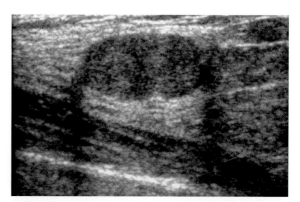

Figure 7.21 Refraction of the ultrasound beam at the steeply oblique margins of solid lesions such as this fibro-adenoma results in characteristic 'edge shadowing'. Note the increased through transmission deep to the lesion indicating that the fibroadenoma is attenuating the sound less than the adjacent normal breast tissue. Longer standing or hyalinized fibroadenomas may attenuate the sound more, giving rise to reduced reflectivity (acoustic shadowing) posteriorly.

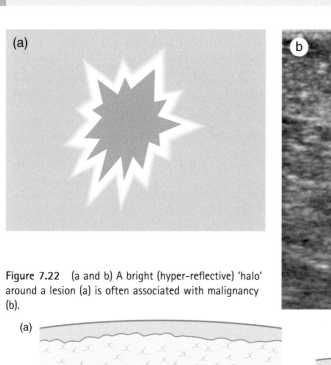

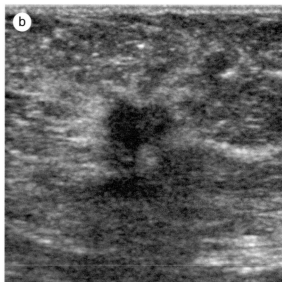

Figure 7.22 (a and b) A bright (hyper-reflective) 'halo' around a lesion (a) is often associated with malignancy (b).

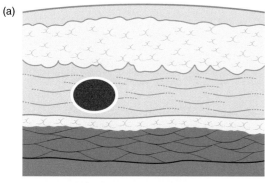

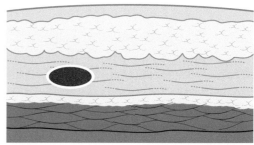

(A) Normal scanning pressure

(B) With additional transducer pressure lesion compresses

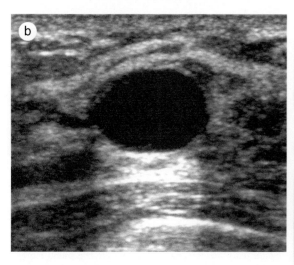

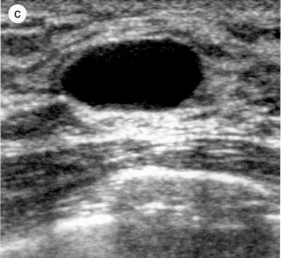

Figure 7.23 (a) Transducer compression will distort the shape of a soft compressible benign lesion. (b) Under normal scanning conditions, a simple cyst is round (c). Since it is a soft, mobile structure, additional transducer pressure will distort its shape.

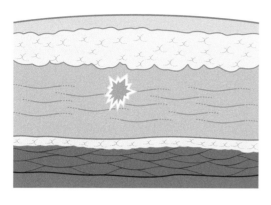 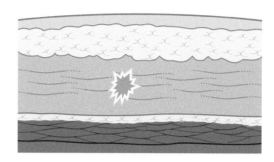

(A) Normal scanning pressure   (B) With additional transducer pressure lesion is displaced

Figure 7.24   If additional transducer pressure is exerted over a malignant lesion, it tends to displace rather than distort, as it is firmer and more adherent to the adjacent breast tissue.

Mobility

Lesion mobility can be assessed both clinically and sonographically, the latter using gentle transducer pressure to determine if there is any relative movement between a focal lesion and its surrounding tissue. Lesions may be described as freely mobile or lacking in mobility, immobile masses appearing fixed or tethered to adjacent tissue.

Architecture of surrounding tissue

It is important to look at the tissue surrounding an area of abnormality and to look at the effect of a focal lesion on adjacent tissue planes and Cooper's ligaments. Normal boundaries between glandular breast tissue and surrounding fibrous and ligamentous tissue are demonstrated on ultrasound as hyper-reflective lines since there is a reasonably large difference in tissue density and/or compressibility. This results in a reasonably large partial reflection of the incident sound beam and thus allocation of a gray-scale value towards the white end of the dynamic range.

Where malignant tumor has invaded the surrounding tissue, the differences in tissue density/compressibility are less marked, with the demarcating tissue boundaries disrupted or appearing discontinuous in the image (Fig. 7.25). Conversely, when a lesion is well encapsulated, the differences in acoustic impedance are preserved and its presence does not destroy surrounding tissue planes. With continued growth, such lesions may eventually exert a *mass effect* on adjacent tissue and raise or displace tissue boundaries from their normal position (Fig. 7.26).

Duct caliber

Lactiferous ducts are considered dilated, or ectatic, when their internal caliber is above 2 mm, although in the subareolar region normal ducts may be up to 8 mm in diameter (Hagen-Ansert 2004). Ectatic ducts are not uncommon, and are particularly associated with benign fibrocystic change. Dilated ducts are echo free when they contain simple serous fluid (Fig. 7.27) and any reflective content should be carefully evaluated. Cellular debris in suspension may be seen to move with the application of additional transducer pressure and will not show any Doppler signal. A single dilated duct is particularly suspicious, and in the presence of intraductal neoplasm (intraduct papilloma) it may be possible to demonstrate Doppler signals in solid tumor material within the duct.

Skin thickening

With good equipment, or using a stand-off device, the thickness of the breast skin layers can be measured, normal skin not usually exceeding 3 mm (Fig. 7.28). Skin thickening may be associated with trauma, irritation, inflammation or malignancy. Focal skin lesions such as sebaceous cysts (Fig. 7.29) are readily demonstrated and localized to the skin layer (Stavros 2004, pp. 325–329).

Nipple changes

Occasionally nipple retraction is congenital, but if acquired may be due to inflammation, periareolar edema or underlying malignancy. The caliber and content of subareolar ducts should be noted and evidence of an underlying focal lesion excluded.

(a)

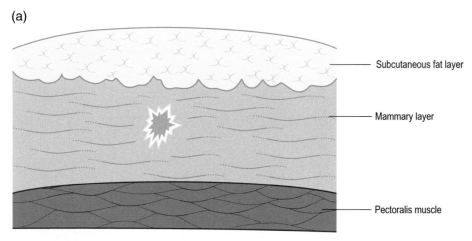

Subcutaneous fat layer

Mammary layer

Pectoralis muscle

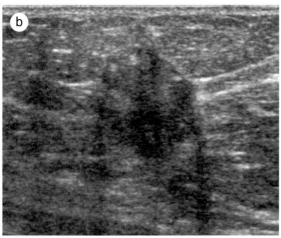

Figure 7.25 (a) Malignant lesions tend to erode and destroy breast tissue planes. (b) On ultrasound images, disrupted (discontinuous) tissue planes are evident adjacent to this carcinoma.

Lymphedema

Severe vascular invasion with aggressive malignant disease may give rise to lymphatic obstruction and lymphedema. Dilated anechoic lymphatic channels can sometimes be visualized in the subcutaneous tissue layer and may be distinguished from blood vessels using Doppler ultrasound (Fig. 7.30). The *halo* immediately surrounding a malignant tumor is sometimes attributed to tumor-filled lymphatics appearing hyper-reflective in comparison with surrounding echo-poor fatty tissues. In addition, a hyper-reflective area may be demonstrated between a malignant lesion and the skin layers since initial lymphatic drainage, and therefore tumor infiltration, is towards the subdermal lymphatic network (Stavros 2004, pp. 640–641).

Lymphadenopathy

Normal lymph nodes are often difficult to differentiate from surrounding fatty tissue, but nodal enlargement is usually readily apparent, particularly in the axilla. Assessment of the size and shape of the lymph node and the degrees of cortical atrophy and hilar fatty infiltration can help distinguish benign reactive enlargement from metastatic infiltration. Size should be assessed using the maximum short axis diameter (Fig. 7.31), 10 mm being the accepted cut-off value for normality (Stavros 2004, p. 855); and shape classified as oval or round. Any cortical thickening should be noted (Fig. 7.32) along with assessment of the severity and its uniform or eccentric distribution (Stavros 2004, p. 858).

Sonographic characteristics—Doppler imaging

Doppler ultrasound is used to look at the number, alignment, configuration and distribution of blood vessels, the orientation and relationship of blood vessels to any focal lesions and the velocity and resistance of arterial blood flow (UKAS 2001, p. 42).

(a)

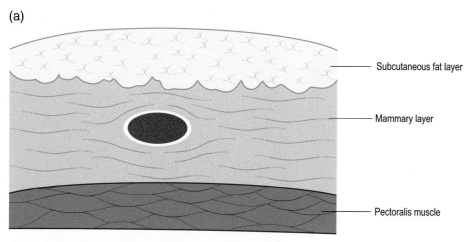

Subcutaneous fat layer

Mammary layer

Pectoralis muscle

Figure 7.26 (a) Tissue planes are conserved and displaced around benign mass lesions. (b) The tissue planes are lifted and displaced around this fibroadenoma—look carefully at the lateral margins.

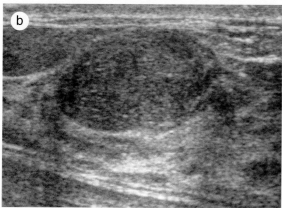

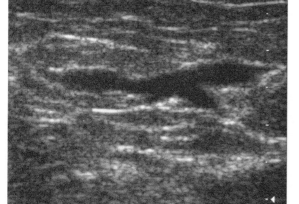

Figure 7.27 Individual ducts are not usually visualized within the breast parenchyma—dilated ducts are demonstrated as echo-free (black) channels.

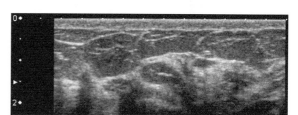

Figure 7.28 Normal ultrasound appearances of the skin layer; its depth is normally no more than 3 mm.

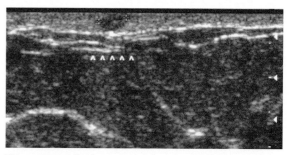

Figure 7.29 A sebaceous cyst has the ultrasound appearance of a hyporeflective (dark gray) focal mass within the skin layer.

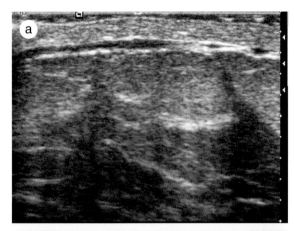

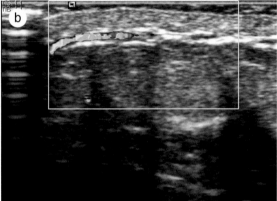

Figure 7.30 (a) Echo-free linear structures just underneath the skin surface may represent dilated lymphatic channels. (b) More usually, however, such channels are superficial veins—blood flow can be confirmed using color flow Doppler mode.

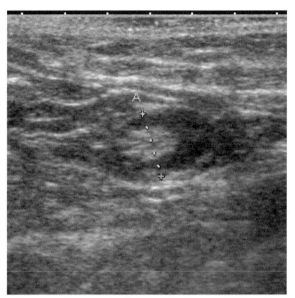

Figure 7.31 Lymph node size should be assessed by measuring the short axis diameter—normally the measurement will be less than 10 mm.

Location, orientation and distribution pattern of vessels

Tumor vessel patterns can be categorized according to vessel location within the tumor and orientation relative to the tumor margin and surrounding normal breast parenchyma (Raza & Baum 1997, Strano et al 2004, Santamaria et al 2005).

Within the tumor, vessels may be peripheral, central or both. A *radial* or *afferent* pattern describes the appearance of 'feeding' vessels entering the lesion from surrounding normal parenchyma and penetrating towards the center of the mass. A *peripheral* or *capsular* pattern describes vessels that are seen only around the margins of a lesion and which do not extend or branch towards the center. When any vessels seen lie within the tumor mass, the pattern is described as *intratumoral*, a benign variant being a *segmental* pattern. A *ramifying* pattern describes uneven branching vasculature with vessels both at the periphery and within the tumor mass.

Most commonly the vessels of solid focal lesions are aligned in a radial penetrating fashion (Fig. 7.34). There is some evidence that the angle at which arteries enter the lesion is a useful benign/malignant differentiating characteristic—with vessels supplying malignant tumors aligned more at right angles to the tumor margin, and vessels into benign lesions being more tangential.

Rapidly growing malignant lesions tend to have a very chaotic pattern of angiogenesis and, as such, a chaotic,

Interpretation of vascular and hemodynamic Doppler information is usually subjective and qualitative for CFM and PD. although it is possible to quantify vascularity and vascular density, and to apply numerical thresholds to try to discriminate between benign and malignant disease.

Spectral Doppler can also be evaluated qualitatively by looking at the shape of the flow velocity waveform and the relative magnitudes of peak systolic and end-diastolic velocities (Fig. 7.33). However, it is more tempting, given the graphical display format, to attempt quantitative assessment. The maximum, minimum and average velocities can be measured or combined to give velocity, resistance and pulsatility indices and, although malignant lesions tend to have high velocity high resistance flow, there is enough overlap in absolute index values with benign lesions to make accurate discrimination unreliable in individual cases.

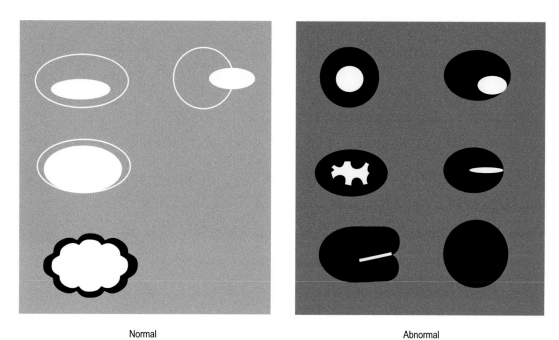

Figure 7.32 Lymph nodes have a hyporeflective (gray) outer cortex and a central hyper-reflective (white) hilum. Evaluation of the relative amounts and distribution of cortical and hilar tissue can help differentiate normal from abnormal nodes.

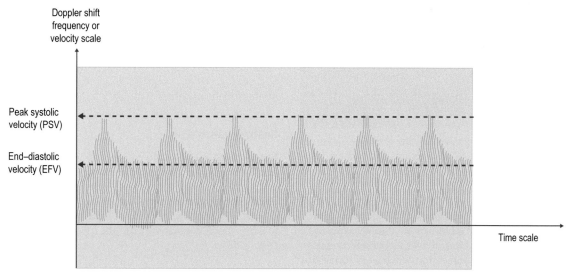

Figure 7.33 Comparison of the peak systolic and end-diastolic velocities demonstrated in the spectral Doppler flow velocity waveform can help differentiate benign and malignant lesions if used in conjunction with the B-mode gray-scale information.

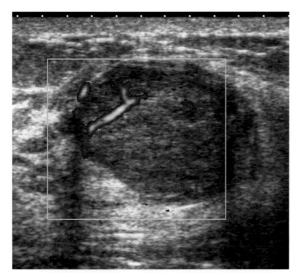

Figure 7.34 Color flow mapping or power Doppler (in the example shown) will demonstrate one or two vessels orientated in a radial pattern in most solid benign lesions.

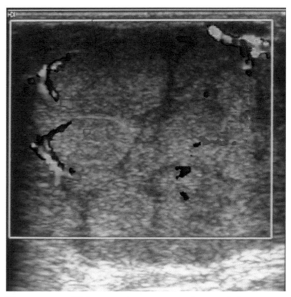

Figure 7.36 If the vessels are arranged around the periphery of a lesion and taper towards its center, the lesion is more likely to be benign.

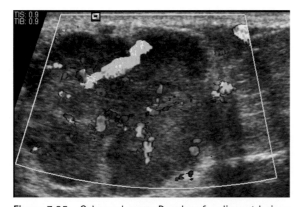

Figure 7.35 Color and power Doppler of malignant lesions are more likely to demonstrate a chaotic arrangement of multiple blood vessels.

irregular, branching (ramifying) CFM Doppler pattern (Fig. 7.35). Slower growing benign lesions have a more organized vascular architecture with a peripheral pattern or one or two gently meandering penetrating vessels that taper towards the center of the mass (Fig. 7.36).

Number

Vascularity describes the number of vessels supplying or within a tumor, malignant tumors tending to have a higher number of vessels (Madjar 2000, p. 233). Vascular density attempts to correlate blood flow volume

within a tumor to the overall tumor volume. According to the number of vessels and relative blood flow volume, lesions may be described as either hypervascular (hyperemic) or hypovascular, compared with surrounding or contralateral breast tissue (Fig. 7.37). A diagnostic level of suspicion would be raised if an equivocal lesion was hypervascular compared with surrounding breast tissue, and the level of suspicion would be reduced if the lesion was noted to be hypovascular compared with surrounding normal breast tissue.

Caliber and shape

Vessel caliber is assessed in comparison with overall mass size. Slow growing tumors demonstrate a more coherent and organized vessel structure with smooth tapering vessels; rapidly proliferating lesions tend to have a more chaotic and irregular pattern with the individual vessels looking large compared with the overall lesion size (Fig. 7.38).

Velocity, pulsatility and resistance

Blood flow velocity, flow velocity resistance and pulsatility indices and ratios (RI, PI and AB ratio) may be measured but are poor discriminating parameters in isolation; typically Doppler parameters show reasonable specificity but poor sensitivity (Hollerweger et al 1997). Inherent practical and technical limitations in measurement tech-

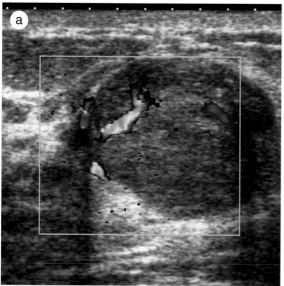

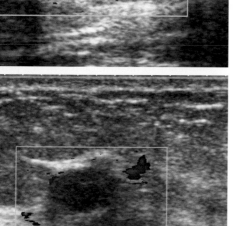

Figure 7.37 (a and b) By including a margin of adjacent breast tissue in the color box, a lesion can be described as either hypervascular (a) if it has more vessels per unit area than the adjacent tissue, or hypovascular (b) if the vessel density is lower (or absent) in comparison with adjacent breast tissue.

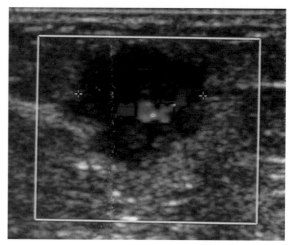

Figure 7.38 Large vessels within a small lesion raise the index of suspicion for malignancy.

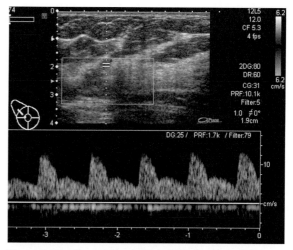

Figure 7.39 Normal blood flow within the breast is low velocity. The color flow sensitivity has been set at 0.06 m s^{-1} to capture this.

nique and in software algorithms render absolute velocity measurements imprecise, and they should be used only with extreme caution.

Normal blood flow velocity within the breast is low, typically around 0.10–0.15 ms^{-1} (Fig. 7.39); the detection of aliasing at default breast pre-set settings will alert the operator to (suspicious) high velocity flow. Where possible, spectral velocity waveforms should be assessed over a number of vessels, on clear waveforms and over at least three cardiac cycles (Fig. 7.40). Typically normal and benign flow is low velocity with relatively low resistance (RI <0.75) and low pulsatility (PI <1.0); malignant lesions tend to have higher RI and PI values (Fig. 7.41) and also show greater variability in Doppler values between peripheral and central vessels (Hollerweger et al 1997, Stavros 2004, p. 882).

IMAGING PROTOCOLS

To take or not to take—that is the question

Unless scans are video-recorded, the person performing the ultrasound examination is the only one who has

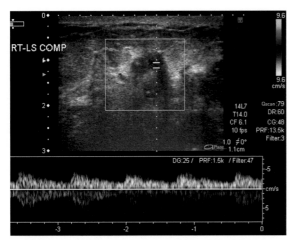

Figure 7.40 Applying a colored hue to the spectral Doppler flow velocity waveform can improve visualization of the trace—at least three cardiac cycles should be used to evaluate resistance and pulsatility characteristics.

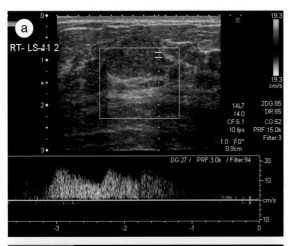

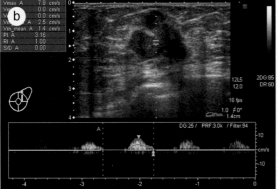

Figure 7.41 (a and b) Benign lesions tend to have low resistance flow patterns with low pulsatility and continuous forward flow in diastole (a). Malignant lesions have higher resistance, high pulsatility waveforms, sometimes with no-end diastolic flow (b).

access to all the potential diagnostic information by virtue of viewing the *real-time* examination in its entirety. The recording of *still* images can at best only ever be representative, and if ill considered has the potential to be misleading.

There are benefits and limitations associated with the recording and storage of retrievable, reviewable 'still' images, these are summarized in Table 7.3.

Any images that are recorded should be retained in line with national and local policies and be readily available, in conjunction with mammography images, according to clinical need (Merritt & Rumack 2003).

The main purposes of image recording, as with the creation of any other medical record, are to:

- Provide evidence of the standard and quality of care afforded
- Facilitate communication between healthcare professionals
- Contribute to the medical record of a patient's diagnosis and treatment
- Promote continuity of patient care between colleagues.

(after Dimond 2002, p. 233).

Most experts advocate that some visual, i.e. *image*, record is made of the information obtained during ultrasound scans. The advantages and disadvantages of doing so need to be balanced in a realistic and pragmatic way with guidance on the number and content of images considered representative of examinations, included in departmental Schemes of Work.

Image recording in 'negative' examinations

An argument can be made for not recording images when appearances are interpreted as normal on the basis that an abnormality might be 'manufactured' at a later date with the benefit of hindsight or by an uninformed observer. However, the recording of at least one image, annotated with the place and date of examination, operator's identity and identifying patient information such as name and date of birth or hospital number, provides evidence that the patient was indeed scanned at a particular location and time, and demonstrates the standard of equipment used and the scan parameters employed by the operator during the examination (Fig. 7.42).

A limited set of standard images produced in accordance with a local departmental protocol provides evidence that a standardized, protocol-driven technique has been followed, with the images being useful for routine audit and quality assurance purposes (Fig. 7.43).

Sometimes true abnormalities are sonographically 'occult', i.e. they do not show up on ultrasound images.

Table 7.3   Advantages and disadvantages of recording images

Advantages of recording images	Disadvantages of recording images
All examinations:	Capital costs of recording equipment
Evidence of compliance with scheme of work	Revenue costs of recording medium and equipment
Record of equipment in use at time of examination	maintenance
	Storage space
Examinations with 'positive' findings:	Available to patients/legal representatives to support claims
Aide-memoire when compiling written report	of incompetence/negligence
Demonstration of findings at clinical meetings	Potential to focus examination on picture taking as opposed
Facilitates comparison with previous/future appearances	to a thorough examination
Allows assessment of progression/resolution	Open to subsequent re- or misinterpretation
Education and training resource	
Available to health care staff/legal representatives to	
defend claims of incompetence/negligence	

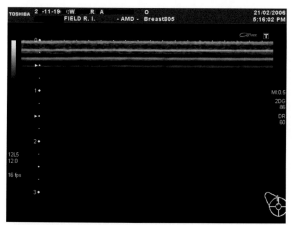

Figure 7.42   All recorded images should include standard patient and examination identification annotation—in this example the patient has been anonymized for illustration purposes. As a minimum, it is good practice to include date, time and location of the examination as well as operator and patient identification details.

If the physical nature of the abnormality means its tissue density and/or compressibility, i.e. its *acoustic imped-ance*, is very similar to that of surrounding normal tissue, there will be no, or only a very subtle, *acoustic boundary* between the tissues; this will render any reflected sound signals below the sensitivity threshold. This is an inherent limitation of the nature of the sound–tissue interaction, and the provision of images of 'normal ultrasound appearances' in such cases serves to illustrate this limitation of the imaging method rather than any limitation of operator technique or error of interpretation (Fig. 7.44).

Imaging when abnormality is present

Recorded images provide permanent/semi-permanent visual documentation of any abnormality detected and have multiple uses (Table 7.3).

Whenever images have been recorded to illustrate abnormal appearances, it is important to remember that the official record of the examination is the written examination report relating to the whole real-time examination, and that the recorded images are only a limited and incomplete record of the examination. Although recorded images are thus only ever representative, they should nevertheless be an accurate and substantiating representation of the examination process and its diagnostic outcome.

The operator will be formulating a conclusion about the image appearances whilst scanning and, once this has been reached, images should be recorded to substantiate the conclusion and demonstrate the salient features that will be described in the written report. When appearances are equivocal and it is not easy to reach a definitive conclusion, representative images illustrating the differentiating sonographic criteria can be objectively and independently considered to reach an informed list of differential diagnoses; they are not, however, a reliable substitute for a 'real-time' second opinion examination in difficult cases.

Any image series should contain at least one global image to show that the whole depth of breast tissue has been well visualized. This should include the skin surface anteriorly and the pleural surface, ribs and anterior chest wall muscles posteriorly (Fig. 7.45).

Additionally, when a focal abnormality is detected, images should be taken to show its location within the breast and its spatial relationships and ultrasound

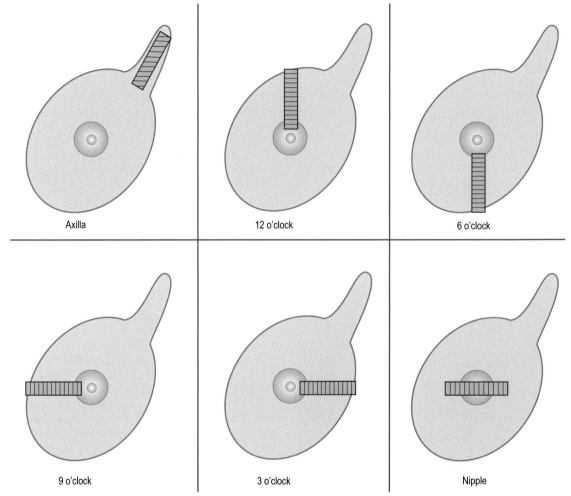

Axilla   12 o'clock   6 o'clock

9 o'clock   3 o'clock   Nipple

Figure 7.43   A minimum record of a whole breast survey examination in a patient with no abnormal findings might include routine images recorded at the 12, 3, 6 and 9 o'clock positions, over the nipple and in the axilla.

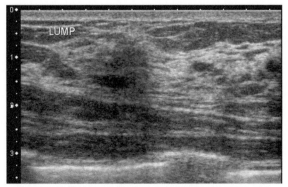

LUMP

Figure 7.44   Even when normal appearances are demonstrated at the site of a palpable lump it is good practice to record one ultrasound image that might be considered representative of the standard of the examination.

characteristics compared with normal breast and surrounding anatomy. Global images will demonstrate the relative spatial relationships of the lesion to the breast skin surface and the underlying chest wall, but magnified images, utilizing the 'depth of view', 'magnification' or 'zoom' controls, will better demonstrate the sonographic characteristics and allow an accurate assessment of lesion size (Fig. 7.46). As a general rule, any feature of interest should occupy approximately two-thirds of the available ultrasound image field of view when detailed evaluation is being performed.

The most important characteristics to demonstrate are lesion border definition and regularity, and the effect of the lesion on surrounding tissue architecture. Maximum lesion diameter is an important factor influencing subsequent clinical management, and at least one

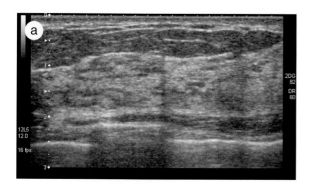

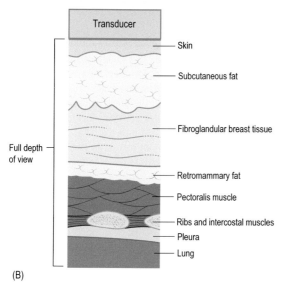

(B)

Figure 7.45 (a and b) Always record at least one image (a) to demonstrate that you have been able to visualize the whole depth of the breast from the skin surface anteriorly to the anterior chest wall posteriorly (b).

Figure 7.46 (a) A full depth of view image shows the relative size and location of superficial focal lesions—in this case a lymph node. (b) Reduced depth of view should be used to magnify superficial structures for full evaluation of their sonographic characteristics.

image showing calliper placement for the measurement of maximum lesion diameter should be recorded (Fig. 7.47).

Image annotation

All images should be annotated to allow them to be correlated with a specific examination of an individual patient at a particular location and point in time, and to allow precise anatomical location of the displayed scan plane and any detected pathology. A summary of essential annotation is given in Box 7.2. It is important that breast annotation is standardized and that terminology is uniform across disciplines within any multidisciplinary service (Tot et al 2002, p. 32).

As an absolute minimum, image annotation should include identifying patient information, usually patient name and date of birth or hospital number and the date the examination took place. In addition, it is good practice to include the institution (or department) name, and some practitioners like to include personnel identification such as the operator's initials.

It is imperative that the operator develops a habit of clearing on-screen patient identification details from the ultrasound machine at the end of each individual examination and refreshes the patient identification at the beginning of each new examination. Most ultrasound machines have the facility to select '*New patient*', with this option clearing all patient identifying information and resetting scan parameters to the default pre-set

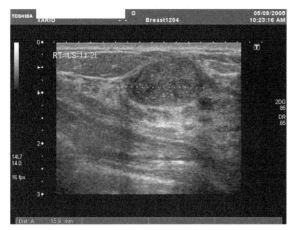

Figure 7.47 One image of this fibroadenoma is all that is required to demonstrate its diagnostic sonographic features: size, definition and regularity of margin, effect on adjacent tissue planes and posterior reflectivity.

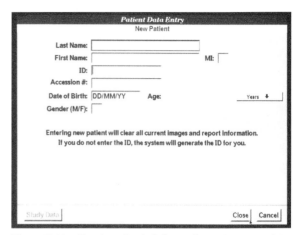

Figure 7.48 Starting afresh. It is good practice to get into the habit of using the facility for selecting a 'new patient' at the beginning of each ultrasound examination—this clears all the data relating to the previous patient from the scanner and reduces the risk of incorrect image annotation. In addition, you should also get into the habit of re-selecting the examination application pre-set at the start of each new examination; this restores all the scanning parameters to the default settings.

Box 7.2   Annotation to be included on breast ultrasound images

General information

- Place of examination—hospital +/− department name
- Date of examination
- Identity of person performing examination (name/initials/ID number)
- Patient identifying information
  - full name
  - date of birth
  - hospital number

Information specific for each individual image (text or pictogram)

- Breast laterality—right or left
- Scan plane orientation—LS/TS/radial/antiradial
- Scan plane location
  - Position in breast
    - quadrant if non-specific
    - clock face segmentation for focal abnormality
  - Distance from nipple (in cm)

Merritt & Rumack (2003)

(Fig. 7.48). It is good practice, and much heartache due to incorrect annotation will be avoided if practitioners get into the habit of using this facility as early as possible in their breast imaging career.

Individual images within an examination series should be additionally annotated to describe their correlating spatial location within the breast.

Invariably ultrasound equipment has a facility to add an overlay of textual annotation to the anatomical image, and most equipment specifically set up for breast imaging will have breast *pictograms* to allow visual annotation of the scan plane location (Fig. 7.49). Careful attention must be paid to image annotation—an incorrectly annotated image is positively dangerous, and of less value than no image at all. During training, operators must develop an examination technique that incorporates an instinctive routine of checking and annotating each individual image after freezing it and before recording it.

Standard formats for image annotation have been proposed (Stavros 2004, p. 48). The minimum information required for identifying the position of a lesion is identification of laterality (right or left), radial location (1–12 clock face segmentation) and distance from nipple (in centimeters). Thus annotation of:

R 4 3

relates to a position 3 cm from the nipple in the 4 o'clock segment of the lower inner quadrant of the right breast.

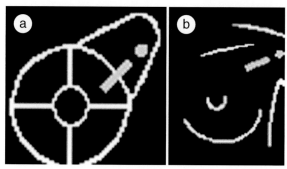

Figure 7.49 (a and b) Breast laterality and scan plane orientation can be annotated directly onto recorded images using breast pictogram functions.

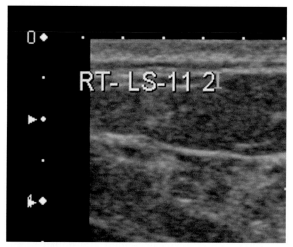

Figure 7.50 Some operators prefer to annotate images using standard nomenclature—as a minimum, laterality (RT = right), scan plane orientation (LS = longitudinal section) and scan plane location (11 = 11 o'clock segment; 2 = 2 cm from nipple) should be recorded.

Scan plane information such as radial (RAD) and antiradial (AR), or LS (longitudinal scan) and TS (transverse scan), can be added to describe the scan plane orientation (Fig. 7.50).

Some formats include information on the depth of the lesion with reference to superficial (A), central (B) and deep (C) zones; this can be particularly useful when the skin and chest wall are not displayed on magnified images.

Thus:

R 4 3 A LS

further indicates that the lesion lies superficially (A) and that the image was achieved using a longitudinal scan plane.

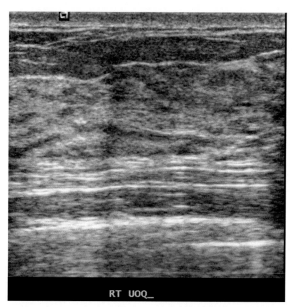

Figure 7.51 When diffuse benign change is observed and no focal lesion is demonstrated, the scan plane location on a global representative image may be broadly annotated as *UOQ*.

In the absence of a focal mass, three-letter acronyms describing the breast quadrant, e.g. UOQ (upper outer quadrant), LIQ (lower inner quadrant), in addition to R or L, for laterality, can be used to annotate a randomly selected image deemed by the operator to be representative of globally normal observed ultrasound appearances (Fig. 7.51).

REPORTING

A written report is an integral component of any ultrasound examination and should be compiled as soon as possible after the examination (UKAS 2001, p. 12). The examination report may be a record of both the conduct and the outcome of the scan, and is a vehicle for communication of this information between all healthcare professionals caring for a patient. The written examination report should be placed in the patient's medical record as the permanent and legal record of the examination (DH 1999, RCR 1999, AIUM 2002).

Breast ultrasound examinations are performed by a variety of healthcare professionals, and a significant number are undertaken by non-medically qualified practitioners. The person who actually performs the scan has the benefit of all the dynamic real-time information available, is in the best position to give an informed and complete interpretation and should therefore be the one to compile the report (UKAS 2001, p. 12); third-party reporting is to be discouraged.

Various professional organizations have issued guidance on what should be included in breast ultrasound image reports (Box 7.3), but the exact content, scope and phrasing of the ultrasound report will necessarily reflect the professional background, training, knowledge and competence of the person compiling it. It is important that the name and qualifications of the person generating the report are clearly stated (UKAS 2001, p. 12). If the person issuing a final report of the examination is not the person who performed the scan, then both personnel should be explicitly identified.

Reports provided by non-medically qualified personnel may contain observations and informed clinical comments relating to ultrasound appearances (CoR 2005); however, responsibility for diagnosis and medical interpretation remains with a medical practitioner unless explicitly delegated or referred under an agreed Scheme of Work (UKAS 2001, p. 2, RCR 1998).

The use of examination worksheets (Fig. 7.52), a standard reporting format (Box 7.4) or locally agreed templates that cover the most common findings will minimize the risk that essential information is omitted and ensure consistency of style and content across several operators, between individual patients and between serial examinations of the same patient. Report standardisation also has the additional benefit of facilitating data extraction for audit or research purposes.

In most cases, the ultrasound report will be of a qualitative, narrative nature, although increasingly, a summary quantitative category, similar to those used to categorize mammography and clinical findings, is also being allocated (Table 7.4).

As general guidance, ultrasound examination reports should:

- Be accurate, explicit and informative
- Be concise, clear and easily understood
- Avoid ambiguous phraseology
- Avoid use of technical or acoustic 'jargon'
- Avoid the use of unnecessary abbreviations and acronyms.
  (RCR 1998, UKAS 2001, Dimond 2002:234)

The negative scan

Not all abnormalities will be apparent on ultrasound images. Tissue interfaces between normal breast and lesions with similar density and compressibility characteristics will not give rise to reflected echo signals and will thus not be discernible in the image; similarly, small structures such as microcalcification may be below the resolution threshold and not displayed. Report terminology should acknowledge the possibility that sonographically 'occult' pathology is present, with phraseology such as 'normal *ultrasound* appearances' and 'no abnormality demonstrated' precisely reflecting both examination findings and limitations of the technique.

The positive scan

Use of a standard reporting template (Box 7.4) will minimize reporting time, particularly if available as either a preprinted or electronic *pro-forma* into which individualized details are inserted for each specific examination.

When an abnormality is detected, the ultrasound report should describe its discriminating sonographic characteristics, maximum dimension(s) and its precise location within the breast in terms of clock face notation and distance from the nipple. Reference should be made to any corresponding clinical or mammographic findings. Where appearances are consistent with a specific diagnosis, this should be stated (UKAS 2001, p. 12).

Box 7.3 Information to be included in breast ultrasound reports

- Location and extent of area examined
- Reference to clinical indication for examination
- Description of sonographic characteristics of a focal lesion including:
  - maximum diameter/extent (mm)
  - precise location within the breast
    - clock face notation and distance from nipple (cm)
- Correlation with clinical and/or mammographic findings
- Summary conclusion/diagnosis/clinical interpretation/list of differential diagnoses in order of likelihood
- Indication of clinical significance of findings
- Recommendations/suggestions for further investigations if appropriate
- Suggestions for clinical management if appropriate

Madjar et al (1999), UKAS (2001), AIUM (2002), Merritt & Rumack (2003)

Hospital NHST
Diagnostic Imaging Dept.

Breast Ultrasound

Patient details

Hospital number

Radiology number

Date of examination

Age of patient _____ yrs

Previous history of Breast Ca   **Y / N**

Family history of Breast Ca   **Y / N**

HRT   **Now / Previous / Never**

Clinical presentation

Palpable lump

Nodularity

Pain

Mammographic lesion

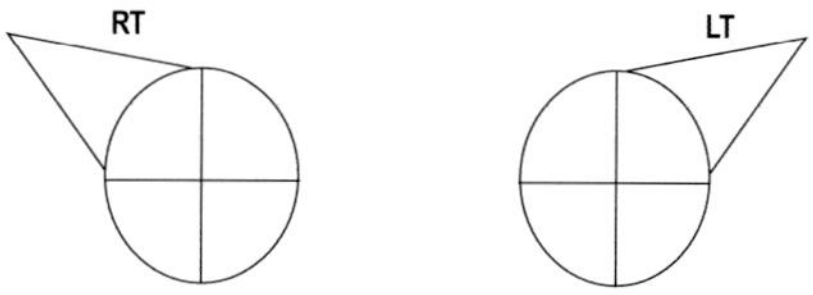

RT   LT

Clinical diagnosis _____   **FNA** done   **Y / N**

Ultrasound findings

Presenting abnormality:

NAD   BBC   CYST   SOLID FA / CA / Indet   OTHER
                                                                    (state)

Intervention

ASPIRATION   BIOPSY

COMMENTS / REPORT

Ultrasound Practitioner: _____   Date: _____

Report confirmed: _____

Figure 7.52   The use of an examination worksheet will help to standardize scanning and reporting practice between multiple operators within a service, and will facilitate audit and research data collection and extraction.

Box 7.4 Standard reporting template

Normal appearances

Ultrasound (right/left) breast: (upper/lower half; upper/lower, inner/outer quadrant/xxx o'clock segment).

No abnormality demonstrated at the site of the (palpable lump/mammographically detected lesion) at the (xxx) o'clock (xxx) cm position.

Abnormal appearances

Ultrasound (right/left) breast: (upper/lower half; upper/lower, inner/outer quadrant/xxx o'clock segment).

The (palpable lump/mammographically detected lesion) at the (xxx) o'clock (xxx) cm position is a (xxx) mm (well/ill) defined (hyper/hypo/iso) reflective mass that exhibits (increased through transmission/posterior acoustic/edge shadowing).

Appearances are (equivocal/those of/consistent with/suggestive of) a (clinical diagnosis/suspicion/mammographic features) of (a simple cyst/a fibroadenoma/malignancy).

(Aspiration/biopsy/interval clinical/ultrasound follow-up) (suggested/recommended/required) to (confirm/exclude/clarify).

Table 7.4 Quantitative categorization of ultrasound findings

Quantitative categorization	Narrative ultrasound interpretation
U1	Normal ultrasound appearances No abnormality detected
U2	Benign
U3	Indeterminate
U4	Suspicious
U5	Malignant

Where uncertainty exists, a list of differential diagnoses should be offered in order of likelihood, and recommendations or suggestions made for further investigations or clinical management (UKAS 2001, p. 43).

When the report is generated by non-medically qualified personnel, the nature of the report should be descriptive and may include an informed professional opinion of the meaning of such descriptions. Responsibility for *clinical* interpretation of the findings may be assumed and included in the report if appropriate local referral protocols exist; interpretation of the *medical significance* of the information and instigation of any subsequent medical action remains the responsibility of the medically qualified referring clinician in charge of the patient to whom the report is directed (GMC 1998, RCR 1998, CoR 2005).

Some suggestions for report wording are given in Table 7.5.

SUMMARY

Accurate ultrasound image interpretation is a dynamic process involving the reliable and consistent application of sonographic criteria to displayed image appearances. With increasing practitioner expertise, highly sensitive and specific breast diagnosis is possible, and as such the need for invasive diagnostic procedures can be minimized.

The recording of representative still images of the examination facilitates communication of examination findings between healthcare professionals and allows monitoring of professional standards and service quality.

Responsibility for providing a permanent and legal record of the examination in the form of a written report should lie with the person performing the ultrasound examination. The report is a formal component of the patient's official medical records and must comply with professional guidance and statutory requirements.

The accurate interpretation, recording and reporting of breast ultrasound examinations is a complex process that requires thorough initial training and regular practical experience underpinned by continuing professional education and clinical case follow-up. This is most appropriately achieved where ultrasound practitioners work to well-defined evidence-based Schemes of Work within effective multidisciplinary healthcare teams and where good communication and rigorous systems of clinical, radiological and pathological correlation operate.

Table 7.5 Suggested report proforma

Clinical indications	Findings	Suggested report format
Patient complains of palpable mass in the upper outer quadrant of the right breast.	Negative	Ultrasound UOQ right breast. No abnormality detected at the site of the palpable lump indicated by the patient.
?? Palpable mass in lower inner quadrant of left breast, site marked by clinician.	Negative	Ultrasound LIQ, left breast. Normal ultrasound appearances demonstrated at possible site of palpable abnormality as marked.
Palpable mass centrally upper half right breast.	Positive—cyst	Ultrasound upper half right breast centrally. The palpable lump at the 12 o'clock 3 cm position is a 24 mm well-defined anechoic mass showing increased posterior through transmission. Appearances are those of a simple cyst.
Mammographically detected spiculate mass in left breast with enlarged lymph nodes.	Positive—malignant with metastatic lymph nodes	Ultrasound left breast and axilla. Corresponding to the mammographically detected lesion, at the 4 o'clock 3 cm position there is a 4 mm irregular ill-defined solid mass showing posterior acoustic shadowing. The internal arterial vessels show high resistance, high velocity flow. The axillary lymph nodes are enlarged, round and uniformly hyporeflective. Appearances are those of malignancy with lymph node involvement. Needle core biopsy of the lesion required for confirmation.
34-year-old presenting with mobile lump in left breast.	Positive—benign	Ultrasound left breast. The palpable lump at the 3 o'clock 2 cm position is a 15 mm well-defined solid mass with increased through transmission and edge shadowing. Appearances would be consistent with a clinical diagnosis of fibroadenoma. Histological confirmation suggested.

References

AIUM 2002 Standard for the performance of breast ultrasound examination. Laurel, MD: American Institute of Ultrasound in Medicine.

Chen D-R, Chang R-F, Huang Y-L 1999 Computer-aided diagnosis applied to US of solid breast nodules by using neural networks. Radiology 213:407–412.

CoR 2005 Medical image interpretation and clinical reporting by non-radiologists: the role of the radiographer. London: College of Radiographers.

DH 1999 For the record: managing records in NHS Trusts and Health Authorities. HSC 1999/053. London: Department of Health.

Dimond BC 2002 Legal aspects of radiography and radiology. Oxford: Blackwell.

GMC 1998. Good medical practice. London: General Medical Council.

Hagen-Ansert S 2004 Sonographic evaluation of the breast. Online. General Medical Systems, Ultrasound Online CME Courses. Available at: http://gemedical-systems.com/rad/us/education/msucmebr.html Accessed 19 January 2004.

Hollerweger A, Rettenbacher T, Macheiner P et al 1997 New signs of breast cancer: high resistance flow and variations in resistive indices evaluation by colour

Doppler sonography. Ultrasound in Medicine and Biology 23(6):851–856.

Hong AS, Rosen E, Soo MS et al 2005 BI-RADS for sonography: positive and negative predictive values of sonographic features. AJR American Journal of Roentgenology 184:1260–1265.

Madjar H 2000 The practice of breast ultrasound. New York: Thieme.

Madjar H, Rickard M, Jellins J, Otto R (eds) 1999 IBUS guidelines for the ultrasonic examination of the breast. European Journal of Ultrasound 9:99–102.

Merritt CRB, Rumack CM 2003 ACR practice guideline for the performance of a breast ultrasound examination. Reston, VA: American College of Radiology.

Rahbar G, Sie AC, Hansen GC et al 1999 Benign versus malignant solid breast masses: US differentiation. Radiology 213:889–894.

Raza S, Baum JK 1997 Solid breast lesions: evaluation with power Doppler US. Radiology 203(1):164–168.

RCR 1998 Inter-professional roles and responsibilities in a radiology service. BFCR(98)6. London: Royal College of Radiologists.

RCR 1999 Good practice for clinical radiologists, BFCR(99)11. London, Royal College of Radiologists.

Santamaria G, Velasco M, Farre X et al 2005 Power Doppler sonography of invasive breast carcinoma: does tumour vascularization contribute to prediction of axillary status? Radiology 234:374–380.

Stavros AT 2004 Breast ultrasound. Philadelphia: Lippincott, Williams and Wilkins.

Stavros AT, Thickman D, Rapp CL et al 2005 Solid breast nodules: use of sonography to distinguish between benign and malignant lesions. Radiology 196:123–134.

Strano S, Gombos EC, Friedland O et al 2004 Colour Doppler imaging of fibroadenomas of the breast with histopathological correlation. Journal of Clinical Ultrasound 32(7):317–322.

Tot T, Tabar L, Dean PB 2002 Practical breast pathology. New York: Thieme.

UKAS 2001 Guidelines for professional working standards—ultrasound practice. London: United Kingdom Association of Sonographers.

Chapter **8**

Benign breast disease

David S. Enion and Anne-Marie Dixon

INTRODUCTION

Benign breast disease is very common and accounts for most of the workload of, particularly symptomatic, breast clinics. Typically, patients with diffuse benign disease are relatively young and present with pain and textural abnormality (nodularity). Symptoms may be bilateral and generalized, unilateral, localized (often to the upper outer quadrant) or specifically focal, and are often cyclic in nature, being most pronounced premenstrually. Discrete focal benign masses also predominate in younger women, but are less likely to be associated with pain or cyclical change in texture. Benign breast disease might be considered as one end of a spectrum of proliferative change in breast tissue—malignancy being the opposite end of the spectrum.

When a benign process is suspected, ultrasound is the imaging method of choice (RCR 2003) as it is safer, i.e. it is not associated with radiation hazard, and it has higher sensitivity and specificity than mammography in the dense breast. Accurate and consistent application of sonographic criteria allows reliable differentiation of cystic and solid masses and a reasonably high level of discrimination between benign and malignant lesions (see Chs 6 and 7). When imaging appearances are equivocal or indeterminate, ultrasound-guided needle core biopsy is a quick and relatively simple technique for obtaining a diagnostic tissue sample, vacuum-assisted procedures offer the opportunity for minimally invasive excision (see Ch. 12).

BENIGN BREAST CHANGE AND FIBROCYSTIC DISEASE

The above terminology is used, somewhat interchangeably and non-specifically, to describe a range of clinical, imaging and pathological features associated with hormonally stimulated ductal and lobular epithelial pro-liferation. The term benign breast or fibrocystic *change* might be used when characteristic features are observed in the normal asymptomatic patient, with the nomencla-ture '*disease*' being reserved for those patients presenting with troublesome clinical signs and symptoms. In addi-tion, the term fibrocystic might be used when discrete cystic lesions are apparent as opposed to when there is only subtle diffuse parenchymal change.

Benign breast change results from disruption of normal physiological cyclical tissue proliferation and involution; it is characterized by global or localized areas of duct ectasia and cystic dilatation due to imbalances in apocrine cell secretion and reabsorption. Clinical symp-toms include fullness, tenderness and pain, which vary during the menstrual cycle. Any clinician palpating the breast may find vague areas of nodularity or thickening or even a well-defined palpable nodule—there is not usually a clinical distortion of breast architecture. The condition is often bilateral and found in increasing numbers of women in their mid to late 30s; it is most common in the premenopausal years, but may present in adolescents during primary breast development. Fibro-cystic change also occurs in the breast as a result of age-related degeneration of glandular breast tissue and perimenopausal hormonal imbalances, and is therefore relatively common in screening populations.

Mammography will generally show overall increased glandular breast density and, as such, sensitivity for detecting malignant lesions is reduced (Fig. 8.1). Focal densities (discrete cysts) may be apparent as well-defined soft tissue masses (Fig, 8.2)—such lesions are often multi-ple and/or bilateral and may be associated with calcifica-tions. Small, less than 2 mm (micro)cysts are not demonstrated.

Ultrasound is an important adjunct to mammography for two reasons. In the dense breast, the technique has higher sensitivity for detecting malignant lesions, and in addition it will confirm the cystic nature of a mammo-graphic or palpable focal abnormality and exclude the presence of a solid lesion.

In BBC ultrasound will classically show normal breast architecture, but the breast parenchyma is usually hyper-reflective and the ductal anatomy prominent—this often gives rise to a 'honeycomb' appearance particularly in the young patient (Fig. 8.3). In the older patient, increased fibrosis results in dense attenuating tissue which renders the deeper tissues difficult to demonstrate adequately (Fig. 8.4). Increased transducer compression to reduce breast thickness, increased acoustic output power and reduced transducer frequency might be employed in an attempt to overcome this limitation—if unsuccessful, such difficulties, and therefore reduced exclusion value, should be noted in the examination report.

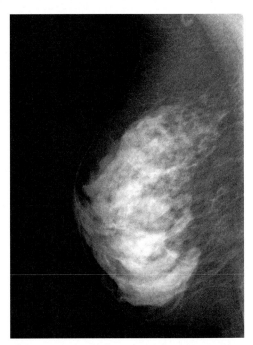

Figure 8.1 Benign breast disease is associated with diffusely increased mammographic density, making it difficult to identify isolated focal abnormalities. (Image courtesy of Dr Erika Denton, Norfolk and Norwich University Hospital.)

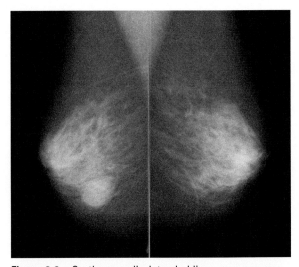

Figure 8.2 On these medio-lateral oblique mammograms, a discrete cyst can be seen as a reasonably well defined oval area of increased radio-opacity in the lower half of the right breast overlying the edge of the dense parenchymal tissue shadow.

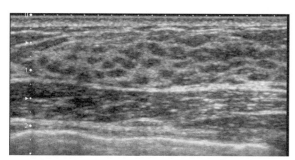

Figure 8.3 Benign breast change in the young patient gives rise to a 'honeycomb' appearance.

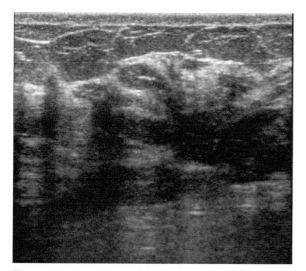

Figure 8.4 In an older patient, dense attenuating fibrotic tissue can make it difficult to demonstrate the deeper structures. In some cases, the reduced exclusion value might have to be reported.

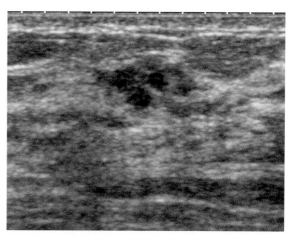

Figure 8.5 Clusters of small cysts can look like hyporeflective masses; however, with modern high resolution equipment, it should be possible to demonstrate discrete echo-free cysts as small as 2–3 mm diameter.

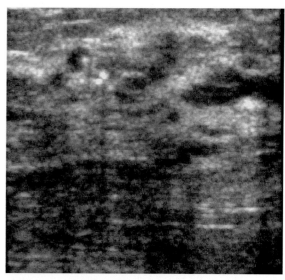

Figure 8.6 Punctate microcalcifications are sometimes seen sonographically. Although other reassuring features of benign breast change may be present, unlike mammography appearances there are no characteristic differences between benign and malignant microcalcifications on ultrasound images.

Increased parenchymal reflectivity without posterior shadowing may represent the presence of microcystic disease. With modern high resolution equipment, individual, and clusters of, tiny cysts as small as 2–3 mm diameter are readily demonstrated (Fig. 8.5). Occasionally punctuate microcalcifications are also demonstrated sonographically and their association with other features of benign breast change, rather than a solid focal mass, is reassuring (Fig. 8.6).

Focal areas of reduced reflectivity often correlate with a palpable abnormality (Fig. 8.7); sometimes these have ill-defined margins and mimic malignant masses while others are well defined and look 'benign'. Invariably biopsy of such areas gives rise to a histological diagnosis of adenosis or adenomatoid change describing hyperplasia and hypertrophy of glandular elements—terminology such as blunt duct, sclerosing and microglandular is used to describe their precise histological features.

Dilated ducts (3–5 mm internal caliber) are easily differentiated from small cysts by demonstrating their tubular nature using radial scan planes (Fig. 8.8). Simple duct ectasia is characterized by smooth-walled echo-free

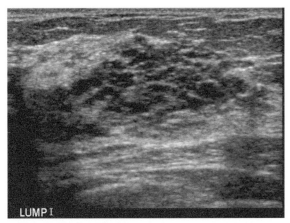

Figure 8.7   Non-specific areas of reduced reflectivity associated with palpable lumps are often diagnosed as 'fibroadenosis' at histology.

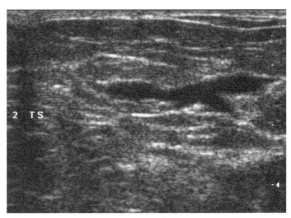

Figure 8.9   In simple duct ectasia, the dilated fluid-filled ducts are seen as tapering echo-free (black) channels with smooth hyper-reflective (white) walls.

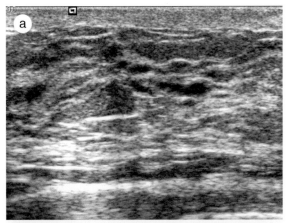

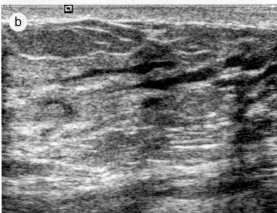

Figure 8.8   (a and b) Dilated ducts may look like small cysts when imaged in cross-section (a). Turning the transducer into a radial scan plane will demonstrate the linear nature of ducts (b).

(fluid secretion-filled) peripherally tapering channels (Fig. 8.9).

Histologically, fibrocystic disease is graded I–III according to the degree of cellular proliferation and the presence of atypia. Proliferative forms of the condition are more likely to be associated with the presence of discrete cysts and ducts of variable caliber that contain solid material—color flow Doppler can be used to differentiate inspissated secretions from intraduct tissue proliferations.

INTRADUCT PAPILLOMA

Five to ten percent of patients referred to symptomatic breast clinics complain of nipple discharge. The patient typically presents with episodes of bloody nipple discharge involving one or more ducts—the usual cause is a solitary intraduct papilloma, although such lesions can be multiple.

Solitary papillomas usually occur in women in and around the climacteric; multiple lesions are more common in younger patients and are also then more likely to be in peripheral rather than in the subareolar ducts. In the adolescent, the condition juvenile papillomatosis is characterized by a localized mass of dilated ducts containing multiple papillary areas of epithelial proliferation—its multicystic appearance gives rise to its alternative name 'Swiss cheese disease' (Rosen et al 1980).

Papillomas are not usually visible mammographically, but occasionally they calcify and produce a non-specific cluster of microcalcifications. On ultrasound examinations, duct ectasia may be demonstrated and sometimes it is possible to localize a focal intraluminal soft tissue

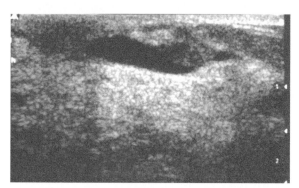

Figure 8.10   Intraduct papilloma: a soft tissue intraluminal mass is outlined by fluid in a central dilated duct.

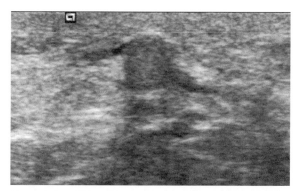

Figure 8.11   This solid mass is also an intraduct papilloma but is only associated with minimal duct dilatation. Intraduct papilloma should be considered as a differential diagnosis whenever a small solid mass is demonstrated in close proximity to the nipple–areola complex.

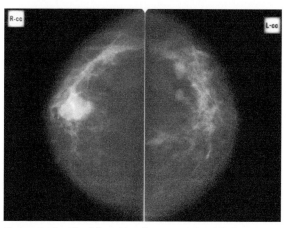

Figure 8.12   The bilateral radio-opaque focal lesions demonstrated in these medio-lateral oblique mammograms represent simple cysts.

lesion (Fig. 8.10). Most often the mass is obviously within a duct and may extend for a variable length along the lumen. Sometimes, however, a well-defined round solid slightly hyporeflective mass lesion is demonstrated in close proximity to the nipple–areolar complex—clinical signs and lesion location may prompt a diagnosis of intraduct papilloma even in the absence of frank nipple discharge (Fig. 8.11).

If left, a benign intraduct papilloma can progress to a more complex lesion and may even become malignant. Up to 5% of patients with solitary nipple discharge have an underlying carcinoma at presentation. Diagnostic, preferably ultrasound-guided, needle core biopsy should be performed when any focal solid lesion is demonstrated. With papillomas, histology often shows usual or even atypical ductal hyperplasia—the lesion is then described as being of uncertain significance, and a microdochectomy (duct excision) is indicated for further evaluation.

CYSTS

Breast cysts are extremely common and occur in up to 20–50% of women of reproductive age, with peak incidence in premenopausal women aged 40–50 years. The essential patho-physiology of a cyst is duct obstruction and localized fluid accumulation. Links to exogenous hormones are not proven, with lower dose oral contraceptives appearing to reduce incidence and hormone replacement therapy not precipitating increased incidence.

In the adolescent, abnormal ductal development or secretory activity imbalance during thelarche can result in subareolar cysts that present as palpable nodules with or without inflammation and pain. Ultrasound is appropriate for diagnosis and monitoring in such patients to avoid the risk of trauma and developmental impairment associated with invasive diagnostic or therapeutic intervention.

Cysts are the most common pathological finding in women presenting with a palpable breast lump. Clinically the typical large cyst is a reasonably firm, smooth and relatively mobile mass, but they have incredibly variable presentation and it is not always clinically obvious that the lump is benign. If the fluid within the cyst is under tension, the mass feels very hard; small cysts and even very large flaccid cysts may not be palpable. Cysts may be associated with localized pain. Overall, signs and symptoms tend to be non-cyclical.

Isolated simple cysts appear on mammography as slightly opaque (soft tissue density) masses, and it is not unusual for additional clinically occult lesions to be demonstrated in the ipsi- or contralateral breast (Fig. 8.12). The mammographic finding of a clearly defined margin around the lesion's whole perimeter suggests benignity, although it is not possible to differentiate its cystic nature from that of a solid benign mass. Whilst cysts are mammographically conspicuous in the involuted 'fatty' breast, they may be masked by dense fibro-glandular tissue in younger women. Sometimes cyst walls contain areas of calcification.

Sonographically, cysts are easily detected and are demonstrated as round or (horizontally) oval, anechoic (black) masses that have smooth, thin, well-defined margins, with the sides exhibiting posterior edge shadowing (Fig. 8.13). Care must be taken to use appropriate overall gain settings, turning the gain up (or employing the color Doppler function) to ensure that the lesion is not a very hyporeflective solid mass. Since the simple cyst is filled with serous fluid which does not attenuate sound as much as adjacent solid tissue, the structures deep to a cyst appear hyperreflective; demonstration of this increased through transmission phenomenon is a characteristic feature of cysts. With modern high resolution equipment, punctate microcalcifications may be demonstrated along the cysts wall; sometimes extensive mural calcification results in prominent acoustic shadowing.

Cysts may have a complex appearance. They can be multilocular, or septated (Fig. 8.14) or may appear to contain low-level reflective material (Fig. 8.15)—it is important to differentiate a cyst from a solid lesion and to exclude the presence of a solid intracystic, mucinous or necrotic tumor.

Reverberation artifact is often seen in a cyst, immediately deep to its anterior margin—this can be eliminated by reducing the time gain compensation at the corresponding level and/or by moving the focal zone deeper (Fig. 8.16). True acoustic reflections from material within a cyst are caused by inspissated cellular or hemorrhagic fluid (Fig. 8.17); sometimes this makes it look like a solid lesion. Patient movement, increased acoustic power and color flow Doppler can be used to try to initiate particle movement, but sometimes aspiration is required for diagnostic clarification.

A layering effect or the demonstration of 'fluid levels' within cysts is caused either by gravitational sedimentation of inspissated fluid (the solid material settles to the

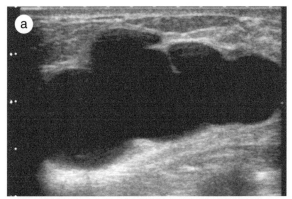

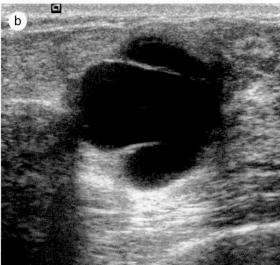

Figure 8.14   (a and b) Multilocular or septated cysts have a slightly more complex lobulated outline—the septation membranes will not be well demonstrated (a) unless they are parallel to the transducer footprint (b).

Figure 8.13   Sonographically, simple cysts have a characteristic appearance—a smooth well-defined margin, a spherical or ovoid shape and an anechoic (black) center. Because their fluid content has very low attenuation, they exhibit marked increased through transmission—they have a 'bright' stripe below them.

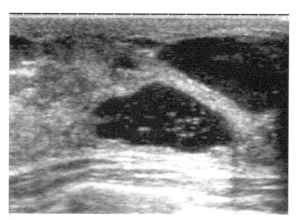

Figure 8.15 Cellular or hemorrhagic debris within a cyst gives rise to low level echoes internally—often these can be seen to move with gentle balloting or use of higher power, e.g. color flow Doppler mode.

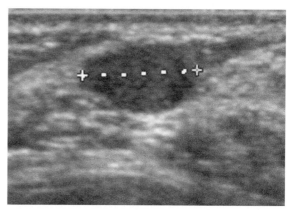

Figure 8.17 Small lesions with fine homogeneous echo texture and reflectivity may represent either cysts containing very thick fluid or small solid fibroadenomas. Absence of a color Doppler signal should prompt an attempt at aspiration to confirm a lesion's cystic nature; if this is unsuccessful, or color Doppler confirms internal perfusion, the lesion is more likely to be solid and a needle core biopsy is required to clarify its exact nature.

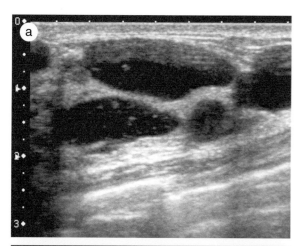

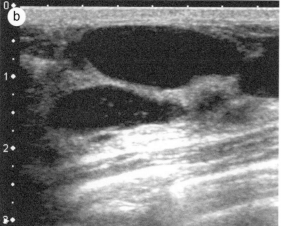

Figure 8.16 (a) Reverberation artifact is common just below the anterior margin of superficial cysts. (b) Reverberation artifact can be eliminated by reducing the near gain and placing the focal zone deeper in the breast.

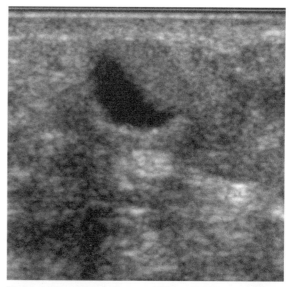

Figure 8.18 This small cyst exhibits a fluid level due to layering of immiscible fluids—the aqueous (black) part lies below the oily component. Remember that the orientation of the fluid level in the image will reflect the effect of gravity on the breast and will not necessarily be horizontal.

cyst floor) or by layering of immiscible oil and water fluid constituents—the hyper-reflective oily component rising above echo-free aqueous fluid (Fig. 8.18).

Aspiration of the sonographically simple (thin walled and anechoic) cyst is not routinely indicated and should only be employed as a therapeutic measure to relieve patient pain or discomfort. Normal serous cyst fluid is aqueous and straw colored, although it may be brown or green. There is no need to send aspirated fluid for cytological analysis unless it is blood-stained.

When reporting breast cysts, it is important to make a note of the number, size, uni- or multilocular nature and to describe and interpret the significance of their internal characteristics. When there are multiple cysts, only the largest, the symptomatic and any unusual ones need be reported. Since cysts are usually round, a single diameter is recorded; for oval cysts, a long axis measurement is recorded. Specific clarification is also required if giving an unusually large measurement when the cyst is shallow and flaccid (Fig. 8.19).

Although cysts are benign and not inherently associated with increased risk of malignancy, occasionally careful evaluation of a cyst wall will show lesions complicated by focal irregularity, thickening or solid excrescences. In such cases, intracystic papilloma and papilliary carcinoma need to be excluded by tissue sampling—surgical excision is usually preferred to avoid the difficulty of subsequently localizing a percutaneously sampled (and therefore aspirated) lesion.

Careful sonographic evaluation of intervening parenchymal breast tissue in the multicystic breast is important due to reduced mammographic sensitivity and distortion of sound propagation.

GALACTOCELE

This milk-filled retention cyst develops in pregnancy or during lactation. Occasionally they occur in neonates if natural re-absorption of 'witch's milk' is impaired. Galactoceles usually present as palpable nodules and have to be differentiated from hormonally stimulated enlarging solid lesions. Ultrasound is an appropriate and accurate first-line investigation, and can be used to guide diagnostic aspiration—milky fluid aspirate being pathognomonic. The classic ultrasound appearance is that of a well-defined but internally complex cyst; high fat content gives the fluid a hyper-reflective and patchy or particulate echo texture, fat/fluid levels may be seen (Fig. 8.20).

FIBROADENOMA

The fibroadenoma is the most commont benign solid breast tumor and the most commonly diagnosed breast tumor in women younger than 30 years of age. Fibroadenomas most often present in the 20–35 years age group, but occur and can be diagnosed at any age, their prevalence being approximately 8–10% in women older than 40 years of age.

The fibroadenoma is a benign tumor that forms due to a hyperplastic or proliferative process in a single terminal ductal unit. Some believe they are an aberration of normal development. Most fibroadenomas are self-limiting and only reach 20–30 mm diameter; many involute spontaneously, lesion regression being common in postmenopausal women. Conversely, however, fibroadenomas may grow rapidly during pregnancy or start to re-grow during hormone replacement therapy.

A particular variant of fibroadenoma, the juvenile (giant) fibroadenoma, occurs in female adolescents. Typically, these grow profusely and rapidly exceed 10 cm in diameter. They are often bilateral, may contain areas of

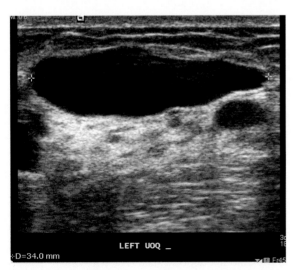

Figure 8.19 Large flaccid cysts will have a ovoid shape, and even very large ones may not be palpable.

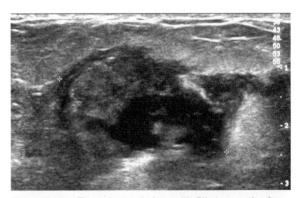

Figure 8.20 The galactocele is a milk filled cyst—the fatty fluid content gives rise to a complex internal appearance. Aspiration of milk is pathognomonic. (Image courtesy of Dr B. Dall, United Leeds Teaching Hospitals.)

atypical ductal hyperplasia and thus have malignant potential. Excised lesions may be locally recurrent, the surgical challenge being adequate excision with preservation of enough parenchymal tissue for subsequent normal breast development.

Histologically the fibroadenoma consists of both stromal and epithelial elements. They have varied pathological appearances depending on whether they arise from intralobular stroma containing lobules of major ducts surrounded by myxomatous stroma, or from intralobular stroma composed of dense fibro-connective tissue mixed with adipose and elastic fibers. Fibroadenomas belong to a family of benign proliferative lesions named according to their histological tissue composition (Table 8.1). In practice, these invariably present and appear on imaging with 'benign' but non-specific features and require tissue sampling for definitive diagnosis.

On clinical examination, fibroadenomas are usually oval, rubbery and extremely mobile, the latter accounting for their characterization as a 'breast mouse'. Fibroadenoma size can vary from smaller than 10 mm up to greater than 15 cm in the giant form, although the latter is very unusual.

Table 8.1   Histological nomenclature for benign lesion classification

	Tissue type and composition
Prefix (commonly used name)	
Fibro-	Connective tissue
Adeno-	Glandular tissue
Lipo-	Fatty tissue
Fibroadenoma	Mixed stromal and glandular—more stromal than glandular
Hamartoma	Mixed stroma, glandular and fatty
Fibroadenolipoma	More stromal than glandular or fatty
Adenolipofibroma	
Adenofibrolipoma	More glandular than fatty or stromal
Lipofibroadenoma	
Rare lesions	
Leiomyoma	Smooth muscle
Neurofibroma	Peripheral nerve sheaths
Chondroma	Mesenchymal cells
Osteoma	Mesenchymal cells
Myoblastoma	Neurogenic—Schwann cells
Angioma	Blood vessels

Since fibroadenomas usually occur in young women, ultrasound is the preferred first-line imaging method and this spares young patients the hazard of mammographic radiation exposure. Clinically occult long-standing fibroadenomas, however, are often detected in population mammographic screening programs. On the mammogram, the fibroadenoma is usually demonstrated as well-defined lobulated soft tissue opacity, and is thus often indistinguishable from a cyst. As they involute, they become hyalinized and may exhibit a classic 'popcorn' calcification pattern (Fig. 8.21).

On ultrasound images, the typical fibroadenoma is a focal mass lesion encapsulated by a thin smooth hyper-reflective margin that exhibits edge shadowing (Fig. 8.22). Internally the reflectivity and echo texture are slightly hyporeflective and homogeneous (heterogeneity may be associated with proliferating or regressing lesions) and there is increased posterior through transmission, with the tissues immediately deep to the lesion looking 'brighter' than adjacent tissue. The lesion is invariably oval—its long axis being parallel to the chest wall—and is usually very well defined; frequently gentle lobulations are present (Fig. 8.23). Fibroadenomas are not particularly compressible but are notoriously mobile, making small ones difficult to biopsy!

Whilst these above appearances are classic and characteristic, unfortunately some malignant lesions look exactly the same (Fig. 8.24). Histological confirmation of an image-based fibroadenoma diagnosis is mandatory in all but the smallest lesions in low risk patients—a closely monitored clinical and imaging follow-up regime might be considered appropriate in such cases.

It is not unusual for patients to have more than one fibroadenoma and, although not routinely indicated, if performed, whole breast ultrasound (WBUS) will often reveal additional clinically occult lesions. The value of WBUS in this context is debatable, with some claiming that it leads to unnecessary investigation of clinically insignificant benign disease (multiple biopsy or follow-up examinations) and others suggesting it is a useful patient management tool particularly if surgery is being contemplated.

PHYLLODES TUMOR—CYSTOSARCOMA PHYLLODES

Phyllodes tumors are rare, usually benign tumors of the breast, but approximately 16% have malignant components. They account for about 0.3% of all breast tumors but are the most common non-epithelial breast tumor. They occur almost exclusively in females, usually in the mid-40s age range, i.e. about 15–20 years after the median age for fibroadenomas, the most common differential diagnosis. Phyllodes tumors are rapidly

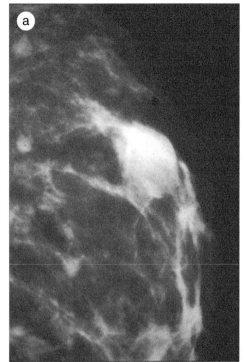

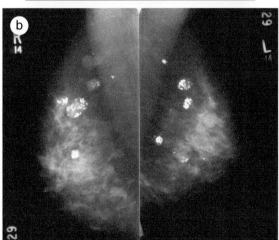

Figure 8.21   (a) The reasonably well defined radio-opaque lesion demonstrated on this medio-lateral oblique mammogram represents a fibroadenoma. (b) Partially calcified fibroadenomas have a characteristic 'popcorn' appearance on mammograms.

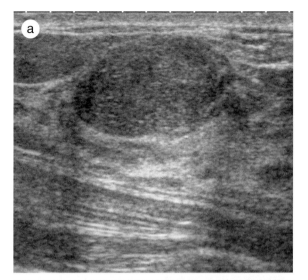

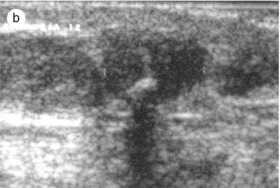

Figure 8.22   (a) On ultrasound images, the classic fibroadenoma is a well-defined smooth margined homogeneous focal lesion that exhibits edge shadowing and slightly increased through transmission. (b) Posterior shadowing can be seen deep to the (popcorn-type) calcification in this fibroadenoma.

enlarging lesions, their average size at presentation being 50 mm. Histologically they are heterogeneous and may contain areas of both benign and malignant tissue; this makes percutaneous core biopsy susceptible to both over- and underdiagnosis.

The patient usually presents with a firm, mobile, well-circumscribed, non-tender breast mass that has increased in size relatively rapidly in the weeks leading up to presentation. It is extremely rare for patients to present with metastatic symptoms or with skin alteration. Mammographically, phyllodes tumors are very similar to fibroadenomas, i.e. round soft tissue densities, usually well defined; occasionally calcifications are seen (Fig. 8.25).

On ultrasound, the phyllodes tumor is well circumscribed with a smooth margin and oval shape—although the latter can be difficult to determine given its size and the relatively small field of view of conventional breast ultrasound transducers (Fig. 8.26). Extended field of view software or a curvilinear transducer can be used to

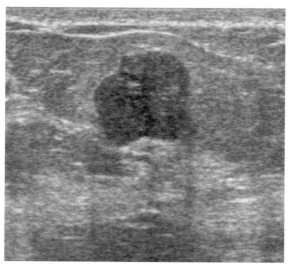

Figure 8.23 Some fibroadenomas have a lobulated margin—again the lesion margin is smooth and well defined.

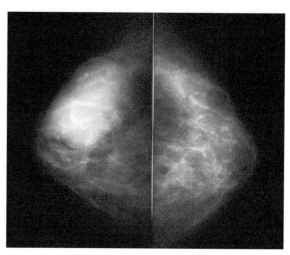

Figure 8.25 The well-defined area of increased density on these cranio-caudal mammograms is due to a large phylloides tumor in the outer half of the right breast.

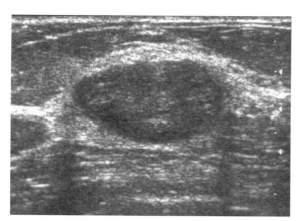

Figure 8.24 This invasive carcinoma exhibits ultrasound appearances usually associated with a fibroadenoma. Because of this 'overlap' in sonographic features, 'fibroadenomas' should be biopsied to confirm their benign nature—occasionally an unexpected malignant diagnosis will be obtained.

demonstrate and accurately assess their full extent (Fig. 8.27). There is often a cystic component to the lesion and they appear slightly more heterogeneous than fibroadenomas. Heterogeneity is thought to correlate with a higher likelihood of the presence of malignant components. Frequently hyper-reflective septations are seen within the mass, and color Doppler shows marked hypervascularity (Fig. 8.28).

Predominantly due to their size, but also in view of their heterogeneity and malignant potential, wide local excision is usually recommended. Local recurrence is common, and patients need a significant period of follow-up. Recurrent lesions tend to be more aggressive than the original tumor and are more likely to become malignant, the lung being the most common metastatic site, with less frequent spread to the skeleton and heart.

LIPOMA

Lipomas are common, occurring in 1% of the population; they are slow growing benign tumors that can arise in fatty soft tissue anywhere in the body. They are usually lobulated soft tissue masses enclosed in a thin fibrous capsule. Many lipomas are asymptomatic and remain undetected; when identified in the breast they must be differentiated from other, clinically significant tumors.

The lipoma may present as a palpable mass, most often if located in the subcutaneous fat layer between the skin and superficial fascia. Typically, they have a soft fluctuant feel, are well defined, oval or lobulated, and are often mobile. Simple lipomas are seldom detectable on mammograms since their fatty content allows normal passage of X-rays. Sonographically the superficial lipoma is usually a subtle but reasonably well defined mass lesion that is invariably more reflective (slightly brighter) than adjacent subcutaneous fat (Fig. 8.29)—if surrounded by glandular tissue, the lipoma will appear hyporeflective (darker than adjacent breast parenchyma).

A combination of clinical and imaging findings frequently allows these lesions to be satisfactorily diagnosed

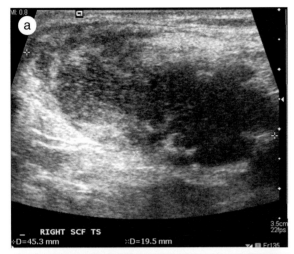

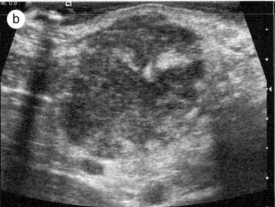

Figure 8.26   (a) Phylloides tumors are usually large at presentation. This makes it difficult to demonstrate their margins and assess the overall size with linear array transducers—a 'trapezoid' extended field of view technique has been used here to include the whole lesion in the field of view. (b) Typically the phylloides tumor is a large well-defined mass with a smooth margin and a heterogeneous echo texture.

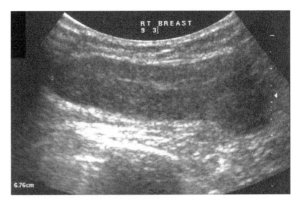

Figure 8.27   A curvilinear array transducer has a diverging field of view that enables visualization of the full extent of a large mass and a reasonably accurate estimate of its maximum diameter—in this case 6.8 cm.

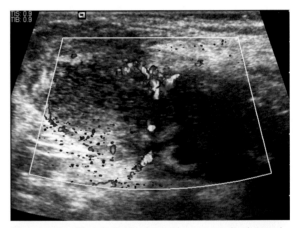

Figure 8.28   The phylloides tumor has a complex internal appearance with both solid components and cystic spaces. Color flow Doppler usually shows marked hypervascularity.

without recourse to core biopsy or excision. Lipomas may, of course, be excised for cosmetic reasons or if there is clinical doubt about the diagnosis. Occasionally a pseudolipomatous appearance is seen around a scirrhous carcinoma due to the desmoplastic reaction.

HAMARTOMA

The hamartoma is an uncommon benign breast lesion resulting from localized but variable overgrowth of glandular, adipose and fibrous tissue; a variety of alternative names exist to reflect their varied differential histological

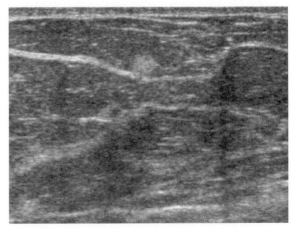

Figure 8.29   Characteristically the lipoma is a hyper-reflective mass localized to the subcutaneous fat layer.

compositions (see Table 8.1). Hamartomas generally occur in women over the age of 30 years, and even though often large are commonly asymptomatic. They may be picked up at screening mammography as well-circumscribed masses of soft tissue density (Fig. 8.30). Often the hamartoma has a thin radio-opaque pseuduo-capsular margin; internal histological variation is reflected in mammographic density variation.

Hamartomas occasionally present as a soft, rubbery palpable mass, typically in the retroareolar region or upper outer quadrant of the breast.

Sonographically, the hamartoma is usually well defined with a clear margin (Fig. 8.31). Although usually hypo-reflective and reasonably compressible like most solid benign lesions, they may be isoreflective with adjacent tissue, heterogeneous, appear septated or contain calcification. They have a variety of reflectivity and echo texture appearances in view of their varied tissue composition. As with other similar lesions, definitive diagnosis and exclusion of malignancy is only possible with tissue sampling.

TUBULAR OR LACTATING ADENOMA

The term adenoma describes a predominantly epithelial lesion containing lobulated masses of acini densely packed together with scarcity of intervening stroma. The terms tubular and lactating are used to differentiate the same type of lesion in two different physiological states; the lesion has also been described as a hamartomatous malformation.

The lactating adenoma is uniquely associated with pregnancy and lactation but is otherwise similar to, and therefore difficult to differentiate from, other benign focal lesions at clinical examination and on imaging appearances.

PSEUDOANGIOMATOUS STROMAL HYPERPLASIA (PASH)

This is a rare phenomenon almost exclusively occurring in premenopausal women but occasionally sometimes in men (Polger et al 1996). It is thought that an abnormal cellular proliferation in response to progesterone stimulation results in benign focal overgrowth of stromal tissue (Kirkpatrick et al 2000). Histologically the lesions show stromal hyperplasia and have anastamosing slit-like spaces outlined by flat bland spindle cells; appearances must be differentiated from those of the phyllodes tumor or an angiosarcoma. The condition usually presents with a clinically palpable painless mass. Rarely it can present with a peau d'orange change in the overlying breast skin mimicking an inflammatory breast carcinoma.

Like many benign lesions it can be mammographically invisible—isodense with glandular tissue—but is more usually seen and best described as an ill-defined indeterminate soft tissue mass; its dimensions vary but are generally between 10 and 20 mm.

Sonographically, PASH nodules have a variety of appearances; they may be occult, very subtle or more obvious. Frequently they are identified as fairly well-defined but non-specific areas of altered reflectivity, often

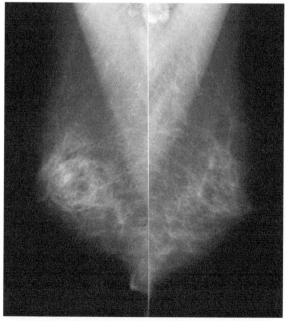

Figure 8.30 These medio-lateral oblique mammographic projections demonstrate a hamartoma in the right breast behind the nipple–areola complex.

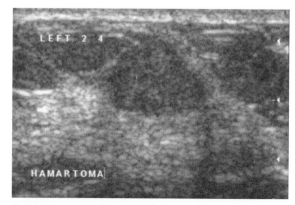

Figure 8.31 This histologically diagnosed hamartoma appeared as a well-defined homogeneous mass having a sonographic appearance similar to that of a fibroadenoma.

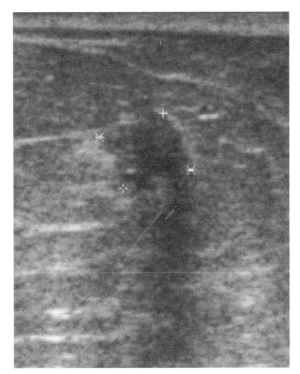

Figure 8.32   The ultrasound appearances of pseudoangiomatous stromal hyperplasia (PASH) are variable and non-specific and as an 'indeterminate' focal mass, a histological diagnosis is required.

producing acoustic shadowing (Fig. 8.32), but they may exhibit typical fibroadenoma features. Essentially PASH is diagnosed through biopsy of an indeterminate mass lesion.

INFARCT

Any of the above solid lesions and indeed regions of hypertrophic breast tissue may undergo total or partial infarction. The etiology is believed to be vascular insufficiency related to significantly increased metabolic demand—the condition is therefore mainly seen during pregnancy and lactation.

The infarct may manifest as a pre-existing mass suddenly increasing in size, or an apparently 'new' mass may appear where nothing was previously palpable. Sometimes the lesion presents with bloody nipple discharge and this, together with a rapid increase in lesion size, often raises suspicion of malignant change.

Lesion infarction may result in an ill- or well-defined mass that can feel tethered to adjacent breast tissue; they may be associated with tenderness and skin fixation. As with other new or rapidly growing solid mass, differen-tiation of a benign from a malignant lesion is difficult, and generally a needle core biopsy is required.

RADIAL SCAR

Radial scars or complex sclerosing lesions are generally asymptomatic and most often detected incidentally at mammographic screening (Fig. 8.33). Histologically, the lesions consist of a single or multiple areas of adenosis around a fibro-elastic center—there is cellular proliferation and hyperplasia and the lesion may contain areas of frank atypia or malignancy. On the mammogram, there is architectural distortion, and in many cases a discrete small central irregular/spiculated mass. The appearance can vary according to the projection—sometimes they are associated with non-specific microcalcifications.

Sonographic features may be non-specific and occasionally mimic malignancy, but most often no sonographic change is apparent at the site of such lesions. Since it is impossible to differentiate the imaging appearances reliably from those of a breast carcinoma, biopsy is required. Though considered a benign entity, in a significant number of cases radial scars are associated with tubular carcinoma, ductal invasive carcinoma or the precursors of such lesions (DCIS, LCIS and atypical hyperplasia) and often, ultimately, excision is performed.

INFECTION AND INFLAMMATION (MASTITIS)

Breast infections can afflict females of any age, may be localized or affect the whole breast, and may or may not be associated with systemic signs and symptoms. The most common route of microbial entry is via the mammary ducts, and most are staphylococcal infections. Breast infection is easily divided into lactational (associated with breastfeeding) and non-lactational types; lactational infections can occur within a few days of commencement of breast feeding and are directly related to this process. Non-lactational infections are subdivided into periareolar and peripheral infections—periareolar infections tending to affect young patients, with an increased risk observed in cigarette smokers. Peripheral breast infections are less common and may be associated with diabetes, rheumatoid arthritis, steroid treatments or trauma. Iatrogenic infection may follow therapeutic breast surgery or prosthesis implantation. Rarely, neonates and juveniles develop breast inflammation and infection in the first few weeks of life or at thelarche, with retained secretions in the developing breast being the underlying cause.

Ultrasound is useful for demonstrating a diffuse acute inflammatory process that may well respond to antibiotic

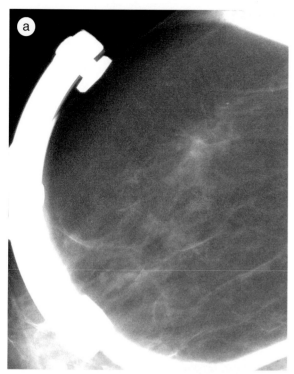

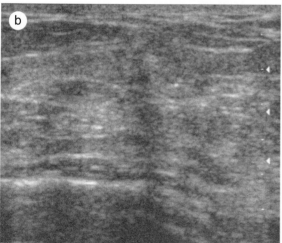

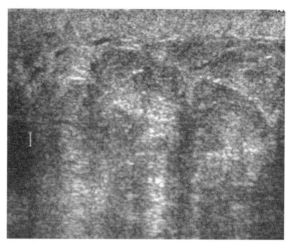

Figure 8.34   Inflammation in the breast results in pronounced thickening of the skin layer and dilation of superficial lymphatics.

Figure 8.33   (a) This magnified coned compression mammogram demonstrates a 'radial scar'. (b) The ultrasound appearances of a radial scar are non-specific—this lesion simply showed some equivocal tissue plane disruption and posterior shadowing.

therapy, and differentiating this from progressive tissue destruction, liquefaction and frank abscess formation. If a discrete abscess forms, surgical excision may be required, although a large percentage, some authorities believe up to 90%, can be treated conservatively with antibiotics and/or needle aspiration. Recurrence, however, is common particularly with multifocal and multilocular collections. Of note, at presentation, diffuse benign inflammatory change in the breast cannot be differentiated from inflammatory carcinoma, and failure to respond to antibiotic therapy should prompt tissue sampling.

Infection typically presents clinically with pain, swelling and erythema, periareolar infection also being associated with nipple discharge and possible nipple retraction. When breast sepsis is suspected, clinically there is no immediate need for mammogram—and indeed the technique is likely to produce suboptimal images, effective compression being difficult in view of tissue edema and pain. However, once the initial and presenting infection has resolved, mammography is indicated in the older patient to ensure that there are no persistent underlying signs of malignancy.

Ultrasound is the imaging investigation of first choice, being useful for both confirming and monitoring infection, and for detection of an underlying focal lesion. Ultrasound will readily show increased fluid retention within the breast tissues, in particular the edematous skin is thickened, the superficial lymphatic channels may be dilated (Fig. 8.34), often there are enlarged 'reactive' lymph nodes in the axilla and any underlying fluid collection in the breast is readily demonstrated. The composition and size of a fluid collection should be assessed, with ultrasound also allowing real-time guidance of needle placement for diagnostic aspiration or therapeutic drainage.

Sonographically, an abscess is a reasonably well-circumscribed complex mass with thick hyperaemic walls

(Fig. 8.35). Tissue liquefaction causes a central fluid component that exhibits increased posterior through transmission. As the abscess resolves, its walls become thinner, peripheral vascularity reduces and the internal structure becomes less complex, any residual fluid collection eventually becoming completely echo free. Due to their complex shape, abscesses and fluid collections should be measured and documented in three diameters, with images including accurate scan plane annotation recorded to allow effective serial monitoring.

Sometimes abscesses become encapsulated or may form a sinus track to the breast surface. When the patient has an open wound, risk of cross-infection can be minimized by adaption an aseptic technique to protect both patient and operator. The operator should wear sterile examination gloves, should cover the transducer with a sterile sheath and should use sterile acoustic coupling gel on the (broken) skin surface. At the end of the examination, effective hand-washing and hard surface decontamination regimes should be followed.

Very rarely, deeper thoracic cavity infections can traverse the anterior chest wall and manifest as a breast mass—empyema necessitatis (Fig. 8.36) (Dixon 1998).

LYMPHOCYTIC LOBULITIS (DIABETIC MASTOPATHY)

This is a relatively rare autoimmune reaction occurring predominantly (but not always) in women with insulin-dependent diabetes (Williams et al 1995). The clinical and imaging features are essentially those of carcinoma—a palpable, usually central mass that gives rise to asymmetric increased mammographic density (Fig. 8.37) and an ill-defined area of heterogeneous dense attenuating parenchymal tissue on ultrasound (Fig. 8.38).

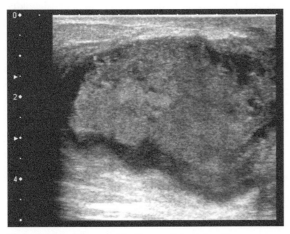

Figure 8.35   Sonographically, an abscess has the appearance of a thick-walled complex mass.

TRAUMA

Accidental and iatrogenic trauma to the breast can result in scarring, tissue necrosis and the formation of fluid collections such as hamatoma, seroma, occlusion and oil cysts and lymphocele.

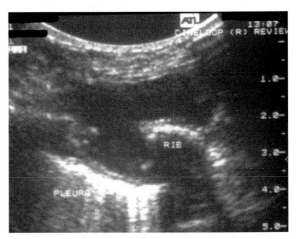

Figure 8.36   Empyema necessitatis is a rare condition—this case presented through a symptomatic breast clinic as a breast mass. Ultrasound demonstrated a retromammary fluid collection communicating with the pleural cavity through the intercostal space.

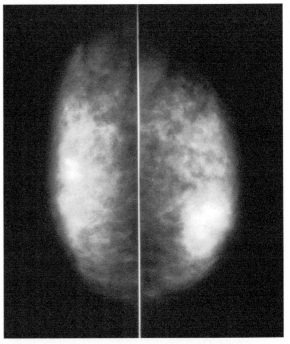

Figure 8.37   The mammograms of this patient with lymphocytic lobulitis demonstrated a non-specific area of increased density in the lower half of the left breast.

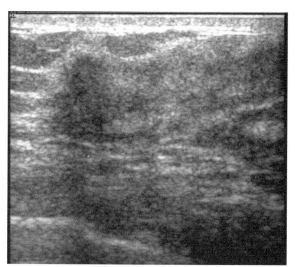

Figure 8.38   Sonographically, lymphocytic lobulitis has malignant features—an irregular hyporeflective mass that exhibits posterior acoustic shadowing.

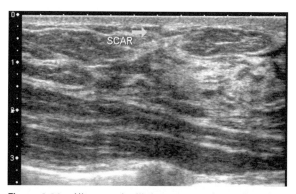

Figure 8.39   Ultrasound will demonstrate tissue plane disruption correlating with skin incision scars at the site of previous surgery.

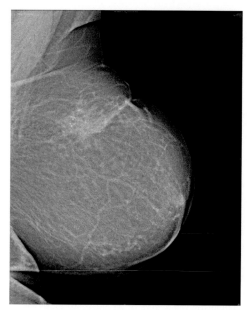

Figure 8.40   Surgical excision scars leave mammographic abnormalities that are indistinguishable from a malignant lesion. (Image courtesy of Dr P. Britton, Addenbrooke's Hospital, Cambridge.)

Postoperative scarring causes parenchymal deformity and alters the way in which both X-rays and ultrasound pass through tissue—these features impair image interpretation since they give rise to appearances that can both mimic and mask malignancy. Although imaging abnormalities due to scarring obviously correlate with skin incision sites (Fig. 8.39), particularly following breast conservation surgery there is a diagnostic challenge to differentiate benign scar tissue from residual, recurrent or de novo tumor.

Clinically, scarring may cause pain (or loss of sensation) and is associated with variable amounts of skin retraction and disfigurement. On mammograms, the parenchymal distortion and spiculate increases in density associated with scar tissue have the same appearance as a classic carcinoma (Fig. 8.40). Similarly, with ultrasound, fibrotic scar tissue causes acoustic shadowing and may look like an irregular, hyporeflective mass—again a classic malignant appearance (Fig. 8.41). With severe skin disfigurement, transducer contact can be a problem; gentle pressure and additional coupling gel help to ensure good sound transmission and thus reduce acoustic shadowing.

To differentiate acoustic shadowing due to malignancy from fibrotic shadowing, color flow Doppler might be employed to show hypervascularity in a 'real' lesion, absence of vascularity reducing the level of suspicion of recurrence in the postoperative patient. Transducer compression can be applied to reduce tissue thickness and attenuation so that normal architectural anatomy can be demonstrated in regenerating tissue. Over time, as tissues regenerate naturally, imaging abnormalities become less conspicuous, but in the early postoperative phase appearances are often equivocal if not overtly suspicious, and tissue sampling cannot be avoided in high risk patients.

The irradiated breast is also a diagnostic challenge, skin thickening, tissue edema and fibrosis again impairing image interpretation and exclusion of recurrent lesions. The irradiated breast will be hyporeflective when edematous and becomes increasingly hyper-reflective as

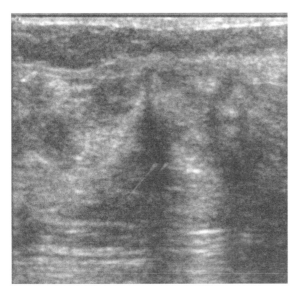

Figure 8.41 Sometimes wide local excision scars give rise to acoustic shadowing of an apparent 'mass'—these ultrasound appearances mimic recurrent malignancy.

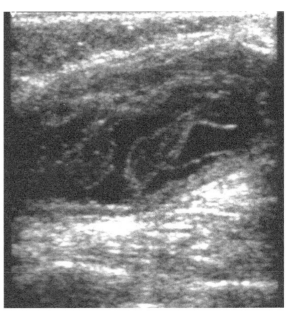

Figure 8.42 Resolving hematomas have a complex appearance—whilst the fluid content is black—organizing hematoma produces internal stand-like echoes. Note the increased through transmission characteristic of fluid-filled lesions.

fibrosis sets in; the skin is invariably thickened, recurrent disease and inflammation being difficult to exclude.

Hematomas and seromas are relatively common in the postoperative period. Small ones will resolve spontaneously, larger ones might require aspiration (which may be image guided); more complex, persistent and infected collections require surgical evacuation. Sonographically, fluid collections have a well-defined but sometimes irregular outline, the center being anechoic (black) if it is simple viscous fluid. Hematoma has a variable time-dependent appearance, but its general fluid nature always gives increased posterior through transmission—a brighter appearance to the structures underneath it on the ultrasound image. Initially the fluid (particularly if still within the tissues) looks hyper-reflective (bright); fluid containing diffuse hemorrhagic debris has homogeneous low-level reflections within it (Fig. 8.42). As the hematoma begins to resolve and become more organized, it starts to appear complex and heterogeneous, and liquefaction results in the presence of anechoic (black) fluid (Fig. 8.43); solid areas of clot retraction may sometimes be seen adherent to the internal walls of the 'mass'. If scanned for the first time at this stage, the appearances are similar to those of an intracystic or necrotic tumor; although a relevant clinical history might exist, and interval imaging will show change in a resolving hematoma, color Doppler and diagnostic tissue sampling should be considered to avoid a false negative, and delayed diagnosis.

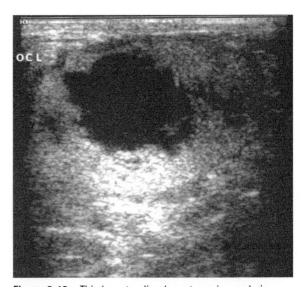

Figure 8.43 This longstanding hematoma is anechoic (black), representing its simple fluid content following liquefaction. If this was the first time this lesion had been visualized sonographically its irregular margins would raise suspicion, and 'cystic' malignancies, e.g. mucinous carcinoma, would need to be excluded from the list of differential diagnoses.

Oil cysts and fat necrosis develop in the breast subsequent to trauma at any age. On mammograms, oil cysts show up as round radiolucent masses with a well-defined capsule (Fig. 8.44); in some instances they have 'eggshell' type calcifications. Ultrasound usually demonstrates a well-defined hyporeflective mass with a thin smooth capsule (Fig. 8.45). Areas of fat necrosis tend to be less well defined and more heterogeneous, having hyper-reflective and fluid (anechoic) areas (Fig. 8.46). Since these abnormalities represent necrotic fatty tissue, sound attenuation through the cyst/area is similar to that in adjacent fatty tissue and the characteristic vertical brighter stripe deep to a normal (serous) cyst or fluid collection is not present. Indeed, oil cysts and areas of fat necrosis may show slight acoustic shadowing, cyst calcification having a pronounced effect. If ultrasound-guided diagnostic cyst aspiration is performed to rule out a small solid lesion, the aspirate is usually thicker and more viscous than that from a standard breast cyst and often has a straw-colored hue.

Granulomas occur if localized hypertropic scarring forms at trauma sites. Their ultrasound appearance is similar to that of a small fibroadenoma, i.e. a well-defined oval homogeneous mass of variable reflectivity.

LYMPHADENOPATHY

Clinical examination of the axilla, although widely practiced, has debateable sensitivity and specificity, with abnormal nodes usually but not always enlarged. Conversely, palpable lymph nodes are not necessarily pathological but can sometimes give rise to physical signs and symptoms that mimic breast pathology.

A lymph node within breast tissue, an intramammary lymph node, may present clinically as a smooth, soft mobile lump. Such lymph nodes are often biologically normal and therefore they exhibit the normal mammographic and ultrasound appearances described in Chapter 5.

On mammograms, lymph nodes may be seen as round or oval soft tissue densities—axillary nodes noted

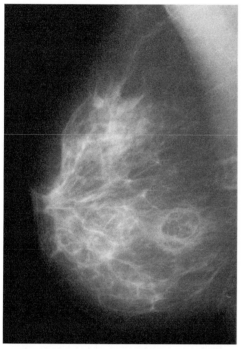

Figure 8.44 Fat necrosis has a characteristic well-defined radiolucent appearance on mammograms.

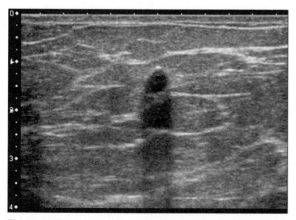

Figure 8.45 Incomplete posterior acoustic shadowing and lack of a hyper-reflective anterior margin differentiate this oil cyst from a simple serous cyst or macrocalcification.

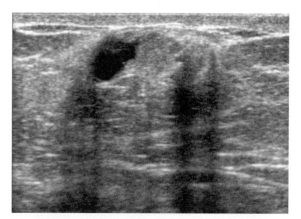

Figure 8.46 Sonographically, fat necrosis has the appearance of a complex heterogeneous mass—typically there are both hyper-reflective and anechoic (fluid) components.

adjacent to, or overlying the pectoralis muscle in the upper inner area of the medio-lateral oblique view (Fig. 8.47). Whilst the majority of lymph nodes are mammographically occult, visualization is a non-specific feature. Occasionally in women treated for rheumatoid disease with gold, small high density particles may be seen within lymph nodes.

Abnormality on both mammography and ultrasound is characterized by enlargement with or without loss of the normal cortico-hilar differentiation (loss of radiolucent hilum on mammograms and loss of central hyper-reflectivity on ultrasound) or by eccentric cortical thickening. Sonographically, since normal axillary lymph nodes are difficult to differentiate from axillary fat, abnormally enlarged hyporeflective nodes are usually readily apparent.

Benign reactive adenopathy is characterized by prominent but otherwise normal lymph nodes, i.e. those that are enlarged, have central hilar hyper-reflectivity preservation and a symmetrical hyporeflective surrounding cortex of functional lymphatic tissue (Fig. 8.48). These features are occasionally associated with non-metastatic malignancy but are more likely to be due to fibrocystic disease or immune, inflammatory and other conditions that stimulate reticulo-endothelial activity (psoriasis, tuberculosis, rheumatoid arthritis, lupus and sarcoidosis). A round (short axis exceeding 10 mm) as opposed to oval shape is particularly worrying, as is loss of hilar reflectivity and eccentric cortical thickening; underlying pathology with these appearances includes lymphoma and metastatic disease. Increased vascularity can occur in both reactive and metastatic lymph nodes, and even when associated with a normal 2D B-mode appearance should be regarded with suspicion.

In older patients, lymph nodes that have undergone repeated infection, scarring and cortical atrophy often have a markedly enlarged hyper-reflective hilum and a very thin surrounding hyporeflective rim (Fig. 8.49); hyper-reflectivity and posterior 'snowstorm shadowing' is often seen in women with silicone implants in situ due either to gel bleed or extracapsular rupture (see Ch. 10).

If the imaging features of a palpable or mammographically detected mass are classically those of a 'normal' lymph node, many practicing physicians would be satisfied and not undertake further investigation; in cases of doubt, surgical excision or image-guided biopsy is required.

SKIN LESIONS

Sebaceous, Montgomery's gland and epidermal inclusion cysts occur when glands within the skin layer become obstructed. They often present as tiny superficial 'pea'-like swellings. High resolution equipment, good near field focusing and sometimes the use of a stand-off gel pad are required to demonstrate them adequately. With careful technique, a well-defined focal mass can usually be demonstrated, its reflectivity being variable according

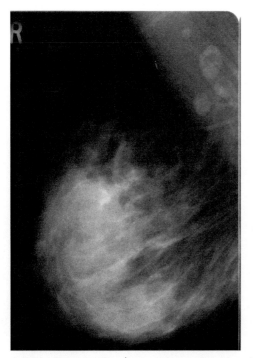

Figure 8.47 Normal axillary/upper outer quadrant lymph nodes can sometimes been seen superimposed over the pectoralis muscle shadow on medio-lateral oblique mammograms.

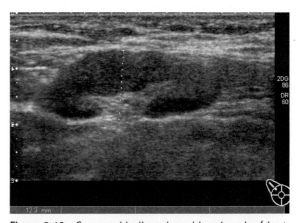

Figure 8.48 Sonographically, enlarged lymph nodes (short axis diameter >10 mm) may be due to infection (this patient had a breast abscess) or other conditions that stimulate reticulo-endothelial activity—a benign process is more likely when the hyper-reflective hilum is preserved.

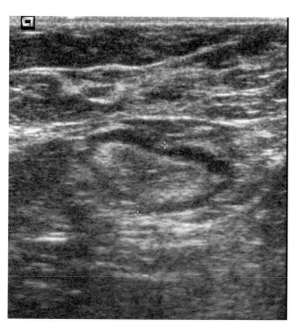

Figure 8.49 Lymph nodes that have undergone repeated infection become scarred and fibrosed—sonographically, their hyper-reflective center becomes more prominent and the hyporeflective rim reduced in thickness.

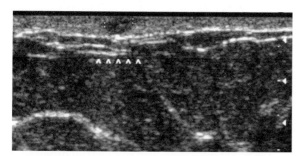

Figure 8.50 A sebaceous cyst is confined to the skin layer. Most present with a superficial pea-like swelling; ultrasound often shows a corresponding small hyporeflective mass lesion.

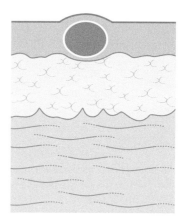

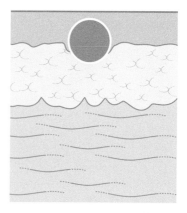

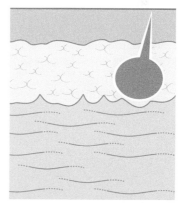

Figure 8.51 Possible sonographic appearances of cysts that arise from the skin layer (after Stavros 2004, p. 326).

to cyst content (Fig. 8.50). Definitive sonographic diagnosis requires demonstration of the lesion's spatial relationship with the skin layer. These cysts lie either entirely within the skin layer or superficially in the subcutaneous layer; in the latter location, skin should be seen dipping down around the edges of the lesion or the gland/hair follicle seen to pass through the skin for a definitive diagnosis (Fig. 8.51).

At areas of localized skin inflammation, the skin is thickened and may have a hyporeflective laminar appearance (Fig. 8.52); occasionally small intra-dermal fluid collections are seen (Fig. 8.53).

DOPPLER ULTRASOUND IN BENIGN DISEASE

Small well-defined lesions with homogeneous low-level echoes may represent solid masses or cysts containing viscous/hemorrhagic fluid. The demonstration of blood vessels within the lesion confirms the lesion to be solid (Fig. 8.54), absence of blood flow indicating that perhaps

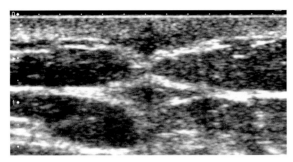

Figure 8.52 Ultrasound may show laminar thickening and reduced reflectivity of the skin layer associated with areas of localized edematous inflammation.

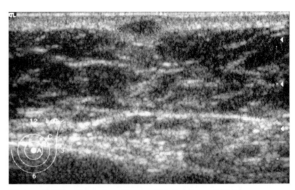

Figure 8.53 Occasionally small intradermal fluid collections are demonstrated.

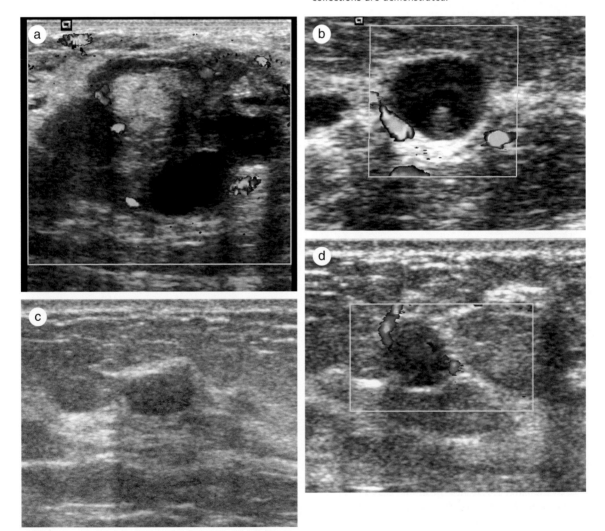

Figure 8.54 (a–d) Color flow mapping Doppler (CFMD) can help to differentiate between complex fluid collections and solid masses. A positive CFM signal (a) confirms the solid nature of this indeterminate lesion; absence of color flow signal (b) suggests that this lesion is essentially fluid filled and the reflective material is likely to be inspissated cellular or hemorrhagic debris. CFM can be used with small equivocal masses (c) to differentiate fibroadenomas and cysts containing viscous fluid; the demonstration of vessels within a mass (d) confirms that it is a solid lesion and not a cyst.

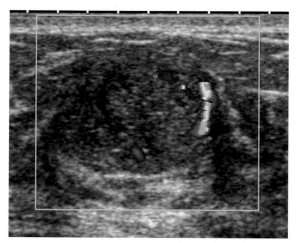

Figure 8.55   CFMD showing the sparse peripheral/radial vessel pattern often associated with benign lesions.

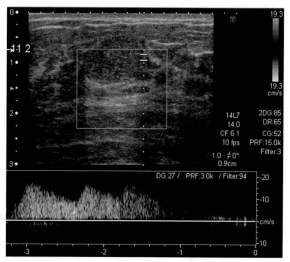

Figure 8.56   Typical benign spectral Doppler flow velocity waveform: low velocity low resistance trace from a fibroadenoma.

fine needle aspiration, rather than needle core biopsy, should be attempted in order to clarify its nature. In some cases, although no vessels are present, use of the color flow mapping function will show pathognomonic fluid movement (streaming) within a cystic lesion as a consequence of Doppler mode operating at higher output power settings.

With modern high resolution ultrasound equipment, careful technique (see Ch. 6) will demonstrate vascularity in the majority of solid lesions. Longstanding stable lesions tend to be hypovascular, with one or two peripheral or radial tapering vessels (Fig. 8.55). There is some evidence that the angle at which arteries enter a lesion is a useful benign/malignant differentiating characteristic, with vessels supplying malignant tumors aligned more at right angles to the tumor margin and vessels into benign lesions more tangential.

Typically, spectral Doppler flow velocity waveforms from the arteries of stable benign lesions show a low velocity, low resistance pattern (Fig. 8.56). Blood flow is increased in both benign and malignant proliferative disease, with pregnancy and lactation, and in the presence of inflammatory processes. Proliferating, enlarging and inflammatory lesions are more likely to have low resistance waveforms than malignant lesions. Assessment of Doppler characteristics, however, is unavoidably subjective and not reliable enough to preclude biopsy in individual cases.

SUMMARY

Most women will experience breast discomfort at some time in their lives, the breast being a hormonally sensitive organ in which cyclical and age-related changes in texture and form are physiological norms. Pathological change in the breast is predominantly caused by benign processes; however, the clinical signs and symptoms for these are often similar to those associated with breast cancer. Accentuated physical change in the breast is worrisome for individual women and presents a diagnostic challenge to their healthcarers—ultrasound is a safe and sensitive diagnostic technique that is increasingly being used early in the patient care pathway.

Benign solid breast masses have a wide variety of underlying histological subtypes which all appear sonographically similar—a mobile reasonably compressible well-defined encapsulated oval or lobulated mass that has an essentially homogeneous and slightly hyporeflective echo texture. An exact definitive diagnosis is perhaps somewhat academic but tissue sampling is nevertheless essential in the majority of cases to identify proliferating lesions and exclude malignancy—of note, mucinous and invasive ductal carcinoma sometimes have this 'benign' appearance.

The ultrasound operator also needs to differentiate reliably true focal masses from transient physiological change and from inflammatory, infective and traumatic abnormality if benign biopsy rates are to be minimized and unnecessary diagnostic surgery avoided.

References and further reading

Dixon AM 1998 Sonographic and radiological features of empyema necessitatis presenting as a focal breast mass. London, British Medical Ultrasound Society. BMUS Bulletin 11:42–43.

Heywang-Kobrunner S, Dershaw DD, Scheer I 2002 Diagnostic breast imaging. 2nd edn. Stuttgart: Thieme.

Kirkpatrick UJ, Burrows C, Loughran CF 2000 Imaging appearances of pseudoangiomatous hyperplasia of mammary stroma. Clinical Radiology 55(7):576–578.

Lister D, Evans AJ, Burrell HC et al 1998 The accuracy of breast ultrasound in the evaluation of clinically benign discrete, symptomatic breast lumps. Clinical Radiology 53(7):490–492.

Madjar H 2000 The practice of breast ultrasound. Stuttgart: Thieme.

Polger MR, Denison CM, Lester S et al 1996 Pseudo-haemangiomatous stromal hyperplasia: mammographic and sonographic appearances. AJR American Journal of Roentology 166:349–352.

RCR 2003 Guidance on screening and symptomatic breast imaging. 2nd edn. BFCR(03)2. London: Royal College of Radiologists.

Rosen PP, Cantrell B, Mullen DL et al 1980 Juvenile papillomatosis (Swiss cheese disease) of the breast. American Journal of Surgical Pathology 4(1):3–12.

Stavros AT 2004 Breast ultrasound. Philadelphia: Lippincott, Wilkinson & Williams.

Tot T, Tabar L, Dean PB 2002 Practical breast pathology. New York: Thieme.

Williams PH, Rubin CME, Theaker JM 1995 Sclerosing lymphocytic lobulitis of the breast. Clinical Radiology 50:165–167.

Chapter 9

Malignant breast disease

Anne-Marie Dixon

CHAPTER CONTENTS

INTRODUCTION

All pathological processes enlarge the terminal duct lobular units (TDLUs) of the breast, producing lesions which at least initially start off as either round, oval or stellate deformities (Tot et al 2002, pp. 26–27). The stellate lesion arises when the TDLUs are destroyed and replaced during the pathological process; this feature is typical of invasive ductal carcinoma (no special type; NST) and tubular carcinomas as well as the pseudomalignant mimic of carcinoma—the radial scar (RS) or complex sclerosing lesion (CSL) (Tot et al 2002, pp. 26–27). When the pathological process distends, expands or distorts the TDLUs, a rounded or ovoid lesion results—this is found in benign lesions and in the more cellular subtypes of ductal carcinoma (Tot et al 2002, p. 26). Rounded lesions are also seen in 'special type' breast cancer such as mucinous (colloid) carcinoma, the rapidly growing grade 3 ductal (NST) carcinoma or medullary-like tumors. As the pathological process progresses, disease extends into the surrounding stromal tissue and lesions become more complex in appearance (Tot et al 2002, p. 27).

Ultrasound imaging is used to assist in determining the presence, size, extent, distribution and location of breast disease, and can provide information which may be indicative of tumor classification and malignant disease stage (Box 9.1) (Tot et al 2002, p. 33). Most malignant lesions present either in symptomatic breast services as a palpable mass or are detected in national mammography-based screening programmes as an asymmetric density; ultrasound is particularly useful in both these contexts.

A variety of terminology for describing breast ultrasound appearances has been described in Chapter 6, and criteria for the interpretation of appearances in characterization and differentiation of breast diseases have been

Box 9.1   Use of ultrasound in malignant breast disease

Diagnosis and surgical planning
Determine

- Tumor size and extent
  - Maximum diameter of largest tumor focus
  - Isolated, multifocal, multicentric, bilateral
- Tumor location—with particular reference to skin, nipple and chest wall
- Lymph node appearances
  - Needle core biopsy guidance
  - Preoperative localization of impalpable lesions

Follow-up

- Adjunct to mammography for screening and surveillance in high risk
- and young women
- Monitoring lesion size and vascularity in response to chemotherapy

Table 9.1   Suspicious clinical and mammographic features

Examination	Features
Clinical examination	New/enlarging palpable abnormality
	Asymmetric thickening
	Pain—unilateral, localized, non-cyclical
	Discharge—single duct, blood-stained
	Unilateral nipple retraction
	Skin changes—retraction, peau d'orange, erythema
	Lymphadenopathy
Mammography	Focal mass
	Irregular or ill-defined outline
	Pleomorphic microcalcification
	Asymmetric density
	Architectural deformity
	Interval change

described in Chapter 7. Through consistent and reliable application of these criteria and the appropriate selection of lesions for tissue sampling, ultrasound can achieve high sensitivity and specificity and good preoperative diagnosis rates for malignancy, this capability being underpinned by expert practice in a 'triple assessment' setting (Lister et al 1998).

The 2D B-mode image is used to evaluate and document disease presence, location and distribution, and to guide tissue sampling. The ultrasound examination should determine the extent of the area of breast involved, ascertaining if disease is localized, multicentric or diffuse, and assess the number and size of any focal abnormalities, localizing them with reference to the nipple and quadrant anatomy of the breast or with reference to clock face annotation (see Ch. 7).

Doppler ultrasound is used to assess blood flow either within a specific lesion or more generally throughout the breast, and although vascularity is increased in both benign and malignant proliferative disease, and with pregnancy, lactation and inflammatory processes (Madjar 2000, p. 231), Doppler can be used to help refine the level of suspicion allocated to lesions that otherwise have equivocal appearances. Color flow mapping can also be used to ensure that a biopsy path avoids large vessels.

This chapter will review classification of malignant breast disease and describe the corresponding range of clinical, mammography and ultrasound appearances.

MALIGNANT BREAST DISEASE

Malignant breast disease is classified as either in situ or invasive disease, and as either ductal (NST) or of special type or mixed in origin on the basis of cytological features and architectural growth pattern.

Most invasive breast cancers are solid lesions and are reliably differentiated from cystic masses with ultrasound, thus sparing women with simple breast cysts further investigation (Jackson et al 1996, Heywang-Kobrunner et al 2001, p. 295). Intracystic papillary carcinomas (a type of in situ carcinoma) can be identified on ultrasound. Solid malignant tumors have diverse morphology and thus a variety of ultrasound appearances. Ultrasound appearances are not diagnostic of any particular histological tumor type; a tissue sample is required before a solid lesion can be dismissed as benign and to characterize a malignant lesion fully (Madjar 2000, p. 163). Ultrasound measurements give a better prediction of histological tumor size than clinical examination or mammography, although there is a tendency to underestimate size, particularly with larger (>30 mm) lesions (Bosch et al 2003, Snelling et al 2004).

Epidemiological factors associated with increased risk of malignancy have been discussed in Chapter 2, and the importance of considering patient history and clinical findings during breast image interpretation has been highlighted in Chapter 7. Sometimes patient demographics, family or previous history, and clinical or mammography findings (Table 9.1) are over-riding factors that result in a decision to categorize sonographic appearances as 'suspicious for malignancy' irrespective of the intrinsic ultrasound features.

ATYPICAL HYPERPLASIA

The natural course of malignant change in the breast is thought to progress through hyperplasia, atypia and in situ stages. Atypical hyperplasia is diagnosed when the tissue exhibits some but not all the histological features of in situ malignancy (NHSCSP & RCP 2005). Atypical hyperplasia has minimal or non-specific clinical and imaging features and is usually diagnosed incidentally when breast biopsy is performed to clarify the nature of 'indeterminate' screen-detected microcalcification. Nevertheless, it is important. Atypical ductal hyperplasia (ADH) is associated with a 2-fold increased lifetime risk of subsequently developing invasive disease, and when there is a strong family history of breast carcinoma in first-degree relatives this risk is doubled and approaches the lifetime risk of ductal carcinoma in situ (DCIS). Thus detection of ADH at 14-gauge biopsy should prompt consideration of 11-gauge vacuum biopsy or excisional biopsy to avoid the risk of disease underestimation; when no malignancy is present, high-risk surveillance, particularly for women with other demographic risk factors, may be appropriate.

NON-INVASIVE MALIGNANCY

Fifteen to twenty percent of breast malignancies (Fig. 9.1) are classified as non-invasive in situ disease where the tumor cells have malignant phenotype but lack the ability to invade surrounding tissue (Dawson 1996, Tot et al 2002). The disease is confined to the glandular tissues, contained within an intact surrounding basement membrane, and has not infiltrated the adjacent stromal tissue (NHSCSP & RCP 2005, p. 50, Tot et al 2002, p. 46). These tumors are classified as either DCIS, lobular carcinoma in situ (LCIS) or intracystic papillary carcinoma in situ. DCIS is further subdivided according to the nuclear size as low, intermediate or high nuclear grade. Traditionally, DCIS has also been typed histologically into comedo, micropapillary, solid or cribriform type, the comedo type more likely to be associated with co-existent or subsequent high grade invasive disease.

Ductal carcinoma in situ (DCIS)

DCIS is the most common non-invasive breast malignancy, and its presence is an important prognostic factor in small (<10 mm) invasive tumors, those with extensive high grade DCIS having a less favorable prognosis (Tot et al 2002, p. 133). Despite its preinvasive nature, DCIS is treated aggressively in view of its malignant potential (Heywang-Kobrunner et al 2001, p. 255). Breast conservation treatments may be successful if disease is well localized, clear surgical margins can be obtained and patients undergo radio- and/or endocrine therapy (Fisher et al 2001, Neuschatz et al 2001, Schwartz 2001).

Histologically, DCIS tumor cells are larger and more cohesive than normal and have a tendency to form gland-like or papillary structures (Tot et al 2002, p. 47). If central necrosis, usually called comedo (as a result of cell death), occurs, necrotic material may calcify in the lumen of ducts (Fig. 9.2) or in the breast acini and render the disease detectable with mammography (Fig. 9.3). The calcification pattern may be described as *casting type* (long branching), *broken needle* clusters or *powdery* (Tot et al 2002, pp. 52–53). Whilst the latter two pat-

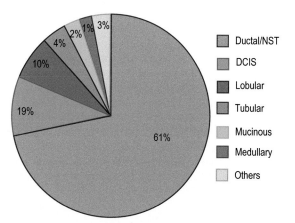

Figure 9.1 Pie chart to show relative prevalence of different cancer types (data from Tot et al 2002, pp. 107–113).

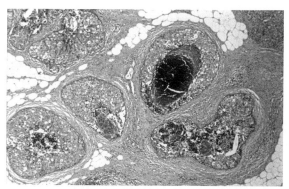

Figure 9.2 Histology appearance of ductal carcinoma in situ. (Image courtesy of Dr J. Lowe, University Hospital of North Tees.)

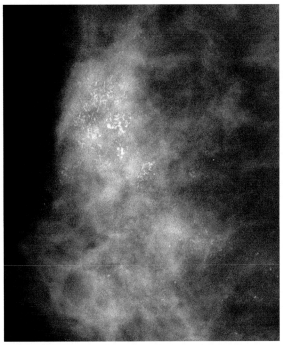

Figure 9.3   DCIS has a characteristic mammographic appearance—irregular clusters of pleomorphic (variable size shape and density) calcifications in a ductal distribution.

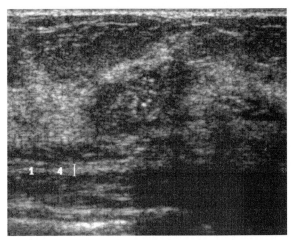

Figure 9.4   Ultrasound will sometimes demonstrate a solid mass in association with a small area of mammographically detected microcalcification. Small hyper-reflective (white) punctate calcifications can been seen within the hypore-flective (dark gray) mass. If a mass is sonographically visible, a needle core biopsy can be done under ultrasound guidance.

terns also occur in benign conditions such as papilloma, fibroadenoma, fibrocystic disease and adenosis, the casting type and a pleomorphic (variable size, shape and density) pattern have high positive predictive value for malignancy.

Most (80%) DCIS is non-palpable and asymptomatic, and is therefore detected in mammography-based population screening programs. Clinically detectable DCIS may be associated with a palpable cystic tumor (intracystic papillary carcinoma), Paget's disease (a chronic eczema-like skin lesion around the nipple and areola), nipple discharge (intraduct papilloma with DCIS or apocrine papillary DCIS) or a palpable stellate lesion (tumor-forming DCIS) (Tot et al 2002, p. 61).

DCIS is graded as low, intermediate or high grade depending on the degree of cellular atypia and growth pattern; low grade is considered to have low invasive potential, with high grade being clinically aggressive and associated with a high probability of local recurrence even after radical excision (Tot et al 2002, p. 62, NHSCSP & RCP 2005, p. 50).

With the excellent spatial resolution of modern high frequency (7.5–13 MHz) ultrasound, small calcifications associated with carcinoma in situ may be demonstrated (Huang et al 1999), but ultrasound is not reliable and appropriate as a screening examination in the general population (Teh & Wilson 1998). Ultrasound is, however, a useful additional examination when apparently isolated microcalcifications are detected on mammography. The ultrasound demonstration of calcification in association with benign breast changes, in the absence of a suspicious focal mass, can reduce the level of suspicion attributed to indeterminate calcifications. When mammographic calcification has a suspicious or overtly malignant pattern, ultrasound will often demonstrate a non-palpable and mammography occult focal mass (Fig. 9.4), particularly when the calcification extends over an area greater than 10 mm diameter (Huang et al 1999); in such cases, core biopsy can be performed under ultrasound, rather than stereotactic mammography guidance.

Sometimes, when an ultrasound examination localized to an area of mammographic abnormality is performed, calcification and hypervascularity can be demonstrated even in the absence of a mass lesion (Fig. 9.5). In such cases, however, tissue sampling should be performed using stereotactic mammography guidance so that it is accurately localized to the area of the originally detected abnormality. Irrespective of whether ultrasound or mammography guidance has been used, biopsy tissue cores should be radiographed to confirm adequate sampling of calcifications (Fig. 9.6).

Lobular carcinoma in situ (LCIS)

LCIS arises in the epithelium in the blunt ducts of the mammary lobules; it is more commonly found in younger

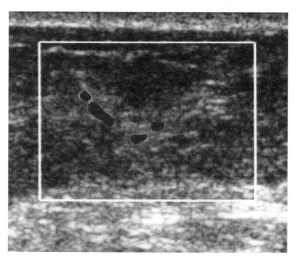

Figure 9.5 Sometimes color flow mapping Doppler ultrasound will demonstrate increased vascularity at the site of a mammographic abnormality although the 2D B-mode ultrasound appearances are essentially normal.

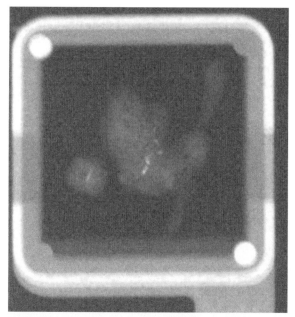

Figure 9.6 Needle core biopsy specimen radiograph. Whenever a needle core biopsy has been performed to evaluate microcalcifications, the core specimens should be radiographed to confirm an adequate yield of calcification.

women of reproductive age and is often multifocal and bilateral (Hagen-Ansert 2004). LCIS is characterized by uniform smallish round nuclei (Fig. 9.7) (NHSCSP & RCP 2005, p. 48), they are less cohesive and never form gland-like or papillary structures (Tot et al 2002, p. 47).

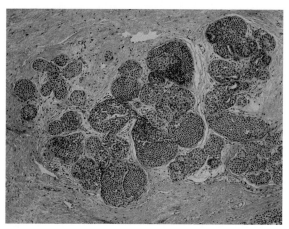

Figure 9.7 Histology appearance of lobular carcinoma in situ. (Image courtesy of Dr P. Carder, Bradford Hospitals Foundation NHS Trust.)

Differentiation of LCIS from atypical lobular hyperplasia (ALH) is subjective and may be problematic; the term lobular neoplasia is now used to encompass both ALH and LCIS appearances (Tohno et al 1994, p. 179, NHSCSP & RCP 2005).

LCIS is a marker lesion for increased risk of subsequently developing invasive cancer (either lobular or ductal) although its natural history is somewhat longer than for DCIS; subsequent invasive lesions may be occult or palpable and may be remote and/or contralateral to the original LCIS site (Tohno et al 1994, Heywang-Kobrunner et al 2001, p. 252, Tot et al 2002, p. 62). Following diagnosis, patients may choose between prophylactic surgery, endocrine therapy or a conservative 'high-risk' surveillance regime (Tohno et al 1994, Heywang-Kobrunner et al 2001, pp. 149, 254).

Since LCIS has no particular macroscopic features, it has no particular clinical or imaging features and is usually occult clinically and on imaging; its detection is usually an incidental finding at breast biopsy (Pope et al 1988, Heywang-Kobrunner et al 2001, pp. 252–253). LCIS is sometimes found when needle core biopsy has been performed for a vague and non-specific clinical, mammographic or ultrasound abnormality; in such cases, LCIS is often associated with DCIS or invasive disease, and these are more likely to be the cause of the abnormality (Heywang-Kobrunner 2001, p. 149). Because of this association, a needle biopsy diagnosis of isolated LCIS requires further evaluation (O'Driscoll et al 2001).

PAPILLARY CARCINOMA

Papillomas develop in the larger central breast ducts, more often in the retroareolar region than peripherally, and may cause serous or blood-stained nipple discharge (Tot et al 2002, p. 84, NHSCSP & RCP 2005).

With careful evaluation, intraduct papilloma can sometimes be demonstrated sonographically as a focal solid lesion within the lumen of a dilated duct (Fig. 9.8) (Tot et al 2002, p. 89). If the duct has become cystically dilated, the lesion is known as an intracystic papilloma (Fig. 9.9), and may be suspected if internal cyst walls are irregular, if solid material can be seen projecting into the cyst cavity (Jackson et al 1996) or when cyst aspiration yields blood-stained fluid (Hagen-Ansert 2004). The solid nature of mural nodules or intraluminal material can be differentiated from hemorrhagic or inspissated debris by using the color flow or power Doppler functions to demonstrate internal vascularity (Fig. 9.10).

Benign and malignant papilloma may have similar clinical and imaging appearances. Patients may, but do not always, present with a palpable mass; mammography may show associated microcalcification and/or sub-areolar duct ectasia (intraduct papilloma) or a well-defined round/oval density (intracystic papilloma), but may be normal. In the past, papillomas were routinely surgically excised to asses the risk of malignancy definitively; however, some now consider a needle core biopsy diagnosis accurate and surgical excision to be unneccesary in some cases (Carder et al 2005). If the epithelial tissue shows metaplastic, hyperplastic or neoplastic change, the lesion may be classified as borderline, in situ or overtly malignant (papillary carcinoma). By definition, these lesions are characterized as in situ disease unless they have penetrated the cyst wall, and they have a very good prognosis (90% 5-year survival) (Heywang-Kobrunner et al 2001, p. 271).

TUBULAR CARCINOMA

Tubular carcinoma is a well-differentiated form of ductal carcinoma (Fig. 9.11) sometimes containing evidence of DCIS or LCIS; they are frequently found in association with a radial scar (see later) (Heywang-Kobrunner et al 2001, p. 272). The tubular carcinoma is invariably classified grade 1 and usually has a very good prognosis (Tot et al 2002, p. 65).

Tubular carcinoma tends to present in middle-aged women and is often a slow growing, stellate tumor that appears on mammography as a small single, although occasionally mutifocal, spiculated radio-opacity (Tot et al 2002, p. 64). On ultrasound (Fig. 9.12), they exhibit many of the typical features of malignancy (Table 9.2).

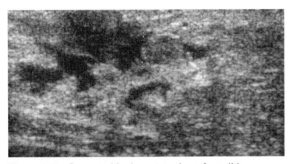

Figure 9.8 Sonographic demonstration of a solid mass within the lumen of a dilated duct suggests the presence of an intraductal papilloma.

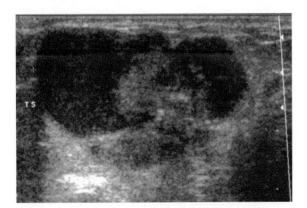

Figure 9.9 Ultrasound image of an intracystic papillary carcinoma—the duct has become grossly dilated and has the appearance of a large complex cyst with the solid papillomatous tumor projecting into its lumen. Note the suspiciously irregular margin and heterogeneous echo texture of the solid component.

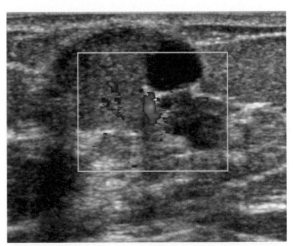

Figure 9.10 Color flow mapping Doppler should be used to evaluate reflective intracystic material—demonstration of blood vessels within the reflective material confirms that it is solid perfused tissue.

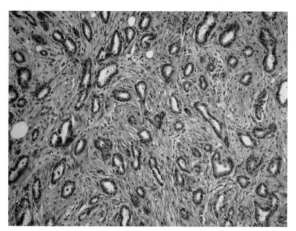

Figure 9.11 Histology appearance of tubular carcinoma. (Image courtesy of Dr P. Carder, Bradford Hospitals Foundation NHS Trust.)

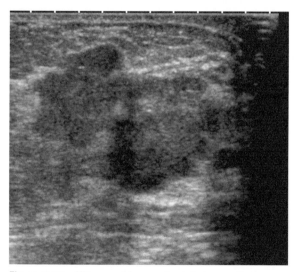

Figure 9.12 Ultrasound image of a tubular carcinoma. This shows typical malignant features—it has an irregular margin, is hyporeflective compared with the surrounding tissue, has a heterogeneous echo texture and exhibits some posterior acoustic shadowing.

MUCINOUS (COLLOID) CARCINOMA

This is a rare slow growing tumor, often found in older women, and usually has a very good prognosis (Tot et al 2002, p. 66). On mammography, these tumors are usually visible as a round or oval area of increased density and whilst histologically the mucinous carcinoma is well circumscribed, on mammography the margins may appear slightly ill defined (Tot et al 2002, pp. 66–67).

Table 9.2 Typical ultrasound features of malignancy

B mode appearances	Irregular shape/contour
	Irregular, spiculated or ill-defined margins
	Hyporeflective
	Heterogeneous echo texture and reflectivity
	Reduced through transmission/posterior shadowing
	Relatively fixed and incompressible
	Depth greater than width
	Discontinuity/destruction of adjacent tissue planes
Doppler features	Hypervascular/increased perfusion
	High vascular density—more than thee internal vessels
	Peripheral and central intratumoural vessels
	Chaotic and branching vessel pattern
	Penetrating and converging pattern
	High flow velocity, RI and PI

Ultrasound often shows a reasonably smooth, well-defined, occasionally microlobulated lesion (Fig. 9.13). The mucinous carcinoma has a gelatinous texture consisting of groups of cells or individual cells floating in larger lakes of extracellular mucin (Fig. 9.14) (NHSCSP & RCP 2005, p. 69). The internal appearance on ultrasound tends to be hypo- or isoreflective compared with adjacent breast tissue, and its fluid nature often gives rise to increased through transmission of sound with a brighter area posteriorly (Heywang-Kobrunner et al 2001, p. 297). Particulate material may be seen to move with patient movement, transducer compression or use of (higher energy) color flow Doppler to induce fluid streaming.

MEDULLARY CARCINOMA

The medullary carcinoma is a rapidly growing highly cellular ductal carcinoma that can occur at any age but is often found in younger and middle-aged women (Heywang-Kobrunner et al 2001, p. 272, Tot et al 2002, p. 68). Medullary or medullary-like carcinomas are important to recognize in view of the increased association with BRCA1 and BRCA2 genes. The 'typical' medullary carcinoma has a smooth well-defined, sometimes lobulated, but non-infiltrating border; large or rapidly

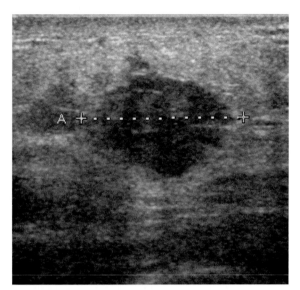

Figure 9.13 Ultrasound image of a mucinous carcinoma. This mass again shows 'malignant' sonographic characteristics—it has an irregular margin, is hyporeflective compared with the surrounding tissue and has a heterogeneous echotexture.

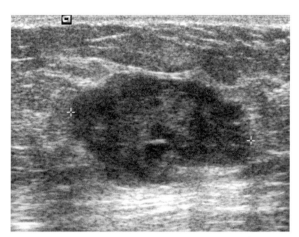

Figure 9.15 Ultrasound image of a medullary carcinoma— the mass has a relatively well-defined margin that is smooth and lobulated, and the mass exhibits increased through transmisison.

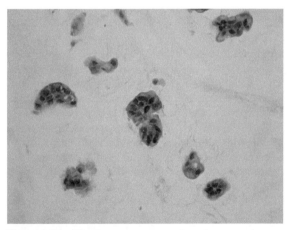

Figure 9.14 Histology appearance of mucinous carcinoma. (Image courtesy of Dr P. Carder, Bradford Hospitals Foundation NHS Trust.)

growing lesions may have a necrotic (fluid) center if tumor growth outstrips perfusion. Medullary carcinomas are usually classified as grade 3 lesions (Denley et al 2001) but they may have a better prognosis than a ductal carcinoma of the same size; atypical lesions that demonstrate an infiltrating border do not have the same prognostic advantage.

The pathologically well-circumscribed border of the typical medullary carcinoma renders it well defined on

both mammography and ultrasound, where it is usually demonstrated as a round or oval solid focal lesion. On mammography, however, its well-defined outline may be masked by overlying normal breast tissue or because of inflammatory infiltration of adjacent tissue.

Sonographically, the medullary carcinoma can look very similar to the benign fibroadenoma with increased posterior through transmission and refractive acoustic shadowing from the lesion edges; sometimes it has a necrotic cystic central component containing calcification (Fig. 9.15). Careful evaluation of the margins in multiple planes may show small suspicious irregularities (Madjar 2000, p. 126).

INVASIVE DUCTAL CARCINOMA (NST)

The majority of invasive breast cancers (up to 75%) do not have more than 50% of the classic features of any of the above 'special type' categories and are classified as being of 'no special type' (NST) (NHSCSP & RCP 2005, p. 61). This classification covers a wide heterogeneous range of ductal adenocarcinoma arising in the TDLU of the breast; individual tumors are subcategorized using morphology-based prognostic indicators as described in Chapter 2 (Tot et al 2002, pp. 76–77).

Most (70%) will present through symptomatic breast services as a palpable mass; about one-third (36%) of these lesions are readily apparent on mammograms as dense spiculated lesions (Fig. 9.16) (Jackson et al 1996), others manifest as reasonably well-defined round or oval densities (Fig. 9.17). Occasionally ductal carcinomas have a diffuse growth pattern with malignant cells per-

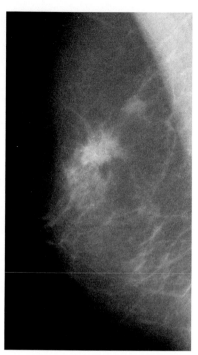

Figure 9.16 Medro-lateral oblique mammography projection of the right breast showing the classic dense spiculated mass associated with an invasive carcinoma.

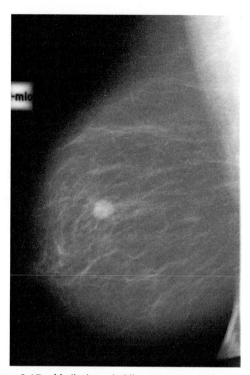

Figure 9.17 Medio-lateral oblique mammography projection showing a well-defined carcinoma centrally in the right breast. Although this lesion appears relatively well defined at first viewing, on closer inspection the margins are noted to be irregular; the patient's advanced age is also a key factor in categorizing this lesion as probably malignant.

meating the breast parenchyma and adipose tissue without forming a discrete mass (Heywang-Kobrunner et al 2001, p. 271). This makes them difficult to recognize on mammography and ultrasound images unless they are associated with microcalcification or local fibrosis and tissue retraction.

Ultrasound will classically demonstrate a solid lesion with an irregular margin (Fig. 9.18) and occasional internal microcalcifications (Fig. 9.19). Often the margins are ill defined (Fig. 9.20); if intraductal extension is seen, the mass has a classic spiculated appearance (Fig. 9.21) similar to that seen at mammography. Some lesions demonstrate a sense of contraction of adjacent tissue planes (Fig. 9.22). The malignant tumor often has a hyperreflective (brighter) rim, or halo (Fig. 9.23), variably attributed to desmoplastic reaction (Jackson et al 1996), multiple echo reflections between the tumor's spiculated edges (Tohno et al 1994) or lymphocytic reaction (Madjar 2000, p. 158).

The dense, hard consistency of these tumors results in attenuation of the ultrasound beam as it passes through the lesion—this gives it a hyporeflective (darker) appearance compared with the surrounding breast and produces the posterior acoustic shadowing phenomenon (Fig. 9.24). The lesion itself is often heterogeneous, and

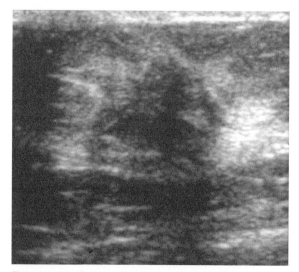

Figure 9.18 Sonographically, invasive carcinomas typically have irregular margins, are hyporeflective and heterogeneous, and they exhibit posterior acoustic shadowing.

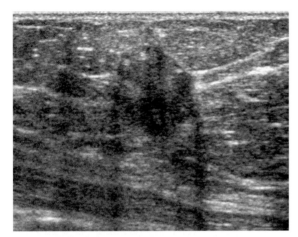

Figure 9.19   Ultrasound image of an invasive carcinoma containing microcalcifications—bright white dots.

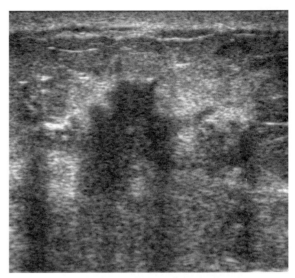

Figure 9.21   Sometimes ultrasound will show a spiculated lesion with hyporeflective tumor mass extending along and expanding the ducts adjacent to the central tumor nidus.

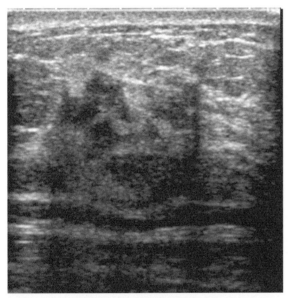
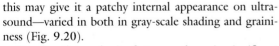

Figure 9.20   This invasive carcinoma did not have an obvious margin—at the site of a palpable mass, ultrasound showed an ill-defined heterogeneous area of reduced reflectivity that was associated with posterior acoustic shadowing.

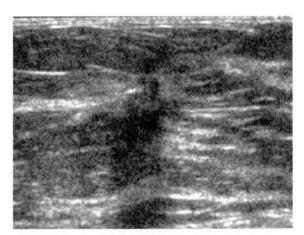

Figure 9.22   This ultrasound image of an invasive carcinoma gives the impression that the tissue planes are being pulled in centrally towards the tumor—this would correlate with a spiculate appearance at mammography.

this may give it a patchy internal appearance on ultrasound—varied in both in gray-scale shading and graininess (Fig. 9.20).

Despite these classic features, there is significant overlap between ultrasound appearances of benign and malignant lesions. In particular, hypercellular malignancies are often round or oval, have a smooth outline, and increased through transmission and edge shadowing,

giving them a similar appearance to a benign solid lesion such as a fibroadenoma (Fig. 9.25); some lesions may be isoechoic and have no effect on surrounding architecture or posterior reflectivity (Fig. 9.26) (Heywang-Kobrunner et al 2001, p. 301). Although patient history and age might particularly raise the ultrasound practitioner's level of suspicion in such cases any iso- or hypo-reflective solid lesion must be subjected to aspiration

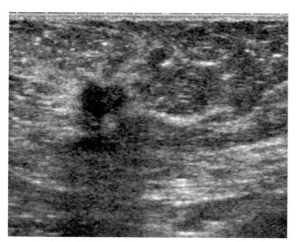

Figure 9.23 A hyper-reflective (brighter) band or 'halo' can sometimes be seen around a malignant lesion—the explanations for this appearance are varied (see text).

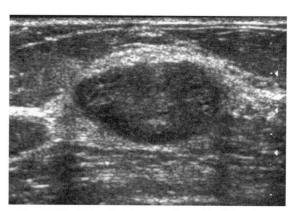

Figure 9.25 This invasive carcinoma does not have any of the classic ultrasound features associated with malignancy and might reasonably be categorized as a U2, i.e. probably benign, lesion. This case illustrates why a histological diagnosis should be obtained for all hyporeflective solid masses.

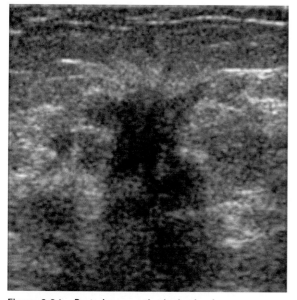

Figure 9.24 Posterior acoustic shadowing is a characteristic feature of most malignant lesions—this pathological shadowing is due to higher attenuation of sound in the tumor compared with the surrounding tissue.

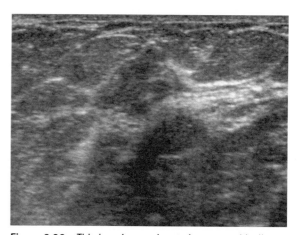

Figure 9.26 This invasive carcinoma is sonographically isoreflective—its gray-scale level is similar to that of the surrounding breast tissue. The most important sonographic characteristic is its irregular margin and the suggestion at the lower right edge that the lesion is expanding and extending along a duct.

and/or biopsy to clarify its nature and to obtain a definitive diagnosis.

INVASIVE LOBULAR CARCINOMA

This is the second most common type of invasive breast cancer, accounting for 12–15% of breast cancers in women (Giordano et al 2004). Invasive lobular carcinoma is notoriously difficult to diagnose clinically and with imaging (Heywang-Kobrunner et al 2001, p. 272). Commonly the tumor does not form a mass but produces an ill-defined 'thickening' on palpation.

The histological appearances are varied, with the 'classic type' invasive lobular carcinoma containing files of small monomorphous lobular cells (Fig. 9.27); solid, alveolar, tubulo-lobular and mixed variants exist (Tot et al 2002:73). Some lobular carcinomas form a stellate

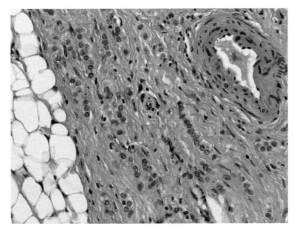

Figure 9.27 Histology appearance of invasive lobular carcinoma. (Image courtesy of Dr. N Dutt, King's College Hospital, London.)

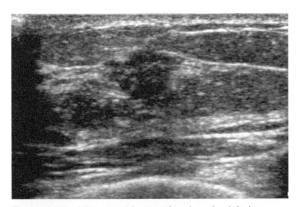

Figure 9.28 Ultrasound image of an invasive lobular carcinoma. This one again has typical malignant sonographic characteristics, i.e. a hyporeflective focal mass with an irregular margin and some posterior acoustic shadowing; however, lobular carcinoma can be sonographically subtle or even occult.

tumor body, but more commonly they grow in a diffuse manner and permeate normal tissue over a wide area without disturbing the normal breast architecture; sometimes a non-specific abnormality is detectable clinically or with ultrasound without it being apparent on a mammogram (Fig. 9.28).

Invasive lobular carcinoma tends to be larger at presentation and has a high risk of multifocality and bilaterality. Patients are more likely to require mastectomy to achieve clear resection margins, but breast conservation (and adjuvant therapy) is sometimes possible; invasive lobular and ductal carcinomas have similar recurrence, and disease-free and overall survival rates (Molland et al

2004). Metastatic lobular carcinoma usually has a diffuse pattern of spread, but lesions are nearly always estrogen receptor positive and patients respond well to endocrine therapy.

CARCINOMA IN THE PEDIATRIC PATIENT

Adenocarcinoma of the breast is extremely rare under the age of 18 years (Office for National Statistics 2003), but invasive ductal, invasive lobular, signet-ring and secretory lesions have been reported (Corpron et al 1995). Ultrasound is the indicated first-line investigation in the pediatric patient with a breast mass, sonographic appearances being similar to those seen in adults, with ultrasound-guided needle core biopsy feasible in most cases. The 'juvenile secretory' type of carcinoma is particularly associated with the pediatric patient and has a more favorable prognosis than other histological types (Ashikari et al 1977). Surgical and adjuvant therapy regimes similar to those employed in the adult population are required for effective disease control (Karl et al 1985, Murphy et al 2000, Rivera-Hueto et al 2002).

INFLAMMATORY CARCINOMA

Inflammatory carcinoma may be found in association with any type of breast malignancy and is characterized by the presence of tumor emboli in the dermal lymphatics. The disease is often metastatic at presentation and, although it may be surgically managed following chemo- or radiotherapy, has a uniformly poor prognosis.

On clinical examination, the breast has typical inflammatory features, being diffusely hard, odematous, erythematous and hyperthermic (Heywang-Kobrunner et al 2001, pp. 272–273). Mammography shows diffuse skin thickening and the affected breast often requires increased exposure dose to achieve adequate penetration. Ultrasound also shows marked skin thickening, thickened Cooper's ligaments and dilated superficial lymphatic channels (Fig. 9.29). It is often difficult, if not impossible to demonstrate the underlying tumor focus; however, tissue diagnosis is achieved with skin biopsy.

Inflammatory carcinoma is clinically indistinguishable from simple inflammation (mastitis) without biopsy; both are associated with axillary lymphadenopathy, with nodes losing their normal cortico-hilar differentiation. Inflammatory carcinoma and lymph node abnormality persist and progress despite antibiotic therapy.

SARCOMA

Sarcoma in the breast is rare, but more common in women than men; it can occur at any age but often presents in middle-aged women (Heywang-Kobrunner

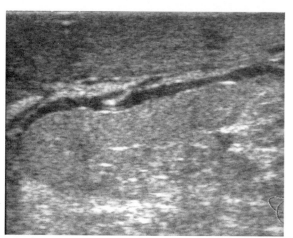

Figure 9.29 In inflammatory carcinoma, ultrasound shows marked skin thickening and dilated lymphatic channels.

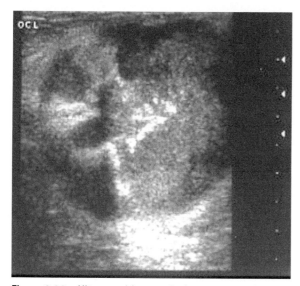

Figure 9.30 Ultrasound image of a large osteogenic sarcoma—it has a well-defined smooth margin and a heterogeneous internal echo texture.

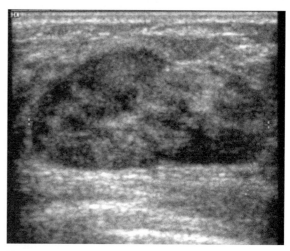

Figure 9.31 Ultrasound image of a large lymphoma—again this has a smooth well-defined margin. Its reflectivity is generally lower than that of the surrounding breast tissue but it is heterogeneous in both reflectivity and echo texture; it exhibits increased through transmission. Lesion size and advanced patient age raise the suspicion for malignancy.

Lesion compressibility, or elasticity varies with tumor subtype, liposarcomas and angiosarcomas being soft and compressible whereas fibrohistiocytomas and fibrosarcomas are firm and less compressible (Heywang-Kobrunner et al 2001, p. 329).

HEMATOLOGICAL MALIGNANCIES

The breast can occasionally be the site of hematological malignancies such as non-Hodgkin's lymphoma, leukemia and, rarely, Hodgkin's lymphoma (Heywang-Kobrunner et al 2001). These tumors may present with diffuse breast enlargement and skin thickening or a focal palpable mass that is invariably soft and mobile. In addition to 'benign' clinical features, the ultrasound appearances may also be those more associated with benign tumors. Typically the mass is a well-defined, smooth-walled lobulated, oval or round lesion that has a homogeneous internal reflectivity and echo texture, is hypo- or isoreflective compared with adjacent normal breast tissue and may exhibit increased through transmission (Fig. 9.31); occasionally, however, infiltration is diffuse and difficult to circumscribe sonographically. In practice, differential diagnosis and level of suspicion attributed to such findings is increased with a pertinent clinical history, large tumor size and hypervascularity; 35% will have regional lymphadenopathy. Although increasing patient age is a noted association, pediatric cases have been reported (Soyupak et al 2000).

et al 2001, p. 328). Sarcomas are rapidly growing tumors that have a well-defined, lobulated or nodular, heterogeneous appearance on ultrasound (Fig. 9.30) (Heywang-Kobrunner et al 2001, p. 329, Hagen-Ansert 2004).

The angiosarcoma is a highly malignant variant forming vascular channels lined with malignant endothelial cells. Clinically the lesion may be ill defined and be associated with skin thickening and nipple retraction. Ultrasound appearances are varied but include a smooth well-defined nodular mass that is generally hyporeflective with hyper-reflective (hemorrhagic) components.

METASTASES

Primary malignancy elsewhere in the body may spread to the breast, most commonly from melanoma, prostate, bronchial, ovarian and renal carcinomas, and from sarcomas (Heywang-Kobrunner et al 2001, p. 335, Hagen-Ansert 2004). In children, breast metastases have been reported in association with rhabdomyosarcoma (Beattie et al 1990, Tamiolakis et al 2004). On ultrasound, the lesions may be solitary or multiple, and usually have a well-circumscribed nodular appearance (Heywang-Kobrunner et al 2001, p. 335). Metastases in the breast tend to be hyporeflective and homogeneous, with no posterior shadowing; some show skin adherence (25%) and many (40%) are associated with axillary lymphadenopathy. Appearances are often indistinguishable from a benign lesion and, although appropriate patient history again can raise the level of suspicion, a definitive diagnosis is obtained with needle biopsy.

LYMPH NODES

Lymph node status is the most important prognostic factor in breast cancer with larger primary tumors, and those with a high number of internal tumor vessels more likely to be associated with positive axillary lymph nodes and therefore poorer prognosis (Santamaria et al 2005). Sonographic assessment of lymph nodes should be performed whenever a focal lesion is classified as indeterminate, suspicious or malignant.

Abnormal-looking lymph nodes, i.e. those that are enlarged (short axis >10 mm), round and/or uniformly hyporeflective (Fig. 9.32) will raise the level of suspicion when the index lesion is indeterminate or suspicious, whereas the demonstration of morphologically normal lymph nodes might reduce the level of suspicion for indeterminate lesions in the low-risk patient. The detection of abnormal lymph nodes, in particular ones that have lost their hyper-reflective center and show eccentric cortical widening, has good predictive value for metastatic spread, although the negative predictive value is not high enough to exclude micrometastases in an overtly malignant-looking index lesion (Clough et al 2005).

In addition to assessing the morphology of the lymph nodes, Doppler ultrasound allows assessment of lymph node vascularity (Fig. 9.33). Increased vascularity can occur in both benign reactive and metastatic lymph nodes but, even in the absence of an abnormal 2D B-mode appearance, should be regarded with suspicion.

The isolated finding of abnormal axillary lymph nodes in the absence of a demonstrable focal lesion in the breast, systemic lymphoproliferative (leukemia, lymphoma) or other known malignant or autoimmune

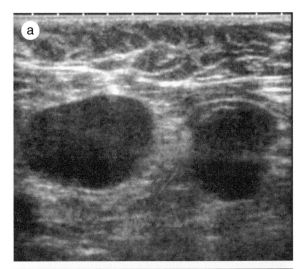

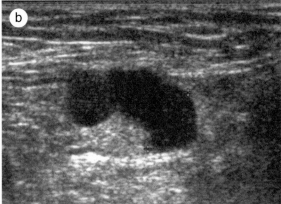

Figure 9.32   (a) Enlarged lymph nodes that are round and uniformly hyporeflective are invariably metastatic—note the loss of a hyper-reflective central hilum. (b) Some metastatic lymph nodes have a preserved hyper-reflective hilum—their cortical tissue is thickened and the hilar and overall margins are irregular.

disease should be regarded with suspicion and prompt consideration of lymph node biopsy and/or further imaging investigations to locate a primary tumor focus.

RECURRENT DISEASE

Ultrasound can be used to examine patients who present with a clinical abnormality at the site of previous breast surgery or in the regional lymph node fossae. In the postmastectomy patient, solid recurrent tumors are readily demonstrated on the anterior chest wall, but appearances can be non-specific in the early postoperative phase. Following wide–local excision, differentiating

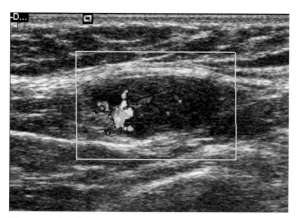

Figure 9.33   Enlarged lymph nodes due to both inflammation and metastatic tumor spread will show increased vascularity on color flow mapping Doppler.

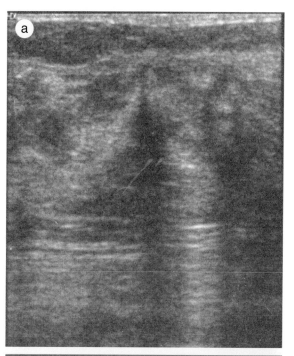

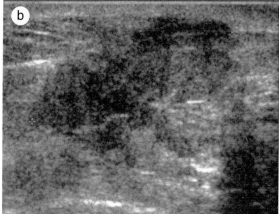

between scar tissue and recurrent or residual disease within the breast parenchyma may be difficult as both may exhibit heterogeneous hyporeflectivity and posterior acoustic shadowing (Fig. 9.34). The presence of color flow Doppler signals increases the level of suspicion, but absence does not exclude malignancy. Magnetic resonance imaging (MRI) is a more sensitive and specific examination for evaluation of potential recurrent disease, but its value is also limited in the early postoperative phase. In most cases of suspected recurrence, diagnostic biopsy cannot be avoided.

MULTIFOCAL, MULTICENTRIC AND BILATERAL BREAST CANCER

Multifocal is the term used to describe the presence of multiple tumor nodules, usually closely spaced in the same ductal system and therefore within the same breast quadrant, arising from a single primary tumor; multicentric describes multiple independent primary lesions usually at a distance of 4–5 cm separation in the same breast; bilateral breast cancer describes the presence of independent primary tumors in each breast (Dawson 1996, Madjar 2000. p. 151).

Up to 40% of patients diagnosed with breast cancer will have ipsilateral multifocal/multicentric disease (Zonderland et al 1999, Wilkinson et al 2005) and approximately 3% of women will have bilateral disease (Kollias et al 2001, Wilkinson et al 2005). In 2.5% of women, bilateral disease is evident at diagnosis (synchronous disease) and in a smaller number (0.5%) it becomes apparent following initial diagnosis and treatment (metachronous disease) (Kollias et al 2001). Detection of multiple tumor nodules (Fig. 9.35) has a significant impact on disease management, most notably making breast

Figure 9.34   (a) Post-operative scarring sometimes has the ultrasound appearance of an irregular focal mass with posterior shadowing. This can be difficult to differentiate from tumor recurrence. (b) Ultrasound image demonstrating extensive recurrent tumor at the site of a previous wide local excision. Characteristic malignant features are similar to those of primary malignancy—an irregular, ill-defined outline, overall reduced reflectivity compared with the surrounding breast tissue and a heterogeneous internal echo texture.

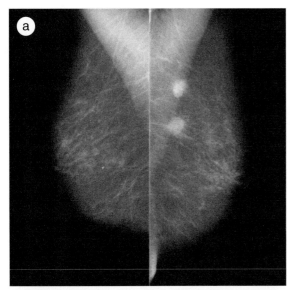

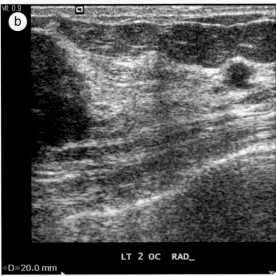

Figure 9.35   (a and b) Multifocal malignancy can be demonstrated both mammographically (a) and sonographically (b).

conservation options less likely to achieve adequate local control or acceptable cosmetic result (Heywang-Kobrunner et al 2001, p. 270).

Increasingly, evidence is emerging that the inclusion of bilateral whole breast ultrasound 'screening' at diagnosis and during successive routine surveillance of malignant disease increases detection of additional lesions and has a positive influence on patient management (Kolb et al 1998, Buchberger et al 2000, Wilkinson et al 2005).

Whole breast ultrasound is particularly worthy of consideration when the original malignancy is not, or not well demonstrated at mammography. Women with a positive family history are more likely to suffer bilateral and early onset disease. Given the reduced sensitivity of mammography for such women, in view of their average lower age and therefore the tendency to have dense breasts, bilateral whole breast ultrasound may be indicated in family history screening regimes, although such practice might be associated with an increased benign to malignant biopsy rate.

When ultrasound has been used as the primary investigation, in young women for instance, and focal lesions exhibiting 'malignant' characteristics are detected, bilateral mammography and whole breast ultrasound 'screening' should be performed to look for further lesions and microcalcifications before any interventional procedure is undertaken (Jackson et al 1996).

FOLLOW-UP OF MEDICALLY MANAGED BREAST CANCERS

Ultrasound can be used to monitor disease response to endocrine or chemotherapy, with the technique allowing accurate serial measurements of lesion size and vascularity. Reduced tumoral blood flow following chemotherapy often predates any change in physical size of the tumor and is thus a more sensitive indicator of tumor response to treatment than anatomical measurement (Madjar 2000, p. 240, Svensson 2006).

MALIGNANT VARIANTS OF BENIGN LESIONS

The 'phyllodes tumour', cystosarcoma phyllodes or giant fibroadenoma, is a rare epithelial–stromal tumor similar to the fibroadenoma but with more cellular and mitotically active stromal tissue; the tumor may be classified as benign, 'borderline malignant' or overtly 'malignant' depending on the number of mitoses and the presence of cellular atypia at histological examination (Tot et al 2002, p. 82).

Clinically, phyllodes tumors are rapidly enlarging lesions that may quickly occupy a large area of the breast (Fig. 9.36). Occasionally they have been reported in the adolescent female (Martino et al 2001, Agarwal & Sparnon 2005, Gojnic et al 2005). On ultrasound, they have the appearance of an oval lobulated mass with a well-defined margin (Fig. 9.37); they are generally hypo-reflective but heterogeneous with hyper-reflective dividing segmentations and some central cystic spaces. They

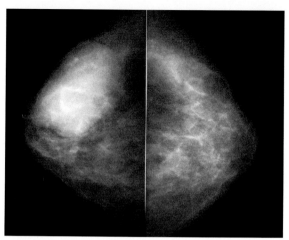

Figure 9.36 The phylloides tumor is usually large at presentation—this one occupies most of the outer half of the right breast; its mammographic appearance is that of asymmetrically increased density.

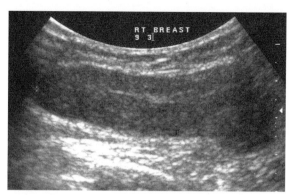

Figure 9.37 On ultrasound, the phyllodes tumor is typically large, with a well-defined smooth margin. The internal characteristics vary and do not particularly contribute to a differential diagnosis. Histologically, phyllodes tumors are heterogeneous, and excision biopsy is required to ascertain their malignant potential fully.

exhibit increased posterior through transmission and are dramatically hypervascular (Hagen-Ansert 2004).

Stromal components of phyllodes tumors may contain areas of liposarcoma, rhabdomyosarcoma or osteosarcoma, and the epithelial components can have areas of DCIS, LCIS or invasive carcinoma (Tot et al 2002, p. 82). This heterogeneity makes adequate needle sampling a challenge, with the potential for both under- and over-estimation of malignant potential (Tot et al 2002, p. 83). Due to their size, progression rate and histological heterogeneity, excision is recommended and usually requires a generous wide local procedure if not mastectomy (Heywang-Kobrunner et al 2001, p. 326). If not widely excised, both benign and malignant variants may recur, any metastatic spread being hematogenous.

Radial scars are small (<10 mm) benign lesions consisting of tubular structures radiating out from a central fibro-elastic zone (NHSCSP & RCP 2005). Radial scars are usually detected at mammography and are difficult to differentiate from invasive carcinoma both histologically and on imaging. Mammography shows a stellate lesion, often with a lucent (black) star-shaped central nidus on a dense (white) background; ultrasound features may also mimic those of a malignant lesion if any abnormality is visible at all (Stavros 2004, pp. 704–705). The presence of low-grade cancer cells (atypical ductal or lobular hyperplasia or carcinoma in situ) in the corona surrounding the central sclero-elastic core or an associated tubular carcinoma is not unusual (Heywang-Kobrunner et al 2001, p. 272, Tot et al 2002, pp. 93–96); because of such lesion heterogeneity, radial scars are often excised.

SUMMARY

Clinical, imaging and pathology correlation are fundamental to collaborative multidisciplinary diagnosis of malignant breast disease and to the planning and management of surgical intervention and oncology therapy.

Breast ultrasound has an important role in the detection and follow-up of malignant disease by virtue of its excellent sensitivity and specificity when performed by experienced practitioners within a 'triple assessment' context. Careful ultrasound technique and consistent and reliable application of sonographic criteria to lesion evaluation, combined with comprehensive practitioner knowledge of breast anatomy and pathology, will optimize the contribution ultrasound can make to a breast care service.

Breast lesions exhibiting clinical or imaging features that render them indeterminate, suspicious or malignant are selectively referred for histological analysis to confirm or exclude malignancy, to delineate in situ and invasive disease and to provide additional prognostic information.

Despite the selective use of MRI in addition to routine mammography and ultrasound, a finite number of malignant lesions will exhibit no abnormal imaging findings. Where the clinical examination findings raise suspicion, negative imaging does not obviate the need for histological evaluation.

References

Agarwal P, Sparnon AL 2005 Benign breast lesions in adolescent girls: an overview with a case report. Pediatric Surgery International 21(5):381–382.

Ashikari H, Jun MY, Farrow JH et al 1977 Breast carcinoma in children and adolescents. Clinical Bulletin 7(2):55–62.

Beattie M, Kingston JE, Norton AJ et al 1990 Nasopharyngeal rhabdomyosarcoma presenting as a breast mass. Pediatric Hematology and Oncology 7(3): 259–263.

Bosch AM, Kessels AG, Beets GL et al 2003 Preoperative estimation of the pathological breast tumour size by physical examination, mammography and ultrasound: a prospective study on 105 invasive tumours. European Journal of Radiology 48(3):285–292.

Buchberger W, Nichoff A, Obrist P, DeKoekkoek-Doll P, Dunser M 2000 Clinically and mammographically occult breast lesions: detections and classification with high-resolution sonography. Seminars in Ultrasound CT MR 21(4):325–336.

Carder PJ, Garvican J, Haigh I et al 2005 Needle core biopsy can reliably distinguish between benign and malignant papillary lesions of the breast. Histopathology 46(3):320–327.

Clough GR, Truscott J, Haigh I 2005 Can high frequency ultrasound predict metastatic lymph nodes in patients with invasive breast cancer? Radiography 12(2):96–104.

Corpron CA, Black CT, Singletary SE et al 1995 Breast cancer in adolescent females. Journal of Pediatric Surgery 30(2):322–324.

Dawson PJ 1996 Bilateral and multifocal breast cancer. Online. Cancer Control Journal 3(3) Available at: http://www.moffitt.usf.edu/pubs/ccj/v3n3/dept6.html Accessed 17 May 2002.

Denley H, Pinder SE, Elston CW 2001 Pre-operative assessment of prognostic factors in breast cancer. Journal of Clinical Pathology 54:20–24.

Fisher B, Land S, Mamounas E, Dignam J, Fisher ER, Wolmark N 2001 Prevention of invasive breast cancer in women with ductal carcinoma in situ: an update of the national surgical adjuvant breast and bowel project experience. Seminars in Oncology 28(4):400–418.

Gojnic M, Dugalic V, Vidakovic S et al 2005 Breast cancer and borderline ovarian carcinoma in young patients—a case report. European Journal of Gynaecological Oncology 26(5):579–580.

Hagen-Ansert S 2004 Sonographic evaluation of the breast. Online. GE Medical Systems. Available at: http://www.gehealthcare.com/usen/education/proff_leadership/products/msucmebr.html Accessed 30 November 2005.

Heywang-Kobrunner SH, Dershaw DD, Schreer I 2001 Diagnostic breast imaging. Stuttgart: Thieme.

Huang C-S, Wu C-Y, Chu J-S et al 1999 Microcalcifications of non-palpable lesions detected with ultrasonography: correlation with mammography and histopathology. Ultrasound in Obstetrics and Gynecology 13:431–436.

Jackson VP, Reynolds HE, Hawes DR 1996 Sonogrpahy of the breast. Seminars in Ultrasound, CT and MRI 17(5):460–475.

Karl SR, Ballantine TV, Zaino R 1985 Juvenile secretory carcinoma of the breast. Journal of Pediatric Surgery 20(4):368–371.

Kolb T, Lichy J, Newhouse J 1998 Occult cancer in women with dense breasts: detection with screening US—diagnostic yield and tumour characteristics. Radiology 207(1):191–199.

Kollias J, Ellis IO, Elston CW et al 2001 Prognostic significances of synchronous and metachronous bilateral breast cancer. World Journal of Surgery 25(9):1117–1124.

Lister D, Evans A, Burrell H et al 1998 The accuracy of breast ultrasound in the evaluation of clinically benign discrete symptomatic breast lumps. Clinical Radiology 53:490–492.

Madjar H 2000 Practical breast ultrasound. Stuttgart: Thieme.

Molland JG, Donnellan M, Janu NC et al 2004 Infiltrating lobular carcinoma—a comparison with diagnosis, management and outcome with infiltrating ductal carcinoma. The Breast 13:389–396.

Martino A, Zamparelli M, Santinelli A et al 2001 Unusual clinical presentation of a rare case of phyllodes tumour of the breast in an adolescent girl. Journal of Pediatric Surgery 36(6):941–943.

Murphy JJ, Morzaria S, Gow KW et al 2000 Breast cancer in a 6-year-old child. Journal of Pediatric Surgery 35(5):765–767.

Neuschatz AC, DiPetrillo T, Safaii H, Lowther D, Landa M, Wazer DE 2001 Margin width as a determinant of local control with and without radiation therapy for ductal carcinoma in situ (DCIS) of the breast. International Journal of Cancer 96:S97–104.

NHSCSP & RCP 2005 Pathology reporting of breast disease. Publication No. 58. Sheffield, UK: NHS Cancer Screening Programme and London: Royal College of Pathologists.

O'Driscoll D, Britton P, Wishart GC et al 2001 Lobular carcinoma in situ on core biopsy—what is the clinical significance? Clinical Radiology 56(3):216–220.

Office for National Statistics 2003 New cases of cancer diagnosed in England, 2003: selected sites by age group and sex. Online. Available at: http://www. statistics.gov.uk/statbase/Expodata/Spreadsheets/D9096.xls Accessed 16 January 2006.

Pope TL, Fechner RE, Wilhelm MC et al 1988 Lobular carcinoma in situ of the breast: mammographic features. Radiology 168:63.

Rivera-Hueto F, Hevia-Vazquez A, Utrilla-Alcolea JC et al 2002 Long-term prognosis of teenagers with breast cancer. International Journal of Surgical Pathology 10(4):273–279.

Santamaria G, Velasco M, Farre X et al 2005 Power Doppler sonography of invasive breast carcinoma: does tumour vascularization contribute to prediction of axillary status? Radiology 234:374–380.

Schwartz GF 2001 The current treatment of ductal carcinoma in situ. Breast Journal 7(5):308–310.

Snelling JD, Abdullah N, Brown G et al 2004 Measurement of tumour size in case selection for breast cancer therapy by clinical assessment and ultrasound. European Journal of Surgical Oncology 30(1):5–9.

Stavros AT 2004 Breast ultrasound. Philadelphia: Lippincott, Williams and Wilkins.

Soyupak SK, Sire D, Inal M 2000 Secondary involvement of breast with non-Hodgkin's lymphoma in a paediatric patient presenting as bilateral breast masses. European Radiology 10(3):519–520.

Svensson WE 2006 Breast imaging update. Ultrasound 14(1):20–33.

Tamiolakis D, Venizelos I, Nikolaidou S et al 2004 Bilateral metastatic rhabdomyosarcoma to the breast in an adolescent female: touch imprint cytology and implication of MyoD1 nuclear antigen. Onkologie 27(5):460–471.

Teh W, Wilson A 1998 The role of ultrasound in breast cancer screening. A consensus statement by the European Group for Breast Cancer Screening. European Journal of Cancer 34(4):449–450.

Tohno E, Cosgrove DO, Sloane JP 1994 Ultrasound of breast diseases. Edinburgh: Churchill Livingstone.

Tot T, Tabar L, Dean PB 2002 Practical breast pathology. New York: Thieme.

Wilkinson LS, Given-Wilson R, Hall T et al 2005 Increasing the diagnosis of multifocal primary breast cancer by the use of bilateral whole-breast ultrasound. Clinical Radiology 60:573–578.

Zonderland HM, Coerkamp EG, Hermans J, van der Vijver MJ, van Voorthuisen AdE 1999 Diagnosis of breast cancer: Contribution of US as an adjunct to mammography. Radiology 213:413–422.

Chapter **10**

Ultrasound of the augmented breast

Anne-Marie Dixon

INTRODUCTION

Breast prostheses are silicone- and/or saline-filled pouches that are surgically implanted into the breast. Approximately 2 million women in the USA have had implants inserted, and approximately 200 000 procedures are performed annually (13 000 in the UK) (Martin-Moreno et al 2000). Most (70–80%) prostheses are inserted for cosmetic augmentation or remodeling, subsequent improvement in psychological well-being due to self-image enhancement and increased self-confidence being well recognized (Martin-Moreno et al 2000). Breast prostheses are also used to correct congenital or traumatic deformity and for breast reconstruction following therapeutic or prophylactic mastectomy (Scarenelo et al 2004).

Prosthesis design has evolved since their first use in the 1960s to try to reduce the incidence of complications and to improve the cosmetic result (Stavros & Rapp 2004, p. 199). Those in current use may be of either single or double lumen type. Single lumen implants contain either silicone gel or saline solution encapsulated in a thin silicone rubber/plastic (elastomer) shell; the double lumen type have an inner silicone-filled lumen and a smaller outer lumen usually filled with saline solution (O'Toole & Caskey 2000, Hölmich et al 2005). Once implanted, as a consequence of the body's natural immune response to the presence of a foreign body, the prosthesis is surrounded and enclosed within a fibrous connective tissue capsule. Despite improvements in implant materials over the years, the slow diffusion of silicone oil through an apparently intact, but obviously semi-porous, implant shell (gel bleed) is a recognized phenomenon, and silicone migration to both local and remote areas of the body has been observed (Brown et al 1997, Caskey et al 1999, Teuber et al 1999, Breiting et al 2004).

In the postmastectomy patient, implants are positioned either deep to the pectoralis muscle, described as either subpectoral, retropectoral, submuscluar or retromuscular, or superficial to it, described as either prepectoral or subcutaneous (Fig. 10.1). For elective cosmetic augmentation, implants can again be placed underneath the pectoralis muscle, but are usually positioned between the muscle and normal glandular tissue, i.e. prepectoral, retroglandular or subglandular (Fig. 10.2). Of interest to ultrasound practitioners particularly, the diagnostically important tissue thus lies superficial to the implant and is readily accessible to ultrasound evaluation.

There is currently no convincing evidence that the presence of a breast prosthesis increases a woman's risk of cancer or systemic neurological, connective tissue or autoimmune disorder, although associated local complications, such as pain, capsular contracture and implant rupture, are common and well recognized (Brown et al 1997, Martin-Moreno et al 2000, Breiting et al 2004).

IMAGING THE AUGMENTED BREAST

Silicone gel and, to a lesser extent, saline solution are both radio-opaque and this makes mammography suboptimal, with ultrasound the preferred first line investigation for patients with implants in situ (RCR 2003).

Mammography is associated with a small risk of implant rupture and it can be difficult to achieve optimal positioning and adequate compression when the patient is in pain or there is severe capsular fibrosis (Caskey et al 1999). If the implant has been inserted electively for cosmetic purposes and occupies less than 50% of the breast volume, it is possible to achieve mammographic demonstration of at least 70% of the natural breast tissue using a specialized displacement technique known as Eklund views (Fig. 10.3) (RCR 2003); this technique is not practical in patients with a postmastectomy reconstruction. Mammography is of limited value in assessing implant integrity (Robinson et al 1995), and the presence of prostheses most often totally precludes useful assessment of any natural breast tissue (Fig. 10.4). Mammography, however, is the most reliable technique for detecting free residual silicone in the breast after implant removal (Caskey et al 1999).

Magnetic resonance imaging (MRI) is the most sensitive and specific diagnostic imaging technique when implants are present due to its excellent demonstration of both the implant and the surrounding tissue (Caskey et al 1999, Madjar 2000, p. 115). As a relatively high cost examination, MRI is not suitable for routine use and, in a minority of patients, i.e. those with temporary or expander implants that have a magnetic filling valve

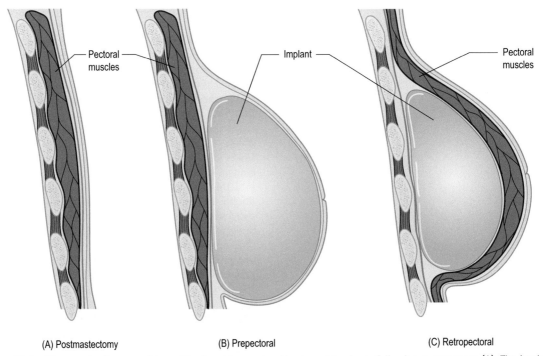

(A) Postmastectomy　　　　(B) Prepectoral　　　　(C) Retropectoral

Figure 10.1 Diagram to show possible positioning of reconstructive breast implants following mastectomy (A). The implant is described as being prepectoral when placed anterior to the pectoralis muscle (B) and retropectoral when placed beneath the muscle (C).

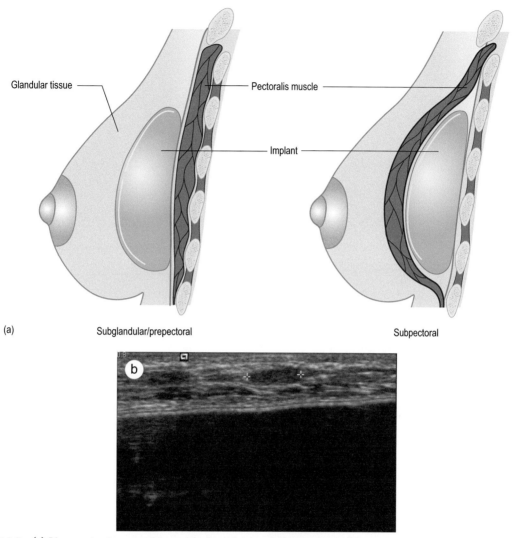

Glandular tissue

Pectoralis muscle

Implant

(a) Subglandular/prepectoral

Subpectoral

b

Figure 10.2 (a) Diagram to show possible positioning of cosmetic (augmentation) breast implants. When placed anterior to the pectoralis muscle, the implant is described as being either subglandular or prepectoral; when positioned beneath the pectoralis muscle, the implant is described as being retropectoral. (b) Ultrasound image of a breast with a prepectoral implant in situ. The functional breast tissue, and a small palpable focal mass, are seen anterior to the implant.

and those with implants that have a metallic identification chip, MRI is contraindicated.

Ultrasound is a clinically useful and a cost-effective alternative to MRI (Liston et al 1994, Netscher et al 1996). In experienced hands, the ultrasound examination is sensitive and specific and has good predictive value for abnormalities of the breast and chest wall tissues and complications related to the implant itself (DeBruhl et al 1993, Harris et al 1993, Liston et al 1994, Venta et al 1996). Routine implant screening is not indicated (Berg et al 1993), and most referrals are patients presenting with an abnormal clinical finding, either a focal palpable lump or a change in the shape, volume or

consistency of the breast. Underlying causes include benign and primary malignant disease of parenchymal breast tissue, recurrent malignant disease and implant leakage or rupture. Occasionally patients present with pain, inflammation or hardening of the breast due to either capsular fibrosis or postoperative infection or hematoma.

ULTRASOUND TECHNIQUE AND NORMAL ULTRASOUND APPEARANCES

It is important to take a careful clinical and implant history before embarking on the imaging investigation

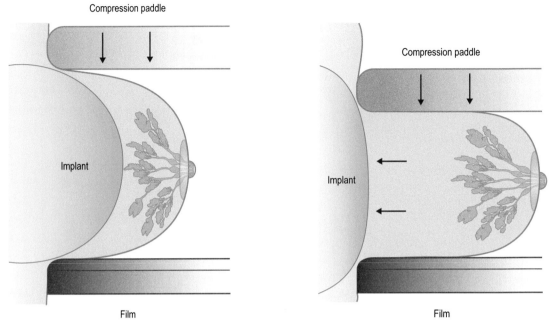

Figure 10.3 Eklund' mammography views involve manual displacement of an implant out of the primary radiation beam to avoid superimposition of implant contents over the natural tissue of the breast.

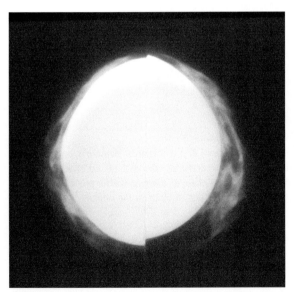

Figure 10.4 With routine mammography technique, implants obscure most of the natural breast tissue and may mask pathology.

in order to aid image interpretation and to improve diagnostic reliability. The ultrasound practitioner should attempt to ascertain the type of implant in situ, the time interval since implantation and if there is any history of complication, additional surgery, removal of previously inserted implants or injection of free silicone (Berg et al 1993, O'Toole & Caskey 2000, Hölmich et al 2005).

The ultrasound examination should always include evaluation of the whole breast (O'Toole & Caskey 2000) and include assessment of both the implant and the surrounding breast and chest wall tissues, with appropriate manipulation of the equipment controls to optimize the settings throughout. In particular, when imaging the implant, the overall gain should be reduced to minimize reverberation artifact, the focal zone placed deeper and the depth of view increased to include the anterior chest wall in the image (Fig. 10.5). When imaging the more superficial breast parenchyma, use of magnification (reduced depth of view) and anterior placement of the focal zone will maximize spatial resolution, thus improving the capability for detection of breast pathology (Fig. 10.6).

Knowledge of the position and type of the prosthesis is important when evaluating sonographic appearances of the implant and those of the surrounding breast and chest wall tissues. Visualization of the upper outer quadrant of the breast allows sonographic identification of the

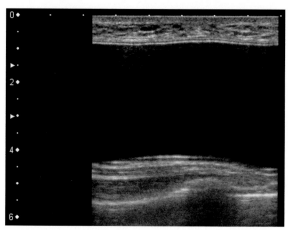

Figure 10.5 In order to demonstrate and evaluate the whole implant and the chest wall anatomy, the ultrasound depth of view will need to be increased to approximately 6 cm.

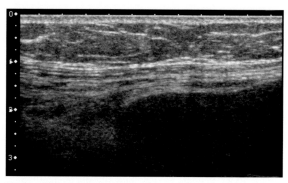

Figure 10.7 Ultrasound imaging in the upper outer quadrant of the breast will allow determination of implant position with reference to pectoralis muscle—this image demonstrates retropectoral placement.

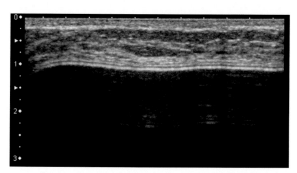

Figure 10.6 Once the implant and anterior chest wall have been assessed, the breast tissue anterior to the implant should be evaluated on magnified images limited to the superficial anatomy—the depth of view should be reduced and the focal zone moved more anteriorly.

implant site and differentiation of retro- or prepectoral location (Fig. 10.7) (Madjar 2000, p. 115). Careful scanning at the periphery of the implant, with the transducer face parallel to the chest wall, may help to identify the implant type, but the various types may appear indistinguishable (O'Toole & Caskey 2000).

Sound attenuation in the saline/silicone implant is minimal, rendering the chest wall readily visible deep to the implant, but implant filling material, in particular silicone, produces several image artifacts. The depth of view of the ultrasound image invariably needs to be increased in order to demonstrate the chest wall, the silicone implant appearing much larger on ultrasound images than it is in reality. Areas deep to the implant

seem to lie at a greater depth from the skin surface than they are in reality and, in addition, the anterior chest wall will appear disrupted and discontinuous across the width of the image (Fig. 10.8 and Fig. 10.9).

These 'misregistration' artifacts occur because the speed of sound in silicone (997 ms^{-1}) is slower than in normal breast tissues (Stavros & Rapp 2004, p. 212). Since the ultrasound machine is calibrated to assume that pulse–echo signals are traveling at the average speed of sound in soft tissue (1540 ms^{-1}), ultrasound signals arising from tissue boundaries where the sound has had to travel more slowly through the implant are plotted at a greater distance from the transducer/skin surface than their true depth (see Ch. 4 for a full explanation). The speed of sound in saline is similar to the average speed assumed by equipment manufacturers for soft tissues in general, and thus saline-filled implants have less anomalous effect on spatial relationships in the image.

Occasionally, a lower frequency (3.5–5 MHz) and a wider diverging field of view (curvilinear array) are needed to evaluate fully the posterior implant margins and anterior chest wall structures (O'Toole & Caskey 2000, Scaranelo et al 2004).

The ultrasound appearance of the implant surface depends on its shape and the degree of fibrous encapsulation that has occurred since implantation. The fibrous capsule is not usually seen separately from the implant's own elastomer shell, the normal capsule–implant surface having a single well-defined smooth hyper-reflective anterior margin (Fig. 10.10). It is not unusual for the anterior margin to have undulations (Fig. 10.11), and indeed these often correlate with a presenting palpable 'abnormality'. The implant appears triangular in shape with its base anterior in the image, and the lateral borders are not well demonstrated due to their parallel

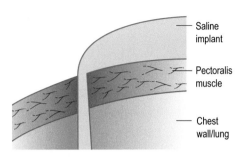

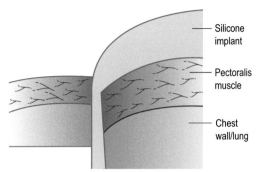

Figure 10.8   Diagram to show how silicone implants cause misregistration of acoustic interfaces. Because the speed of sound in silicone is slower than in soft tissue and in saline, echo signals traveling through the silicone take longer to return to the transducer. Since the scanner is calibrated to assume a speed of sound in normal soft tissue (1540 m s⁻¹), it represents these signals in the image as if they have come from structures further away from the transducer.

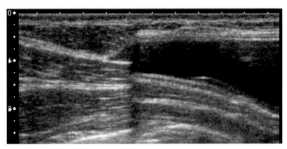

Figure 10.9   Ultrasound image to show misregistration artifact at the edge of a silicone implant.

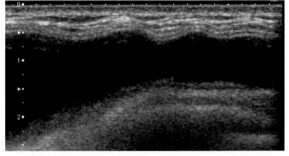

Figure 10.11   It is not unusual to see gentle ripples or undulations in the surface of an implant—these may correlate with palpable lumps.

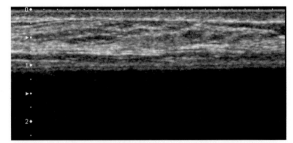

Figure 10.10   Magnified ultrasound image of the interfaces between breast tissue, the fibrous capsule and the implant elastomer shell.

orientation to the ultrasound beam axis and the effect of critical angle artifact (see Ch. 3). The lateral borders, however, are a sensitive location for silicone granuloma detection (Stavros & Rapp 2004, p. 211), and improved visualization can be achieved by placing the transducer more peripheral on the breast and angling the scan plane towards the center, or by using compound imaging software (Fig. 10.12) (O'Toole & Caskey 2000).

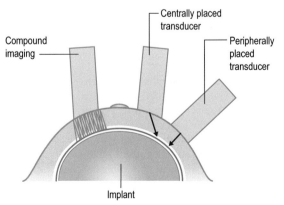

Figure 10.12   Since the edges of implants lie parallel with the ultrasound beam axis, they are not well demonstrated. Compound imaging or angling the ultrasound beam from a peripheral skin contact site can help visualize the side margins of the implant.

Although the connective tissue capsule and anterior margin of the intact implant are closely apposed and not normally visualized separately, a small amount of interposed anechoic fluid can sometimes be seen (Fig. 10.13), particularly in association with any wrinkles or folds that have developed (Heywang-Kobrunner et al 2001, pp. 124–125). This fluid is invariably echo free and should not be confused with silicone leakage. Small anechoic fluid collections around the implant (Fig. 10.14) are also considered to be a normal variant (Berg et al 1993, O'Toole & Caskey 2000).

Internally, the saline and silicone implant content should be echo free, but strong reverberation artifacts are seen, particularly anteriorly within the implant lumen (Fig. 10.15) (DeBruhl et al 1993, O'Toole & Caskey 2000) as a consequence of the large changes in acoustic impedance across the boundaries where sound enters and leaves the implant. Reverberation artifact is exacerbated if the operator exerts too much transducer pressure. This flattens the implant surface, making it parallel to the transducer face (Stavros & Rapp 2004, p. 211).

When the focal zone(s) are positioned just below the anterior surface of the implant, sound energy is concentrated at this level, increasing reverberation signal intensity (Madjar 2000, pp. 107–108). Reverberations can be reduced (Fig. 10.16) by maintaining implant surface convexity, using a single focal zone placed deep within the image, reducing depth gain compensation at the corresponding level, and by employing harmonic and/or compound signal processing functions (see Ch. 4) (Madjar 2000, pp. 107–108, Stavros & Rapp 2004, p. 212).

Since there are wide variety of implant materials and designs in current use, it is useful to examine the contralateral side as a comparative 'control' when evaluating the ultrasound appearances of the implant surface and the internal contents; adjacent display of corresponding sections can be achieved using the 'split' or 'dual' image function (Stavros & Rapp 2004, p. 211).

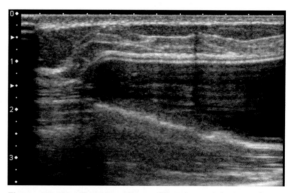

Figure 10.15 Reverberation artifact is seen deep to the anterior surface of an implant and should not be mistaken for intracapsular rupture.

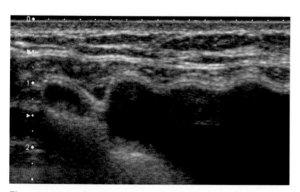

Figure 10.13 Small amounts of fluid between the anterior margin of the implant and the connective tissue capsule, particularly in association with capsular ripples, can be considered a normal finding.

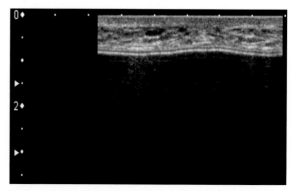

Figure 10.16 Reducing the near gain and placing the focal zone deeper in the image can reduce reverberation artifact.

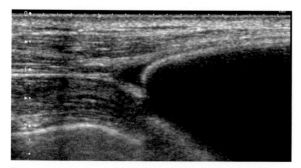

Figure 10.14 A small amount of fluid at the edge of an implant is also common and not clinically significant.

FIBROSIS, SCARRING AND CAPSULAR CONTRACTURE

As with any surgical procedure, prosthesis implantation is unavoidably associated with fibrosis and scar tissue formation, fibrous encapsulation of the implant being a normal immune response. In some cases, the fibrous capsule may undergo partial or total calcification, and some patients, particularly those with prepectoral and single lumen silicone implants, develop capsular hypertrophy. Capsular hypertrophy results in pronounced fibrotic thickening that may progress to painful shrinkage and hardening known as capsular contracture. Capsular hypertrophy is thought to result from a pronounced immune response to the 'gel bleed' phenomenon and, although occurring in up to 50% of patients with older 'smooth shell' implants, is less commonly associated with modern 'textured' implants (Martin-Moreno et al 2000, Breiting et al 2004).

Capsular contracture presents symptomatically with pain, a sensation of hardness, tension or squeezing of the breast, reduced breast/implant mobility and disfigurement, particularly spherical distortion of the breast. Ultrasound in these patients is technically challenging (O'Toole & Caskey 2000) and not particularly useful as there are no specific findings; although contracture is associated with increased implant wrinkling and folding, these are also seen as normal variant appearances (Madjar 2000, p. 109).

In addition to normal fibrotic encapsulation, surgical scarring in surrounding breast tissue may occur. On ultrasound images, scar tissue appears hyporeflective and causes posterior acoustic shadowing that reduces visualization of deeper anatomical structures. As in the non-augmented breast, these appearances are difficult to differentiate from malignancy, and high specificity cannot always be achieved even with the use of transducer compression maneuvers and color flow mapping Doppler techniques. Although of limited use in the early postoperative phase, contrast-enhanced MRI is a more accurate differentiating investigation (Madjar 2000, p. 115) and might thus be considered before contemplating a diagnostic tissue sampling procedure.

SILICONE GRANULOMA (SILICONOMA)

Silicone granuloma is the term used to describe a focal collection of silicone that has accumulated within breast tissue (DeBruhl et al 1993). Although this may be the result of overt extracapsular implant rupture, they may also form as a result of gel bleed (Brown et al 1999, Madjar 2000, p. 113). Ultrasound will differentiate extracapsular silicone and granuloma formation from a simple implant herniation—protrusion of an intact implant through a capsular defect (Stavros & Rapp 2004, p. 205).

Occasionally the silicone granuloma has the ultrasound appearance of a focal hyporeflective lesion, but more commonly it is a hyper-reflective lesion (Caskey et al 1999) similar to that of a fatty lesion such as a lipoma (Fig. 10.17) (O'Toole & Caskey 2000). The lesion characteristically has a reasonably well-defined anterior margin and a fine-grained internal echo texture; posteriorly it is ill defined and exhibits a characteristic white 'noisy' vertical shadow—the 'snowstorm' effect, and obscures structures that lie deep to it (Fig. 10.18) (Harris et al 1993, Brown et al 1997). Careful attention

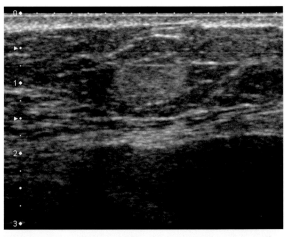

Figure 10.17 Silicone within the breast tissues is usually hyper-reflective and may take the appearance of a well-defined mass.

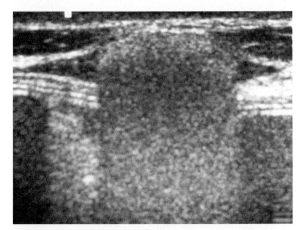

Figure 10.18 Ultrasound appearances of the classic silicone granuloma are pathognomonic—the diffuse 'noisy' posterior shadowing is described as having a 'snowstorm' appearance. (Image courtesy of Dr J. Liston, Leeds Wakefield Breast Screeing Service, Leeds, UK.)

should be paid to differentiate this effect from the classic echo-free posterior acoustic shadowing effect that might be seen deep to capsular calcification (Brown et al 1997). Sometimes, echo-free globules of silicone are seen, but usually the white noisy 'snowstorm' effect can be seen posteriorly rather than the classic increased reflectivity seen deep to a serous cystic lesion (Caskey et al 1999).

IMPLANT RUPTURE

Definitions of the characteristics for diagnosis of implant rupture include the detection of small amounts of silicone attributed to gel bleed (slow escape of silicone oil through a macroscopically intact shell), detection of visible tears in the implant membrane and the presence of complete shell disintegration (Brown et al 1997). Implant failure is a well-recognized, almost inevitable complication of breast prosthesis implantation, with some studies showing evidence of leakage or overt rupture in up to two-thirds prostheses that have been in situ between 10 and 20 years (Robinson et al 1995, Hölmich et al 2004, Scaranelo et al 2004). Although implant ruptures may be associated with trauma (including screening or diagnostic mammography), most occur spontaneously (Hölmich et al 2004), and are a time-dependent phenomenon attributed to age and progressive weakening of the implant shell (Robinson et al 1995, Brown et al 1997). Implant rupture and leakage are not always symptomatic or otherwise clinically apparent (Harris et al 1993, Robinson et al 1995, Netscher et al 1996), but diagnosis is nevertheless important since silicone dissemination and migration can be associated with acute inflammatory and immune responses that may result in severe debilitating tissue damage and neuropathy (Teuber et al 1995, 1999, Brown et al 1997). The effects of rupture of a saline-only implant are purely cosmetic, saline being readily absorbed with no adverse clinical effect (Martin-Moreno et al 2000).

Implant rupture is defined as extracapsular when silicone is found outside the fibrous connective tissue capsule and intracapsular when silicone is present outside the implant shell but confined within the fibrous connective tissue capsule.

Extracapsular rupture is occasionally evident at mammography (Fig. 10.19) as an irregular implant outline or when radio-opaque free silicone is seen within the breast or axilla outside the implant margin (Caskey et al 1999). On ultrasound, free silicone is more readily detected as it exhibits the characteristic 'snowstorm' appearance. With a small silicone leak, the appearance may be of a localized focal lesion, i.e. the silicone granuloma; with more extensive rupture there is a diffuse increase in reflectivity across the image due to widespread dispersion of silicone microglobules throughout breast tissue (Fig. 10.20). In view

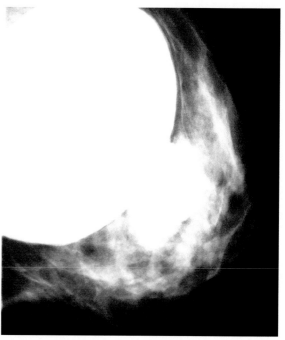

Figure 10.19 Extracapsular rupture can be seen on mammograms. This medio-lateral oblique projection of the left breast shows dense silicone in the breast outside the implant capsule margin. (Image courtesy of Dr J. Liston, Leeds Wakefield Breast Screening Service, Leeds, UK.)

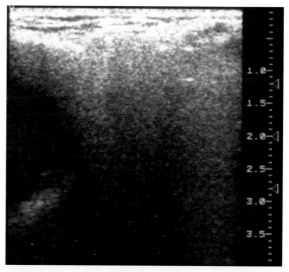

Figure 10.20 Diffuse free silicone in the breast totally degrades the ultrasound image—the 'snowstorm' shadowing effect obscures the underlying native breast tissue and the implant itself.

of the gravity dependence of fluids, the lower half of the breast is the most sensitive location for small leaks (Madjar 2000, p. 113).

Intracapsular rupture is more difficult to diagnose, with mammography invariably looking normal (Brown et al 1997), but both ultrasound and MRI can show a complicated appearance of the implant's internal structure (Berg et al 1993). On ultrasound, since the fibrous connective tissue capsule and the implant shell are normally closely apposed, any significant separation should prompt a careful evaluation for any of the characteristic signs of rupture or leakage.

Low level homogeneous echoes and/or multiple discontinuous linear 'step-ladder' reflections, the latter representing the retracted elastomer shell, may be seen within the normally echo-free implant lumen if the shell is ruptured (Fig. 10.21). However, care must be taken to differentiate this appearance from reverberation artifact due to contour variation or folding of the implant shell (Berg et al 1993, DeBruhl et al 1993, Caskey et al 1994, Venta et al 1996).

In extreme cases, a completely collapsed implant shell can be seen floating freely in the encapsulated saline–silicone liquid mixture which itself may appear either diffusely and homogenously reflective (Fig. 10.22) (Venta et al 1996, Madjar 2000, p. 110) or more heterogeneous, containing both hyporeflective globules and areas of 'snowstorm' shadowing (Scaranelo et al 2004).

Implant rupture has been confirmed where the only unusual sign is that of a bulge in the implant contour, although this is a common and somewhat non-specific finding (O'Toole & Caskey 2000).

MRI is the most sensitive and accurate diagnostic imaging investigation for implant rupture (Everson et al 1994). Non-contrast studies, using a dedicated breast

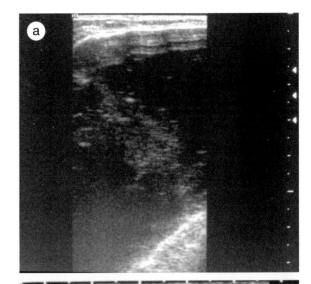

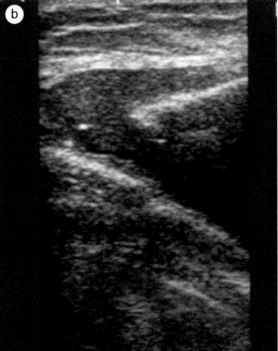

Figure 10.22 (a and b) Intracapsular rupture is also associated with complex heterogeneous echoes within the implant lumen (a); in addition to diffuse increased reflectivity, prominent hyper-reflective edges of the free floating capsule may be seen (b).

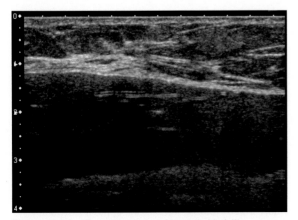

Figure 10.21 The appearance of 'step-ladder'-like reflections within an implant is indicative of intracapsular rupture.

coil and a combination of high resolution scanning sequences including silicone-specific ones, show characteristic appearances. These include the Linguini sign (Fig. 10.23) where the collapsed inner shell is visible as a lower signal (darker) curvilinear structure within the higher signal (white) silicone, and the 'salad oil sign' (Fig. 10.24) where punctuate changes in signal density are seen due to mixing of silicone and saline fluids (Heywang-Kobrunner et al 2001, p. 366, O'Toole & Caskey 2000, Hölmich et al 2005).

SILICONE MIGRATION AND LYMPHADENOPATHY

Extruded silicone can migrate throughout the upper extremity, chest and abdomen, and may be taken up by the lymphatic system (Brown et al 1997, Caskey et al 1999, Teuber et al 1999). Silicone accumulated in axillary lymph nodes (silicone lymphadenopathy) may be demonstrated with mammography but is more reliably detected sonographically (Harris et al 1993). On mammography, affected lymph nodes have a dense, radio-opaque appearance; on ultrasound (Fig. 10.25) they exhibit characteristic hyper-reflectivity and 'snowstorm' posterior shadowing (Heywang-Kobrunner et al 2001, p. 320). It is not unusual to note enlarged axillary lymph

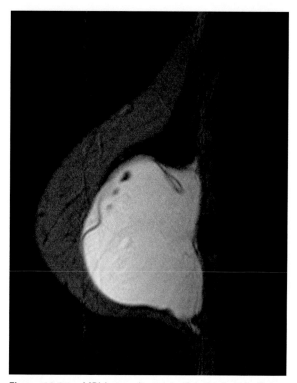

Figure 10.24   MRI image demonstrating the 'salad oil' sign associated with intracapsular rupture. In addition to the collapsed implant shell, droplets of aqueous fluid (saline) are seen floating within the inner silicone. (Image courtesy of Mrs D. Dambitis, United Leeds Teaching Hospitals NHST, UK.)

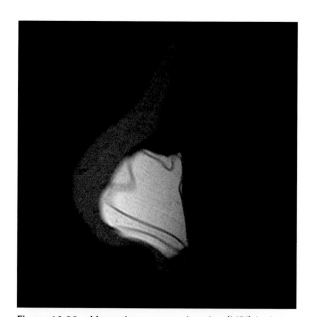

Figure 10.23   Magnetic resonance imaging (MRI) is the best diagnostic imaging technique for evaluating implant integrity. Intracapsular rupture is associated with the 'linguini' sign demonstrated here, the collapsed implant shell looking like a string of linguini pasta! (Image courtesy of Mrs D Dambitis, United Leeds Teaching Hospitals NHST, UK.)

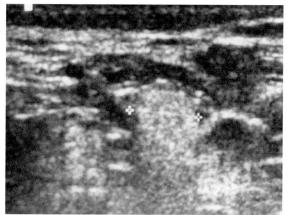

Figure 10.25   Ultrasound appearances of an axillary lymph node in a patient with implants in situ. 'Snowstorm' shadowing indicates the presence of silicone within the node—this may be a normal feature of 'gel bleed' uptake and is not necessarily indicative of implant failure. (Image courtesy of Dr J Liston, Leeds Wakefield Breast Screening Service, Leeds, UK.)

nodes that have a benign 'reactive' appearance in patients with implants in situ.

PALPABLE MASSES

Palpable masses presenting in the breast of a patient with implants in situ may arise from the implant itself or from the surrounding breast and chest wall tissues, and ultrasound can reliably differentiate and characterize these (Shestak et al 1993).

In addition to the silicone granuloma and organic breast or chest wall abnormality, palpable lumps may be due to normal variant change in the implant contour as the outer shell undulates, wrinkles or folds in response to fibrous contracture, underlying physical change in surrounding breast tissue or change in patient position and activity.

Functional parenchymal breast tissue is subject to the same physiological and pathological changes that occur in the non-augmented breast and it is clinically important that women and their healthcarers do not dismiss new palpable lumps as variant implant contour or a simple silicone granuloma. In women who have undergone cosmetic augmentation, a palpable mass may represent normal physiological parenchymal change, benign disease or malignancy, the inherent ultrasound appearances being no different from those described in preceding chapters.

Postmastectomy patients are susceptible to both de novo and recurrent malignant disease, and this is usually located superficial to the implant in the subcutaneous tissue—again appearances are similar to those described in previous chapters.

BIOPSY OF FOCAL ABNORMALITY

As in the non-augmented breast, tissue sampling is required to determine the exact nature of any solid focal lesion; in the breast with a prosthesis, percutaneous needle biopsy techniques are complicated by the risk of procedure-related implant perforation.

Where the clinical and/or imaging index of suspicion is high enough to warrant this risk and lesion location is favorable, the standard ultrasound-guided biopsy technique might safely be employed by an experienced operator. In such cases, the informed consent process should include an explicit warning of the potential risk to implant integrity.

SUMMARY

Although MRI is considered the gold standard diagnostic imaging investigation for patients with breast implants, ultrasound is a reliable and cost-effective alternative investigation for routine clinical practice, mammography being of limited utility. The experienced observer will recognize characteristic normal and abnormal appearances and thus can potentially achieve similarly high sensitivity and specificity to MRI; as such, the more costly and complicated technique might be reserved for equivocal or more unusual cases.

References

Berg WA Caskey CI, Hamper UM et al 1993 Diagnosing breast implant rupture with MR imaging, US and mammography. Radiographics 13(6):1323–1336.

Breiting VB, Hölmich LR, Brandt B et al 2004 Long-term health status of Danish women with silicone breast implants. Plastic and Reconstructive Surgery 114(1):217–226.

Brown SL, Silverman BG, Berg WA 1997 Rupture of silicone-gel breast implants: causes, sequelae, and diagnosis. Lancet 350:1531–1537.

Caskey CI, Berg WA, Anderson ND et al 1994 Breast implant rupture: diagnosis with US. Radiology 190(3):819–823.

Caskey CI, Berg WA, Hamper UM et al 1999 Imaging spectrum of extracapsular silicone: correlation of US, MR imaging, mammographic, and histopathologic findings. Radiographics 19:S39–S51.

DeBruhl ND, Gorczyca DP, Ahn CY et al 1993 Silicone breast implants: US evaluation. Radiology 189(1):95–98.

Everson LI, Parantainen H, Detlie T et al 1994 Diagnosis of breast implant rupture: imaging findings and relative efficacies of imaging techniques. AJR American Journal of Roentgenology 163(1):57–60.

Harris KM, Ganott MA, Shestak KC et al 1993 Silicone implant rupture: detection with US. Radiology 187(3):761–768.

Heywang-Kobrunner SH, Deershaw DD, Schreer I 2001 Diagnostic breast imaging. 2nd edn. Stuttgart: Thieme.

Hölmich LR, Vejborg IM, Conrad C et al 2004 Untreated silicone breast implant rupture. Plastic and Reconstructive Surgery 114(1):204–214.

Hölmich LR, Vejborg I, Conrad C et al 2005 The diagnosis of breast implant rupture: MRI findings compared with findings at explantation. European Journal of Radiology 53:213–225.

Liston J, Malata C, Varma S et al 1994 The role of ultrasound imaging in the diagnosis of breast implant rupture: a prospective study. British Journal of Plastic Surgery 47(7):477–482.

Madjar H 2000 The practice of breast ultrasound. 2000
New York: Thieme.

Martin-Moreno J, Gorgojo L, Gonzalez J et al 2000
Health risks posed by silicone implants in general with
special attention to breast implants. PE 168.396/Fin.
St./rev. Luxembourg: European Parliament.

Netscher DT, Weizer G, Malone RS et al 1996 Diagnostic value of clinical examination and various imaging
techniques for breast implant rupture as determined in
81 patients having implant removal. Southern Medical
Journal 89(4):397–404.

O'Toole M, Caskey CI 2000 Imaging spectrum of breast
implant complications: mammography, ultrasound, and
magnetic resonance imaging. Seminars in Ultrasound,
CT and MRI 21(5):351–361.

RCR 2003 Guidance on screening and symptomatic
breast imaging. 2nd edn. BFCR(03)2. London: Royal
College of Radiologists.

Robsinson OG Jr, Bradley EL, Wilson DS 1995 Analysis
of explanted silicone implants: a report of 300 cases.
Annals of Plastic Surgery 34(1):1–7.

Scaranelo AM, Marques AF, Smialowski EB et al 2004
Evaluation of the rupture of silicone breast implants by
mammography, ultrasonography and magnetic resonance imaging in asymptomatic patients: correlation
with surgical findings. Sao Paulo Medical Journal
122(2):41–47.

Shestak KC, Ganott MA, Harris KM et al 1993 Breast
masses in the augmentation mammaplasty patient: the
role of ultrasound. Plastic and Reconstructive Surgery
92(2):209–216.

Stavros AT, Rapp CL 2004 Non-targeted indications:
mammary implants. In Stavros AT (ed.) Breast ultrasound. Philadelphia: Lippincott, Williams and Wilkins,
pp. 199–275.

Teuber SS, Yoshida SH, Gershwin ME 1995 Immuno-
pathologic effects of silicone breast implants. Western
Journal of Medicine 162(5):418–425.

Teuber SS, Reilly DA, Howell L 1999 Severe migratory
granulomatous reactions to silicone gel in 3 patients.
Journal of Rheumatology 26(3):699–704.

Venta LA, Salomon CG, Flisak ME et al 1996 Sonographic signs of breast implant rupture. AJR American
Journal of Roentgenology 166(6):1413–1419.

Chapter 11

Breast disease in the male patient

Caroline Begaj

INTRODUCTION

Ultrasound examination of the male breast is easy to perform and can be chosen as the first-line diagnostic investigation, after a clinical examination and in preference to conventional mammography, due to the inherent difficulty in obtaining radiographs of a shallow, dense breast and controversy around the accuracy of mammography in this clinic setting (Evans et al 2001). The male breast can be successfully examined in contiguous transverse and longitudinal sections, with radial planes not necessary because the male breast has few, if any, lobes. A satisfactory examination can be achieved with the patient in the supine position, rather than the contra lateral posterior oblique position adopted with women, as there is less breast tissue and less need for immobilization.

It is worth noting at the outset that the majority of men, on finding a breast lump, are often acutely embarrassed, are equally as concerned as women and may experience a range of emotions similar to those reported by women (anxiety, grief, helplessness and hopelessness) on diagnosis of malignancy (Donovan 2003).

PHYSIOLOGICAL DEVELOPMENT OF THE MALE BREAST

Rudimentary male breast tissue is predominantly subcutaneous fat overlying the pectoralis muscle, with the fat supported by connective tissue septae towards the nipple (Sohn et al 1999). Small amounts of glandular tissue can be found extending towards the nipple, and this contains the major subareolar ducts, but there is little secondary branching. Lobular units are rare and, although lobular lesions are therefore rare, all pathology occurring in the female breast may also be encountered in men (Cardenosa 1997).

ULTRASOUND APPEARANCES

Normal male breast parenchyma is mainly hypo-reflective fat with sparse hyper-reflective connective tissue strands and minimal areas of glandular tissue (Fig. 11.1). The skin layer is normally thin with little or no perceptible thickening towards the nipple, the nipple itself being slightly hypo-reflective (Fig. 11.2). The pectoralis muscle is well demonstrated as horizontal hyper-reflective strands deep to the fat layer, the fat layer being of variable depth depending on the size of male breast under examination (Figs 11.3 and 11.4).

BENIGN DISEASE

A variety of benign disorders affect the male breast, by far the most common being gynecomastia. Other causes of palpable benign lumps include lipoma, subareolar sepsis, mastitis, sebaceous cyst, epidermal inclusion cyst, hematoma and fat necrosis (Gunham-Bilgen et al 2002). There is one case report of a hamartoma in a male breast, these being extremely rare and accounting for only 0.7% of female benign breast lesions (Ravakkah et al 2001). Galactoceles have been observed in the newborn male (Rahman et al 2004, Welch et al 2004).

Gynecomastia

Gynecomastia, simple hyperplasia of breast parenchyma (Fig. 11.5), is the primary benign breast condition diagnosed in males and must be differentiated from a simple excess of subcutaneous fatty tissue associated with obesity. The prevalence of true gynecomastia is estimated at 40% of all disorders of the male breast (Sohn et al 1999); it can present as a unilateral, bilateral, symmetric or asymmetric condition and shows peak incidence at puberty and in mid-life (Kopans 1989, Chersevani et al 1995).

Physiological gynecomastia is the most common finding (72%) in the pediatric male patient presenting with a breast mass (Welch et al 2004).

Gynecomastia results from an imbalance in the effects of estrogen and testosterone on the breast tissues (Stavros 2004, p. 713) and it results in breast enlargement due to subareolar duct development with secondary branching and proliferation of the surrounding stroma (Fig. 11.6). Clinically, gynecomastia usually presents as a painful swelling; it has a variety of ultrasound appearances.

Gynecomastia can occur without apparent cause in the adolescent or elderly when it is often a self-limiting condition that resolves spontaneously. More commonly, there is an underlying causative association, in particular gynecomastia is a feature of conditions that increase estrogen or decrease androgen levels (Table 11.1). If a causal mechanism is identified, removing the stimulus

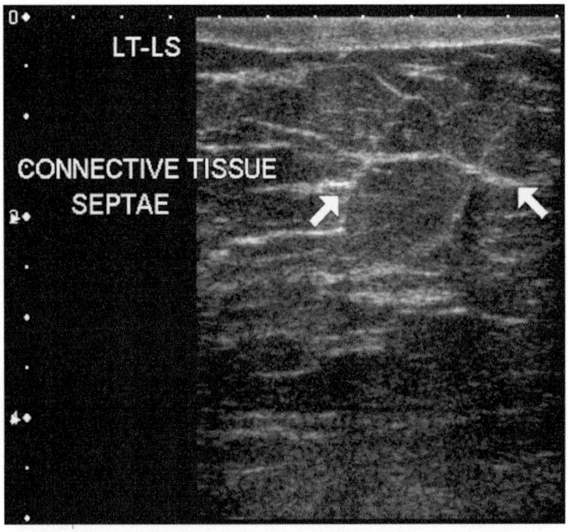

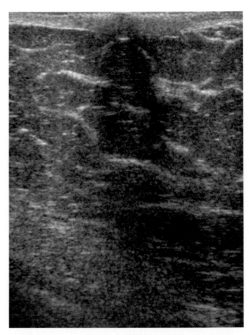

Figure 11.1 Normal ultrasound appearances of the male breast.

Figure 11.2 Normal ultrasound appearances of the male nipple.

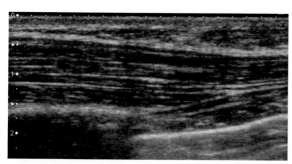

Figure 11.3   Ultrasound image showing a male breast with minimal fat layers: a small disk of breast tissue (minimal gynecomastia) is demonstrated between the skin and striated pectoralis muscles.

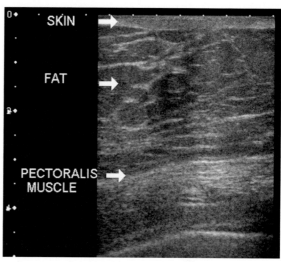

Figure 11.4   Ultrasound appearances when a significant amount of subcutaneous fatty tissue is present—note that there is no hyper-reflective 'parenchymal' layer.

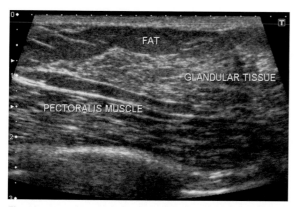

Figure 11.5   Ultrasound appearances in a patient with gynecomastia: There is a prominent hyper-reflective glandular tissue layer between the hypo-reflective subcutaneous and retromammary fat layers.

Table 11.1	Causes of gynecomastia
Common	Puberty
	Drugs—prescription therapy and misuse (spironolactone, cimetidine, digoxin, cyprotrone, steroids, marijuana)
	Alcohol
	Chronic liver disease (especially alcohol-related cirrhosis)
	Lung disease including carcinoma
	Hyperthroidism
Occasional	Hypothyroidism
	Hyperprolactinemia
	Renal disease, hemodialysis and chronic renal failure
	Testicular trauma/orchidectomy
	Testicular and adrenal tumors
Rare	Klinefelter's syndrome
	True hermaphroditism and male pseudohermaphroditism
	Acromegaly
	Hypernephroma and other carcinomas
	HIV therapy and antiviral therapy

Data from Garcia Rodriguez & Fisk (1994), Gewurz et al (2005).

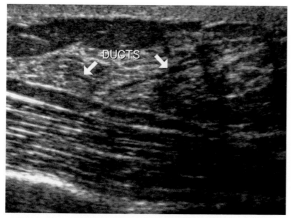

Figure 11.6   Ultrasound image of patient with gynecomastia showing well-developed ductal architecture.

may result in spontaneous regression; however, in some cases, the hyperplastic glandular tissue simply becomes inactive and fibrous. The condition is not reversible once this occurs and the only course of action, if chosen, is surgical excision (Wigley et al 1981).

Gynecomastia has three clinical phases: acute, intermediate and chronic (Kopans 1989). The acute or active phase is associated with proliferation and hyperplasia of ductal epithelial and myoepithelial tissue (Stavros 2004, p. 718). On ultrasound, the normal adipose tissue in the rudimentary breast is replaced by a hypo-reflective area, deep to the nipple, that can appear irregular, ill-defined and spiculate and the normal fat planes are distorted (Fig. 11.7). This appearance can mimic malignancy (Figs 11.8 and 11.9). The application of color Doppler is not a useful adjunct to the procedure due to its lack of specificity and the increased vascularity associated with both inflammatory and malignant change (Buada et al 1997).

In the intermediate (mixed or transitional) phase, histology shows a mixture of proliferative ductal change and some periductal fibrosis (Stavros 2004, p. 718). Sonographically there is a combination of a pronounced hypo-reflective 'mass' appearance deep to the nipple as described above (Fig. 11.10), and the development of a hyper-reflective and heterogeneous glandular ellipse of tissue that has similar ultrasound appearances to those seen in the normal female breast; subareolar ducts and their branches can be identified (Figs 11.11 and 11.12). The tissue may exhibit some posterior shadowing, but this is random and dependent upon transducer position and sound beam angulation, differentiating it from the consistent shadow associated with malignancy (Hashimoto and Bauermeister 2003).

When gynecomastia becomes inactive or chronic, dense collagenous periductal fibrous tissue is laid down (Stavros 2004, p. 718) and the ultrasound appearance is

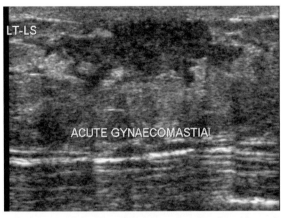

Figure 11.7 The subareolar tissues are often irregular and hyporeflective in acute gynecomastia.

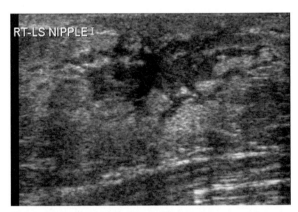

Figure 11.9 Acute gynecomastia—appearances again may be mistaken for an irregular infiltrating mass.

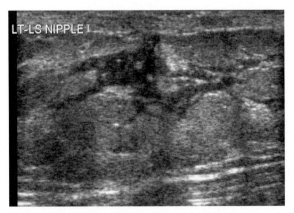

Figure 11.8 Acute gynecomastia—an irregular hypo-reflective area deep to the nipple mimics the appearances of a malignant mass.

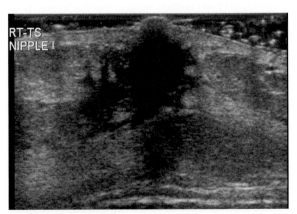

Figure 11.10 Intermediate phase gynecomastia—the central subareolar region is highly attenuating; again this can be mistaken for a focal mass.

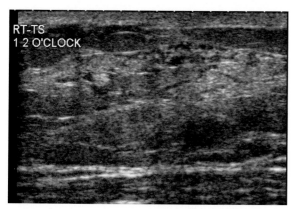

Figure 11.11 Typical ultrasound appearances of the developing glandular tissue in intermediate phase gynecomastia.

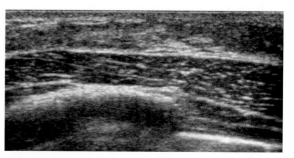

Figure 11.13 Ultrasound appearances typical of chronic gynecomastia—a centrally located hyper-reflective disk of parenchymal breast tissue.

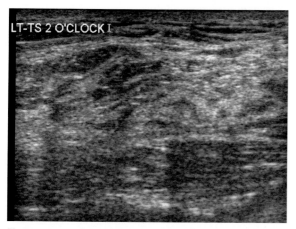

Figure 11.12 Intermediate gynecomastia has a similar appearance to a normal female breast (shown here for comparison with Fig. 11.11).

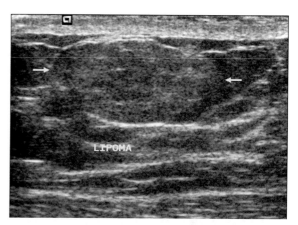

Figure 11.14 The classic ultrasound appearances of a lipoma are similar in men and women: a reasonably well defined slightly hyper-reflective mass in the subcutaneous fat layer.

similar to that of a normal female breast, with glandular tissue, subareolar ducts and their branches readily appreciated (Fig. 11.13). Clinically, the breast is not usually tender at this stage but a hard 'mass' is still usually palpable.

Lipoma

Lipomata can develop in the rudimentary male breast and may be isolated or multiple. Clinically they present as a soft round or ovoid palpable mass (Sohn et al 1999) and on ultrasound have the same appearance as when detected in the female breast; invariably they are demonstrated as a reasonably well defined hyper-reflective focal lesion at a superficial location (Fig. 11.14).

Cysts

In clinical practice, male breast cysts are rarely encountered, but have the same etiology as when occurring in women (Weinstein et al 2000). Complex cysts are more likely to be malignant (papillary carcinoma) in men than women, and those with thick walls or mural excrescences should undergo biopsy (Hashimoto and Bauermeister 2003).

The ultrasound appearance of a simple cyst is characteristically that of a well-defined smooth-walled mass that has no internal echoes and demonstrates increased posterior through transmission (Fig. 11.15).

MALE BREAST CANCER

Although the incidence of male breast cancer appears to be on the increase, it is a rare condition. It occurs in up to 300 men in the UK (1700 in the USA) annually and

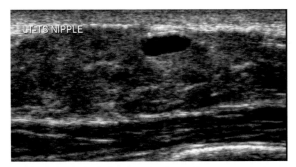

Figure 11.15 Male breast cysts have the same typical ultrasound appearance as in the female breast—a well defined round or oval anechoic mass.

accounts for less than 1% of both the total number of breast cancers reported and the total number of male cancers (Donovan 2003, Giordano 2005). Median age at diagnosis tends to be slightly higher in men than in women, 67 years compared with 62 years and as in women, increasing age is associated with increased risk (Giordano et al 2004). Men can be affected at any age. however, and the incidence in younger men (below the age of 40 years) appears to be escalating.

It was once thought that male breast cancer was inherently more aggressive than female breast cancer, but this is now disputed. Men are generally older than women at diagnosis, tend to have larger tumors and be at a more advanced disease stage (Giordano et al 2004). Men might be considered to have higher death rates due to delay in initial consultation with a doctor, but disease stage-matched relative 5-year survival rates (adjusted for age, gender and race) are in fact similar for both men and women (Giordano et al 2004). Due to the overall low incidence of male breast cancer, researchers are still trying to determine the optimal treatment for men, current regimes being based on extrapolation of data for female breast cancers.

Risk factors that predispose men to breast cancer (Box 11.1) include Klinefelter syndrome, testicular abnormalities, radiation exposure, estrogen administration and diseases which lead to high estrogen levels such as liver cirrhosis (Giordano 2005, Weiss et al 2005). Some men have a genetic predisposition to breast malignancy, BRCA2 mutations being present in 4–14% of male breast cancers (Ford et al 1998).

Male breast cancer types are similar to those encountered in women (Table 11.2); the most common type (93.7%) is invasive ductal carcinoma, but lobular carcinoma is less common in men due to the rarity of lobules in the male breast (Giordano et al 2004). There are occasional case reports of inflammatory carcinoma (Hashimoto and Bauermeister 2003), papillary carcinoma (Kinoshita et al 2005), Paget's disease of the nipple (Petrocca et al 2005), ductal carcinoma in situ (Wadie et al 2005), atypical ductal hyperplasia (Prasad et al 2005), lobular carcinoma (Giordano et al 2002, Sanchez 1986) and breast metastases (Hashimoto and Bauermeister 2003). Most male breast cancers are estrogen receptor positive; however, the exact disease etiology is as yet unknown.

The presenting symptoms of breast malignancy in the male overlap with those of chronic gynecomastia and indeed carcinomas may be obscured by co-existing gyne-

Table 11.2 Relative prevalence (%) of cancer types in men and women

Type	Men	Women
Ductal	76.5	74.3
No special type	17.2	9.3
Papillary	2.6	0.6
Mucinous	1.8	2.2
Medullary	0.5	1.8
Lobular	1.5	11.8

Data from Giordano et al (2004).

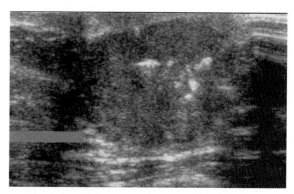

Figure 11.17 Ultrasound image demonstrating calcification in a male breast cancer.

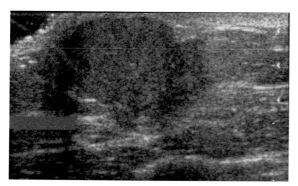

Figure 11.16 Invasive carcinoma in a male: male breast cancers have similar ultrasound appearances to female breast cancers.

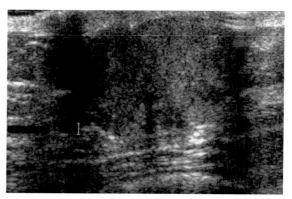

Figure 11.18 This male breast cancer has complex heterogeneous echo texture and reflectivity.

comastia (Sohn et al 1999). Both conditions usually present with a central small and hard palpable lump. The clinical level of suspicion is raised when this is associated with nipple retraction and bloody nipple discharge (Goss et al 1999); malignancy is less likely to be associated with pain (Donovan 2003)

On ultrasound, male breast cancer may exhibit the characteristic malignant features as seen in women: a focal mass lesion that is spiculate in shape, hypo-reflective and associated with a posterior acoustic shadowing. However, this is not always the case. Whilst invasive mass lesions will usually disrupt normal fat planes and interrupt connective tissue septations, they may be reasonably well circumscribed and only minimally hypo-reflective (Fig. 11.16). The presence of calcifications and a heterogeneous echo texture with patchy posterior shadowing should raise suspicion of malignancy (Figs 11.17 and 11.18). The lesions may be deep to the nipple and may invade the posterior skin surface of the nipple (Fig. 11.19) (Giordano et al 2002), but are often slightly eccentric in location (Gunhan-Bilgen et al 2002). Late presentation may be associated with fungation through

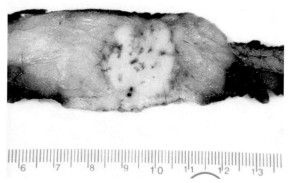

Figure 11.19 Pathological specimen of a male breast cancer involving the nipple.

the skin surface. It is important to examine the posterior aspect of the lesion carefully and determine its relation to the pectoralis muscle as involvement will alter surgical procedure and follow-up treatment. As with women, axillary node metastases can occur, and the ultrasound

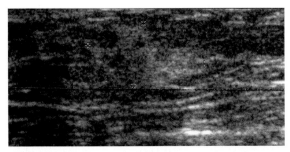

Figure 11.20 This malignant male breast lesion had no particularly suspicious sonographic features—its ultrasound appearance was indistinguishable from that of gynecomastia.

examination should be extended to include the axilla if the clinical or ultrasound-based level of suspicion is high.

Occasionally male breast cancer does not exhibit typical 'malignant' ultrasound appearances and may mimic gynecomastia. Figure 11.20 shows a case that exhibited none of the typical ultrasound features that would have raised suspicion of carcinoma, only demonstrating a localized hyper-reflective region with no architectural distortion; at excision biopsy, this was an invasive ductal carcinoma.

Ultrasound-guided needle core biopsy of an indeterminate, suspicious or overtly malignant-looking lesion is preferred for differential diagnosis, it being a safe and accurate procedure (Westenend 2003a, Janes et al 2006). The cost-effectiveness of indiscriminate needle core biopsy for all male focal breast abnormalities must be weighed against limited human and financial resources and the potential to raise anxiety levels, particularly in the patient with benign disease.

CARING FOR THE MALE PATIENT

Current diagnostic care pathways for males presenting with an abnormality in the breast have come under criticism as there is no standard national protocol for men and not all are afforded the accepted 'gold standard' their female counterparts can expect—rapid access to 'triple assessment' (Hanavadi et al 2005). Diagnostic work-up protocols are inconsistent and vary from a simple clinical examination and needle core biopsy (Westenend 2003a, b, Perkins & Middleton 2003) to mammography without biopsy (Evans et al 2001) or ultrasound with or without biopsy according to image findings (Daniels and Layer 2001). Recent literature suggests that there is a need for a standardized approach to avoid unnecessary surgery and offer better definitive treatment (Westenend 2003b, Perkins & Middleton 2003).

Public awareness of male breast, and indeed other, male cancers is not as high as that of female breast cancer; the disease is invariably perceived as a 'female' condition and there is a noticeable gender bias to clinical and support services provided by both professional and lay organizations (Donovan 2003, Iredale et al 2006). Breast cancer in men is treated in a similar way to female breast cancer and its response to treatment is essentially similar (Giordano 2005). Male mastectomy, although not having the same symbolic significance as in women, is still disfiguring and associated with altered body image; systemic hormonal therapy may result in feminization and sexual dysfunction (Anelli et al 1994, Donovan 2003). It cannot be assumed that men have similar psychosocial needs to women.

Recent studies suggest that men with breast disease are not catered for within existing facilities and that there is a need either to increase the number of gender-specific clinical and support services for men or to ensure that existing support services and resources include information about male disease (Donovan 2003, Iredale et al 2006). Men are less likely to seek investigation and support, and healthcare professionals need to be particularly sensitive to the patient's embarrassment and other pertinent issues such as delay in diagnosis, shock and stigma (France et al 2000).

References

Anelli TF, Anelli A, Tran KN et al 1994 Tamoxifen administration is associated with a high rate of treatment-limiting symptoms in male breast cancer patients. Cancer 74:74–77.

Buada LD, Murakami J, Murayama S et al 1997 Colour Doppler sonography of breast masses: a multiparameter analysis. Clinical Radiology 52:917–923.

Cardenosa G 1997 Breast imaging companion. Philadephia: Lippincott–Raven.

Chersavani R, Tsunoda-Shimizu H, Giuseppetti GM et al 1995 Breast. In Solbiati L, Rizzatto (eds) Ultrasound of superficial structures. Edinburgh: Churchill Livingstone, pp. 141–200.

Daniels IR, Layer GT 2001 Gynaecomastia. European Journal of Surgery 176(12):885–892.

Donovan T 2003 The forgotten few: men get breast cancer, too. Nurse2Nurse 3(11) Online. Available at: http://www.n2nmagazine.co.uk/print. asp?ArticleID=224 Accesssed on 7 August 2005.

Evans GF, Anthony T, Turnage RH et al 2001 The diagnostic accuracy of mammography in the evaluation of male breast disease. American Journal of Surgery 181(2):96–100.

Ford D, Easton DF, Stratton M et al 1998 Genetic heterogeneity and penetrance analysis of the BRCA1 and BRCA2 genes in breast cancer families. The Breast Cancer Linkage Consortium. American Journal of Human Genetics 62:676–689.

France L, Michie S, Barrett-Lee P et al 2000 Male cancer: a qualitative study of male breast cancer. The Breast 9(6):343–348.

Giordano SH 2005 A review of the diagnosis and management of male breast cancer. The Oncologist 10:471–479.

Giordano SH, Buzdar AU, Hortobagyi GN 2002 Breast cancer in men. Annals of Internal Medicine 137(8):678–87.

Giordano SH, Cohen DS, Buzdar AU et al 2004 Breast carcinoma in men: a population based study. Cancer 101(1):51–57.

Goss PE, Reid C, Pintilie M et al 1999 Male breast carcinoma: a review of 229 patients who presented to the Princess Margaret Hospital during 40 years: 1955–1996. Cancer 85:629–639.

Gunhan-Bilgen I Bozkaya H, Ustun EE et al 2002 Male breast disease: clinical, mammographic and ultrasonographic features. European Journal of Radiology 43(3):246–255.

Hanavadi S, Moneypenny IJ, Mansel RE Is mammography overused in male patients? The Breast 15(1):123–126.

Hashimoto B, Bauermeister D 2003 Breast imaging—a correlative atlas. New York: Thieme.

Iredale R, Brain K, Williams B et al 2006 The experiences of men with breast cancer in the United Kingdom. European Journal of Cancer 42:334–341.

Janes SE, Lengyel JA, Singh S et al 2006 Needle core biopsy for the assessment of unilateral breast masses in men. The Breast 15(2):273–275.

Kinoshita T, Fukutomi T, Iwanoto E et al 2005 Intracystic papillary carcinoma of the breast in a male patient diagnosed by needle core biopsy: a case report. The Breast 14(4):322–324.

Kopans DB 1989 Breast imaging. 2nd edn. Philadelphia: Lippincott, Williams and Wilkins.

Perkins GH, Middleton LP 2003 Breast cancer in men. British Medical Journal 327:239–240.

Petrocca S, LaTorre M, Cosenza G et al 2005 Male breast cancer: a case report and review of the literature. Chirurgia Italiana 57(3):365–371.

Prasad V, King J, McLeay W et al 2005 Bilateral atypical ductal hyperplasia, an incidental finding in gynaecomastia—case report and literature review. The Breast 14(4):317–321.

Rahman N, Davenport M, Buchanan C 2004 Galactocele in a male infant with congenital hypopituitarism. Journal of Pediatric Endocrinology and Metabolism 17(10):1451–1453.

Ravakkah K, Javadi N, Simms R 2001 Hamartoma of the breast in a man: first case report. Breast Journal 7(4):266–268.

Sanchez AG, Villanueva AG, Redondo C 1986 Lobular carcinoma of the breast in a patient with Klinefelter's syndrome. A case with bilateral, synchronous, histologically different breast tumours. Cancer 57:1181–1183.

Sohn C, Blohmer J, Hamper U 1999 Breast ultrasound. A systematic approach to technique and image interpretation. Theime: New York.

Stavros AT 2004 Evaluation of the male breast. In Stavros AT (ed.) Breast ultrasound. Philadelphia: Lippincott, Williams and Wilkins.

Wadie GM, Banever GT, Moriarty KP et al 2005 Ductal carcinoma in situ in a 16 year old adolescent boy with gynaecomastia: a case report. Journal of Paediatric Surgery 40(8):1349–1353.

Weinstein SP, Conant EF, Orel SG et al 2000 Spectrum of US findings in paediatric and adolescent patients with palpable breast masses. Radiographics 20(6):1613–1621.

Weiss JR, Moysich KB, Swede H 2005 Epidemiology of male breast cancer. Cancer Epidemiology, Biomarkers and Prevention 14(1):20–26.

Welch ST, Babcock DS, Ballard ET 2004 Sonography of pediatric male breast masses: gynaecomastia and beyond. Pediatric Radiology 34(12):952–957.

Westenend PJ 2003a Core needle biopsy in male breast lesions. Journal of Clinical Pathology 56:863–865.

Westenend PJ 2003b Breast cancer in men. Evidence suggests preoperative work up is suboptimal. British Medical Journal 327(7420):930.

Wigley KD, Thomas JL, Bernardino ME et al 1981 Sonography of gynaecomastia AJR American Journal of Roentgenology 136:927–930.

Chapter **12**

Ultrasound-guided interventional techniques

Anne-Marie Dixon

INTRODUCTION

Minimally invasive percutaneous procedures in the breast are performed either to assist in establishing a diagnosis or to achieve a therapeutic benefit (Table 12.1). Techniques range from the relatively straightforward fine (21-gauge) needle aspiration of serous fluid from a simple cyst to the excision of benign lesions using wide bore (11-gauge) vacuum-assisted biopsy devices. Diagnostic interventional procedures should be embedded within the 'triple assessment' protocol, wherever possible integrated with attendances for diagnostic imaging examinations, and be performed at the same patient visit (Ralleigh & Michell 2002, RCR 2003). Medical imaging is increasingly being used to guide percutaneous interventional procedures.

Table 12.1 Clinical and radiological indications for minimally invasive procedures

Aspiration	Relief of symptomatic cysts—pain/lump
	Confirm cystic nature
	Suspected infection
	Suspected intracystic neoplasm
	Drainage of abscess
Biopsy	Confirmation of benign lesions in high risk patients
	Clarify equivocal/suspicious appearances
	Preoperative confirmation of malignancy
	Confirm multicentric disease
	Evaluation of focal abnormalities in patients with previous history of breast cancer
Localization	Sonographically visible impalpable lesion for excision

When an abnormality is palpable, percutaneous needle procedures can be performed under clinical guidance. Most benign lesions are notoriously mobile, and some malignancies are associated with peripheral desmoplastic reaction, peritumoral edema and central necrosis—this makes such lesions difficult to localize clinically and this reduces sampling accuracy (White 1997, Heywang-Kobrunner et al 2001, p. 132). With a 'blind' clinical procedure, it is impossible to guarantee that benign and normal biopsy findings are truly from a target abnormality of interest and not from adjacent breast tissue (Madjar 2000, p. 187).

Implementation of image-based national breast screening programs has resulted in the detection of many small asymptomatic and impalpable lesions; breast screening programs are associated with challenging targets for benign surgical biopsy and preoperative diagnosis rates, and this has increased the demand for image-guided tissue sampling procedures (NHSCSP 2001, 2003, 2005).

Image guidance is suitable, and indeed preferable, for both palpable and clinically occult abnormalities as it makes the procedure more accurate (Hatada et al 1996, RCR 2003). The use of ultrasound for image guidance has many advantages over mammography or magnetic resonance imaging (MRI) guidance. The principle benefits are:

- Lack of inherent biological (radiation) hazard
- Shorter procedure time
- Enhanced patient comfort
- Continuous *real-time* visualization of needle placement within the breast for positioning and confirmation of sampling location.

Where appropriate operator experience is available and the abnormality can be visualized sonographically, ultrasound imaging is efficient, economical and accurate, and should be used in preference to mammographic stereotactic guidance (Jackson et al 1996, Hauser et al 2000). Stereotactic guidance remains the choice for mammography-detected isolated microcalcification, architectural distortion and focal asymmetry, as these are not reliably correlated with an abnormal ultrasound appearance (White 1997, Harvey et al 2000).

This chapter will describe the procedures for ultrasound-guided interventional techniques. Clinical and radiological indications for undertaking intervention are also considered.

PERSONNEL AND TRAINING

As with general breast ultrasound, the performance of image-guided breast interventional techniques does not lie within the domain of any particular healthcare profession and may be undertaken by suitably experienced and trained medical (Cabaseres 1997), radiographic (Duthie 2001) and, potentially, nursing (Wilkinson et al 2005), staff working within agreed Schemes of Work that reflect local circumstances.

Persons performing ultrasound-guided interventional procedures should be qualified and experienced ultrasound practitioners capable of performing high quality imaging examinations; they must be accomplished in ultrasound image interpretation, have the ability to characterize lesions reliably and be able to select appropriate patients for further investigations (Hauser et al 2000, RCR 2003)

Additional operator training, competence-based assessment in performance of interventional techniques and ongoing audit are required to ensure consistency in accurate positioning of the sampling device, effective tissue retrieval and appropriate management of complications. It is not surprising that technical success rates and diagnostic accuracy improve with increased operator experience, experienced operators tending to have lower inadequacy rates and requiring fewer needle passes to achieve a definitive diagnosis (Brenner et al 1996).

Professional bodies and other special interest organizations have issued guidance on the training requirements for practitioners undertaking minimally invasive ultrasound-guided interventional procedures, although the recommended amount of practical training for achievement and maintenance of competence varies considerably (Table 12.2) (Madjar et al 1999, Hauser et al 2000, RCR 2003, NHSCSP 2005, pp. 22–26). Formal certificated postgraduate training programs are offered by some UK Higher Education Institutions, often in conjunction with NHSBSP centers, although it has been

Table 12.2 Recommendations for training and experience

American College of Radiology	
Initial training	Board-certified/Royal College-accredited radiologists
	Radiologists with 3 months dedicated ultrasound training including breast and interventional procedures
	Physicians with postgraduate training to include 500 ultrasound examinations including breast
	Physicians with 2 years clinical experience of ultrasound to include 500 general ultrasound examinations OR 100 breast ultrasound examinations
Royal College of Radiologists, London	
Gaining and maintaining competence	Employment of at least three (screening) days/one (symptomatic) day in breast imaging
	Undertake minimum of 5000 screening and/or symptomatic or 500 symptomatic cases per year
	Have attended RCR course
	Be involved with assessment as well as screening/image interpretation
	Be experienced in use and interpretation of X-ray and ultrasound procedures
	Have access to pathology and surgical follow-up
	Undertake formal audit of performance
Ideally personnel should	Be involved in both screening and symptomatic work
	Have clinical examination skills
	Participate in approved performance quality assurance scheme for mammography
UK National Health Service Breast Screening Programme	
Minimum monthly experience in training	Full-time specialist—12 months training
	Part-time as breast screening and other duties—6 months training
	300 image interpretations
	80 symptomatic cases including ultrasound
	20 image-guided procedures
International Breast Ultrasound School	
Accuracy and confidence technique and interpretation; improving and maintaining skills	Performance of at least 500 breast ultrasound examinations in a multidisciplinary environment
	Performance of at least 300 cytology/histology correlation cases
	Performance of at least 50 interventional procedures with follow-up

Madjar et al (1999), Hauser et al (2000), RCR (2003), NHSCSP (2005).

suggested that structured in-house training (Table 12.3) may also be feasible (Duthie 2001). A procedure checklist (Box 12.1) is a useful training aid and can be adapted into a criterion-based tool for assessment of *technical* competence (Dixon 2006). Audit of actual clinical practice can be used to demonstrate *clinical* competence, a diagnostic sample retrieval rate of 80% over 30 cases being an appropriate benchmark (Dixon 2006). Subsequent maintenance of competence can be evidenced by continual or periodic pathology-verified individual performance audit.

Although ultrasound is theoretically well suited for intervention guidance, it can be difficult for individual practitioners to coordinate the spatial relationships of patient anatomy, needle device and ultrasound scan plane (Stetten et al 2001). Ultrasound-guided tissue sampling involves good psychomotor skills to enable coordination of the operator's right and left hand movements to ensure continuous alignment of the biopsy device and needle (usually in the right hand) with the ultrasound scan plane (transducer, in the left hand). It is helpful and will increase operator versatility if the technique is practiced using the dominant hand for either function (Harvey et al 2000).

Before practitioners carry out interventional procedures on actual patients, it is advisable to practice with

Table 12.3 Five-stage in-house training scheme

Stage 1	Learn and perform	Aseptic technique
		Subcutaneous injection
		Histology sample documentation
		Disposal of sharps
Stage 2	Observe 10 demonstrated procedures with instructional commentary related to skills and technique	
Stage 3	Practice injection and needle placement skills on a tissue-mimicking phantom	
Stage 4	Undertake 10 procedures on patients with direct supervision	
	Engage in postprocedure reflection and discussion	
Stage 5	Demonstrate independent procedural competence	

After Duthie (2001).

a patient-mimicking phantom (Madjar 2000, p. 190). This can improve technique, accuracy and operator confidence, although practice does not necessarily reduce operator anxiety or procedure duration in vivo (Harvey et al 1997). Commercially produced tissue-mimicking phantoms are available (and expensive), but it is possible to manufacture one *in-house* with no more than a trip to the local supermarket! Stuffed olives placed inside a turkey breast or leg of lamb produce a similar ultrasound appearance to solid breast lesions, and small detergent-filled balls can be used to mimic cystic lesions (Figs 12.1 and 12.2).

Instruction and practice in a protected learning environment gives the operator the opportunity to develop their psychomotor skills and improve hand–eye coordination, in particular it helps them to improve sonographic visualization of the needle shaft and choose a safe needle track (Harvey et al 1997). If the learning environment also simulates the clinical scenario, trainees can become familiar with aseptic technique and use of clinical consumables, and can practice patient communication skills (Dixon 2006).

PATIENT PREPARATION, CONSENT AND CONTRAINDICATIONS

As with any healthcare procedure, the patient should be greeted, unequivocally identified and introduced to all personnel involved in the care episode. The proposed intervention should be fully described and explained, and informed consent obtained (Hauser et al 2000).

Box 12.1 Twenty-five item checklist for performing a needle core biopsy

- Collect and check equipment and clinical consumables
- Review patient's clinical examination and prior imaging results
- Confirm location of interest and plan approach
- Greet patient and confirm identification (ID) information
- Explain procedure and obtain informed consent
- Check for contraindications
- Prepare and position patient, enter ID into ultrasound machine
- Perform baseline ultrasound examination and record control images
- Choose skin entry site to give biopsy track parallel to chest wall
- Wash hands and put plastic apron and sterile gloves on
- Open and prepare consumables and equipment
- Clean patient's skin and infiltrate with local anaesthetic
- Load needle into biopsy device and test fire
- Confirm loss of sensation and perform skin incision
- Insert biopsy needle and advance into prefire position
- Activate biopsy device and sample tissue using horizontal trajectory
- Retrieve sample and compress puncture site
- Repeat sampling up to five times
- Compress wound until hemostasis achieved, then dress with a plaster
- Discard consumables, dispose of sharps, clean equipment
- Remove gloves and wash hands
- Store and document samples—check identification with patient
- Document procedure in departmental records
- Compile the examination report
- When fit, give patient postprocedure information and discharge

(after Skills for Health 2003)

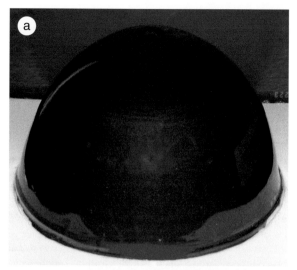

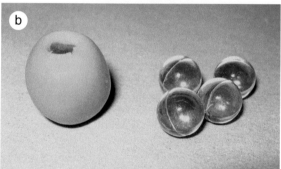

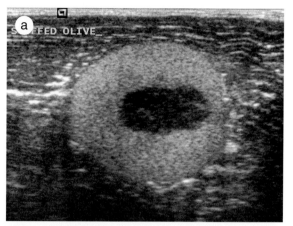

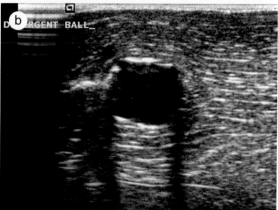

Figure 12.1 (a) A commercially available breast ultrasound biopsy phantom (Model: Gammex 429 available from Gammex RMI Ltd, Nottingham, UK). (b) Stuffed olives and liquid soap balls can be placed inside a piece of 'turkey breast' meat for a 'home-made' breast aspiration/biopsy phantom.

Figure 12.2 (a) The ultrasound appearance of a stuffed olive inside a piece of turkey breast meat simulates a solid focal mass through which a needle core biopsy can be taken. (b) The ultrasound appearance of a liquid soap ball simulates a cystic lesion that can be aspirated.

Explanations should be given in a manner that encourages the patient to relax and cooperate, and their emotional state should be ascertained and responded to appropriately (Skills for Health 2003). The potential benefits of the procedure should be explained to the patient in a way that balances them against the associated limitations, risks and most common potential complications of the procedure, the risks associated with not having the procedure and the relative risks of obtaining the information using an alternative technique (Harvey et al 2000).

Patients should be asked about their past medical and surgical history, if they suffer from any allergies, are currently taking medication or if they have a predisposition or family history of abnormal bleeding (Hauser et al 2000). Anticoagulation therapy, such as aspirin, heparin or warfarin, is not automatically a contraindication to needle intervention although it is prudent to check the patient's coagulation profile before proceeding with wide bore biopsy procedures. Some patients will need longer postprocedure wound compression and possible use of a pressure dressing (Melotti & Berg 2000, Heywang-Kobrunner et al 2001, p. 136). If the procedure is carried out under truly aseptic conditions, patients with prosthetic cardiac valves will not need prophylactic antibiotics (Heywang-Kobrunner et al 2001, p. 136).

The presence of breast implants does not preclude a needle procedure, and real-time ultrasound-guided aspiration can be extremely useful in these patients (Madjar 2000, p. 194, RCR 2003). Where the suspicion of malignancy is high and lesion location is favorable, needle core biopsy (NCB) may also be appropriate, although consideration should first be given to performing MRI.

Verbal consent is adequate for simple fine needle procedures; some centers prefer to obtain formally documented written consent particularly for wide bore biopsies; consent for preoperative localization is often incorporated into the formal surgical consent procedure.

PREPROCEDURE ULTRASOUND EXAMINATION

It is important that a full clinical assessment and all routine imaging studies have been performed before any interventional procedure is carried out (Heywang-Kobrunner et al 2003, RCR 2003). Although the risk is low for experienced practitioners, and particularly for fine needle procedures (Laws et al 2002), if imaging is performed *after* a clinically guided intervention, accuracy of image interpretation may be compromised. For example, postprocedure hemorrhage may be classified as appearances suspicious of malignancy or truly malignant appearances dismissed as postprocedure change.

Prior to starting the intervention, the person performing it should review all the original imaging findings and rescan the patient to identify and localize the area of interest unequivocally, plan a safe needle approach and determine the needle insertion site. It is worth interrogating an area to be biopsied with color flow Doppler to ensure that the intended needle pathway avoids large vessels.

As a general principle, an ultrasound-guided intervention is performed with the target lesion at one edge of the ultrasound image and the needle tip inserted through the skin close to the short edge of the opposite end of the transducer (Fig. 12.3). The needle is then advanced in alignment with the scan plane through the breast towards the lesion, under continuous real-time ultrasound visualization to ensure it remains in line with the transducer footprint (Madjar 2000, p. 187).

PREPARATION OF ENVIRONMENT AND EQUIPMENT

Diagnostic imaging equipment can become a reservoir for disease-causing organisms, and imaging staff are potential vectors for nosocomial (hospital-acquired) infection (Smith & Lodge 2004). Careful adherence to local infection control policies will limit the small but nevertheless finite risk of opportunistic and cross-infection; image-guided interventional procedures should be carried out in an environment in which principles of asepsis can be applied. Most image-guided interventional procedures are undertaken using a 'clean no-touch' technique, although aseptic principles are adhered to as far as possible.

Risk of cross-infection can be minimized with careful technique, the use of disposable equipment where possible, and thorough cleaning and decontamination of all re-usable equipment at the beginning and end of every procedure. Care must be taken when using the ultrasound keyboard during interventional procedures; a suitably trained assistant may be instructed to manipulate the scanning parameters and record images to reduce the risk of cross-contamination.

HAND WASHING

Healthcare personnel should always adopt an effective hand-washing technique (Fig. 12.4) using soap and

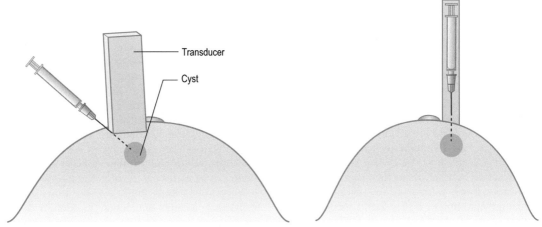

Figure 12.3   Diagram to show the relative positions of the transducer, needle and a cystic lesion for a successful ultrasound-guided aspiration.

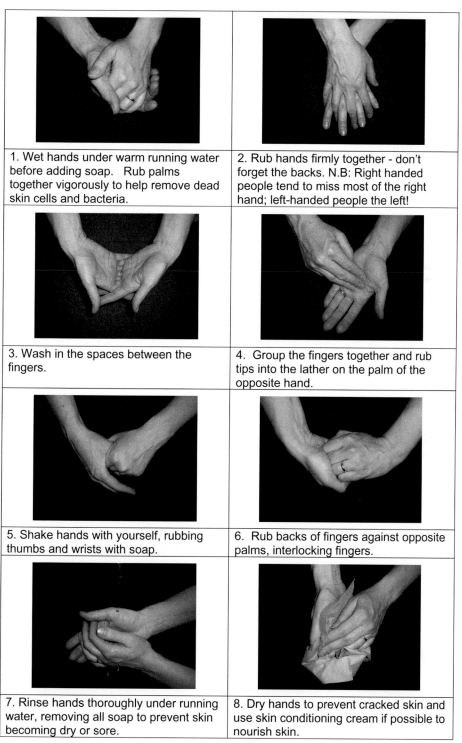

1. Wet hands under warm running water before adding soap. Rub palms together vigorously to help remove dead skin cells and bacteria.	2. Rub hands firmly together - don't forget the backs. N.B: Right handed people tend to miss most of the right hand; left-handed people the left!
3. Wash in the spaces between the fingers.	4. Group the fingers together and rub tips into the lather on the palm of the opposite hand.
5. Shake hands with yourself, rubbing thumbs and wrists with soap.	6. Rub backs of fingers against opposite palms, interlocking fingers.
7. Rinse hands thoroughly under running water, removing all soap to prevent skin becoming dry or sore.	8. Dry hands to prevent cracked skin and use skin conditioning cream if possible to nourish skin.

Figure 12.4   Recommended hand-washing protocol (after RCN 2005).

warm running water for at least 10–15 s between patients; longer washing times are required if hands are visibly soiled. Alcohol hand rubs are suitable for hand cleaning between patients where soap and running water are not available but are not effective for removing visible dirt, bacteria or blood. Cuts and scratches should always be covered with waterproof dressings, and the wearing of rings and wristwatches is discouraged. Examination or surgical gloves should be worn for the performance of all interventional procedures.

SETTING A STERILE TROLLEY

It is the responsibility of the person performing the procedure to check that all the required equipment is available, in working order and compatible, and that pharmaceuticals and sterilized consumables have not passed their expiry date.

The equipment and consumables needed for image-guided interventional procedures (Box 12.2, Table 12.4) should be assembled and opened immediately prior to each procedure. For simple cyst aspirations, the syringe and needle can be opened by an assistant and handed directly to the operator; equipment for biopsy and localization procedures is prepared onto a sterile tray or trolley (Fig. 12.5).

Sterile trays and trolleys should be made of stainless steel and regularly cleaned with soap and water. Immediately before each procedure, the trolley should be sprayed or wiped with an alcohol-based disinfectant and allowed to air dry.

Prior to setting the sterile trolley, the healthcare practitioner should wash their hands using an antibacterial soap product, dry them with a sterile towel and then put on sterile gloves. Care must be taken to avoid touching non-sterile surfaces with washed hands prior to putting on gloves and once sterile gloves are on. An assistant is required to open sterile packs.

The trolley should be covered with a sterile dressing towel. Sterile and non-sterile items are kept on separate areas on the trolley; a non-sterile re-usable biopsy device may be placed in a sterile receiver until ready for use.

FINE NEEDLE ASPIRATION OF FLUID

Cysts

Aspiration of fluid from a sonographically simple (thin walled and completely echo free) cyst is only indicated as a therapeutic measure to relieve patient pain/discomfort or to reduce a palpable mass (Tot et al 2002, p. 107). Aspiration is indicated for diagnostic clarification when the ultrasound appearances of small lesions are equivocal, i.e. a small fibroadenoma may look exactly

---

Box 12.2   Supplies required for departments performing image-guided interventional procedures

Sterile
  Gloves
  Pre-injection swabs
  Cotton wool balls
  Gauze swabs—5-packs 7.5 × 7.5 cm
  Wound dressings
    Small adhesive plasters, hypoallergenic
     dressings, pressure bandaging
  Syringes
    2 ml, 5 ml, 10 ml, 20 ml
  Scalpel blades size 11
  Needles—hypodermic
    Short 25G (orange), 21G (green)
    Long 21G (green), 19G (white)
  Needles—biopsy
    10 cm 14G
  Needles—wire localization
  Transducer covers
  Coupling gel sachets
  Biopsy device
Plastic aprons
Face masks
Adhesive strapping tape
Specimen containers
  Pots containing fixative, e.g. formalin
  Fine mesh envelopes
  Histology cassettes
Pathology request forms and sample bags
Pharmaceuticals
  2% lignocaine hydrochloride, e.g lidocaine,
    xylocaine with epinephrine/adrenaline
Alcohol hard surface/transducer wipes
Sharps bin
Clinical waste bags

---

the same as a small cyst containing viscous fluid, to distinguish complicated cysts or complex fluid collections from solid masses and to exclude intracystic malignancy (Jackson et al 1996).

Simple serous intracystic fluid can normally be aspirated using a 'green' 21G bevel tip hypodermic needle, although a longer needle (70–90 mm) than those routinely used for venepuncture and intradermal anesthetic

Table 12.4   Routine trolley settings

Aspiration		
Sterile	Preinjection swab	
	Long hypodermic needle	21G (green)
	Syringe	2–30 ml range
	Gauze swabs	5-pack: 7.5 × 7.5 cm
Non-sterile	Examination gloves	
	Small adhesive plaster	
	Alcohol transducer wipes	
	Sharps bin	
	Clinical waste bag	
Needle core biopsy		
Sterile	Examination gloves	
	Preinjection swab	
	Gauze swabs	5-pack: 7.5 × 7.5 cm
	Syringe	2 ml
	Scalpel blade	size 11
	Short hypodermic needles	25G (orange), 21G (green)
	Biopsy needle	10 cm 14G
	Biopsy device	
	Transducer cover	
	Coupling gel sachet	
	2% lignocaine hydrochloride with adrenaline	
Non-sterile	Plastic apron	
	Face mask	
	Small adhesive plaster	
	Histology specimen container with fixative	
	Histology cassette/mesh envelope	
	Pathology request form and sample bag	
	Alcohol transducer wipes	
	Sharps bin	
	Clinical waste bag	
Wire localization		
Sterile	Examination gloves	
	Preinjection swab	
	Gauze swabs	5-pack: 7.5 × 7.5 cm
	Syringe	2 ml
	Short hypodermic needles	25G (orange), 21G (green)
	Localization needle	
	Transducer cover	
	Coupling gel sachet	
	2% lignocaine hydrochloride with adrenaline	
Non-sterile	Plastic apron	
	Face mask	
	Adhesive strapping tape	
	Alcohol transducer wipes	
	Sharps bin	
	Clinical waste bag	

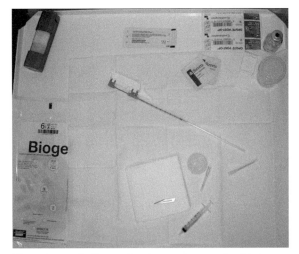

Figure 12.5 Trolley setting for an ultrasound-guided needle core biopsy—see Table 12.4.

infiltration is usually required. More viscous, or particulate fluid will require a larger caliber needle, a supply of long (79–90 mm) 19G 'white' needles should be available. Cyst aspiration technique is summarized in Box 12.3. Cyst wall puncture may be difficult when the lesion is surrounded by thick fibrous tissue or when the wall is soft and deformable (Jackson et al 1996).

Typical cyst fluid that is thin, clear and yellow, green or black in color does not require cytological analysis (White 1997, Tot et al 2002, p. 107). If a suspected cystic lesion appears to have solid components, cannot be completely aspirated or yields blood-stained or thick mucinous fluid, needle-core biopsy is indicated (Jackson et al 1996, White 1997); however, such lesions are more reliably characterized with surgical excision (Tot et al 2002, p. 107).

Abscess drainage

Percutaneous therapeutic drainage is not usually indicated as breast abscesses tend to contain thick particulate fluid, and are often multilocular and thus require surgical drainage; diagnostic fine needle aspiration may be performed prior to antibiotic therapy to obtain material for bacteriological analysis (White 1997).

DIAGNOSTIC TISSUE SAMPLING

Tissue sampling is indicated where a significant clinical or imaging abnormality is present and the diagnosis is considered indeterminate, suspicious or overtly malignant (RCR 2003, p. 12). There is increasing evidence that an experienced operator's image-based *benign* diagnosis may be reliable enough to make conservative

Box 12.3 Cyst aspiration technique

- Clean transducer and patient skin surfaces with antiseptic wipes
- Hold the transducer in one hand and position it centrally over the cyst
- Hold the needle and syringe in the other hand, puncture the skin close to the midpoint of the transducer short edge and advance the needle tip slowly and carefully through the subcutaneous tissue layer
- Identify the needle shaft on the image by aligning the transducer face and needle shaft parallel
- Keeping the needle shaft and syringe in line with the long axis of the transducer, advance the needle tip towards the cyst wall maintaining continuous visualization of the whole needle shaft and tip throughout
- Once the needle tip abuts the cyst, make a sharp 'stab' forwards to puncture the cyst wall
- Position the needle tip centrally within the cyst and then pull back the syringe plunger to aspirate
- Observe the cyst walls collapse—aspirate to dry wherever possible
- Withdraw needle, compress puncture site and cover with adhesive dressing.
- Inspect fluid aspirate—discard or retain as appropriate
- Dispose of sharps and clinically soiled waste safely

follow-up and interval imaging a safe and acceptable management option, particularly in low risk patients (White 1997, Graf et al 2004). However, confidence in such an approach is tempered by a recognized overlap in benign/malignant ultrasound appearances and recognition of a degree of subjectivity in classification of ultrasound appearances (Jackson et al 1996, Lister et al 1998). With the exception of lesions exhibiting the classic features of a normal lymph node or lipoma therefore, most solid lesions are considered 'indeterminate' and are referred for tissue sampling.

Where patients present with palpable abnormalities but mammography and ultrasound show normal breast tissue, it has been suggested that the negative predictive value is high enough to avoid biopsy (Dennis et al 2001). However, up to 6% of malignant lesions remain undetected even with combined ultrasound and mammography imaging (Duijm et al 1997, Kolb et al 1998, Soo et al 2001, Beyer & Moonka 2003). In the presence of a palpable abnormality and negative image findings, the decision to proceed to biopsy requires careful evaluation of clinical examination findings and the patient's risk profile if malignancy is not to be missed (Beyer & Moonka 2003).

Percutaneous tissue sampling reduces the need for open (surgical) diagnostic procedures and provides an accurate, safe and cost-effective alternative that is well tolerated by patients as an outpatient procedure (Parker et al 1993, 1994, Woodcock et al 1998, Hauser et al 2000, Smith et al 2001). In patients with benign disease, image-guided needle diagnosis is expedient and helps avoid unnecessary surgery, cosmetic scarring and future imaging pseudolesions (Parker 1994, Huber et al 2003). In patients with malignant disease a definitive preoperative tissue diagnosis can provide histological and immunohistochemcial prognostic information; this facilitates informed patient counseling and treatment planning, offers the potential for single-stage therapeutic surgery and obviates the need for 'frozen section' (Litherland et al 1996, Harvey et al 2000, Hauser et al 2000, RCR 2003, Vargas et al 2004).

FINE OR LARGE BORE NEEDLE PROCEDURE?

Microscopic analysis may be undertaken on cellular material retrieved using either fine gauge (19–25G) or large bore (8–18G) needles.

Fine needle aspiration cytology (FNAC)/biopsy (FNAB) is a simple and rapid technique that is well tolerated by patients and has a low postprocedure complication rate (Phillips et al 1994). However, many consider the technique to have unacceptably high false-negative and inadequate specimen rates; in addition, the technique has incomplete tumor characterization (typing and grading) capability and as often prohibitive requirement for specialized cytopathological interpretation (Sneige et al 1994, Klijanienko et al 1998, Zardawi et al 1999). Some caution that it is a 'rule in' technique, reliable for confirming a clinical diagnosis of probably benign or suspicious for malignant, but not reliable enough for the evaluation of clinically indeterminate lesions as it has particularly high false-negative rates for lobular and tubular malignancy and for ductal carcinoma in situ (DCIS) (Rubin et al 1997, Tot et al 2002, pp. 103–104).

In experienced hands, high sensitivity and specificity can be achieved, but results vary considerably between operators and centers (Snead et al 1997, Arisio et al 1998, Wells et al 1999, Tot et al 2002, p. 102). UK NHSBSP absolute sensitivity thresholds of 70% have only been met with the increasing substitution of large bore NCB instead of FNAB in many centers (Litherland et al 1996, Britton & McCann 1999, RCR 2003). Substituting NCB improves diagnostic sensitivity and specificity, especially for isolated microcalcifications, small and unusual lesions (Britton et al 1997), but it is not without its drawbacks (Table 12.5).

Where on-site cytopathology expertise is available (Heywang-Kobrunner et al 2001, p. 133), use of FNAB yields a rapid result and enables a truly one-stop diagnostic service to be offered (Laws et al 2002, Litherland 2002), large bore NCB requiring up to 3 or 4 days processing time and a delayed patient re-attendance to obtain the results. Expertise and availability of local personnel, economic and logistic factors, in addition to lesion characteristics, will influence the choice of technique in any particular diagnostic breast service and for each individual patient, but it is becoming increasingly difficult to justify the use of FNAB (Britton 1999, NHSCSP 2001, Litherland 2002).

The large bore NCB technique has the principle advantages of ease of sample collection and preparation, a more complete pathological interpretation and thus definitive lesion characterization and preoperative diagnosis (Britton 1999, Tot et al 2002, p. 105); it is increasingly being used in preference to FNAB. In a large

Table 12.5 Advantages and limitations of 14G needle core biopsy compared with fine needle aspiration biopsy

Advantages	Limitations
More complete lesion characterization	Increased Tissue processing time
Tumor grading	Cost
Tumor typing	Local trauma
Discrimination of in situ and invasive disease	Complication rate
Determination of estrogen receptors, progesterone receptors, Cerb$_2$ status	
Reduced operator variability Aspiration technique Pathological interpretation	Requires skin incision
Reduced inadequate specimen rate	
Improved sensitivity and specificity	

proportion of cases, a successful NCB specimen will yield accurate information about histological tumor type, tumor grade, presence of DCIS and hormone receptor status. Published series show malignancy sensitivity approaching 100% (Schoonjons & Brem 2001), high concordance of tumor grading and type between biopsy and surgical specimens (74%) and high predictive values for estrogen and progesterone receptor status; however, tumor grade and DCIS component underestimation in core biopsy specimens is not uncommon, particularly when the volume of tissue retrieved is small (Heywang-Kobrunner et al 2001, p. 133, Badoual et al 2005).

FNAB TECHNIQUE

Although customized, and therefore more expensive, specialist needles are available, an adequate FNAB can

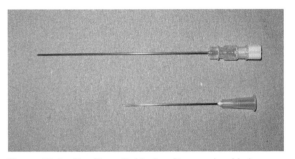

Figure 12.6   Needles suitable for ultrasound-guided aspiration of fluid: the upper (yellow hub) needle is a 10 cm spinal needle, the lower (green hub) needle is a long (70 mm) 20G hypodermic needle.

be performed using a long (70 mm) 20G bevel-tipped hypodermic needle, connecting tubing and 20 ml syringe; spinal needles may be used for deeper lesions (Fig. 12.6), (White 1997, Madjar 2000, p. 190).

FNAB technique is similar to that for a simple fluid aspiration, but once the needle tip is in the center of a solid mass, suction is applied to the syringe by an assistant whilst the operator makes 6–10 repeated small thrusting movements using a corkscrew motion (White 1997, Heywang-Kobrunner et al 2001, p. 136). Suction is maintained until aspirate is noted at the needle hub, indicating that the needle is full. Suction is then stopped whilst the needle is withdrawn from the breast. The syringe is then disconnected from the needle, filled with air and then re-attached to express the needle contents onto a slide or into preservative fluid. Cytology slides are then spread and either air dried or alcohol fixed according to local staining preferences.

Three to five additional aspirations should be performed in a fan-shaped pattern (Fig. 12.7) to sample different areas of the lesion (Madjar 2000, p. 190). Any blood-stained aspirate should be discarded and a fresh needle used for subsequent passes.

LARGE BORE NEEDLE CORE BIOPSY

Parker (1994) first described the technique for ultrasound-guided automated percutaneous large core breast biopsy using a 10 cm, long throw (23 mm) 14G needle in a spring-loaded automated device, and this continues to be the recommended technique (RCR 2003).

A variety of automatic cutting needles and spring-loaded biopsy devices are available on the market, and

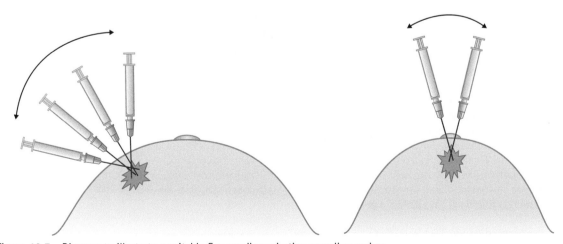

Figure 12.7   Diagram to illustrate a suitable fine needle aspiration sampling regime.

personal preference tends to govern which one is used. Some biopsy systems are totally disposable incorporating an integral spring-activated firing mechanism and a cutting needle (Fig. 12.8) supplied in a presterilized pack for single procedure use. Others systems combine single-use presterilized disposable needles with a re-usable outer housing that is sterilized and/or cleaned between procedures (Fig. 12.9).

Although single-use disposable systems are lightweight and easier to handle than the more robust multiuse devices, early devices were criticized for suboptimal performance. Modern disposable equipment is more effective and preferred by some to reduce risk of cross-infection. Recent innovations in multiuse devices have incorporated lighter weight materials and more ergonomic design to improve operator control and facilitate single-handed deployment.

Automatic cutting needles incorporate a coaxial inner stylet with a short recessed notch to house the tissue specimen, and an outer cutting cannula (Fig. 12.10). Once the biopsy device spring mechanism is activated,

the stylet and cannula are automatically propelled forward in rapid succession to cut and cover a sample of tissue (Fig. 12.11). Some devices have the facility to control deployment of the stylet and cannula independently so that the exact sampling position can be more accurately verified prior to activating the tissue cutting process. Most needles are supplied with integral spacer clips (Fig. 12.12) to facilitate their correct location in a re-usable biopsy device, and care should be taken to ensure that needles purchased for use with re-usable devices are compatible. Some manufacturers use surface scoring or coating of the needle tip to increase reflectivity and make it easier to detect in the ultrasound image; the expense of these additions can be avoided with good ultrasound technique.

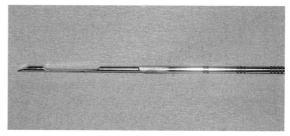

Figure 12.10   Photograph of a 14G automatic cutting needle showing the tissue sampling notch.

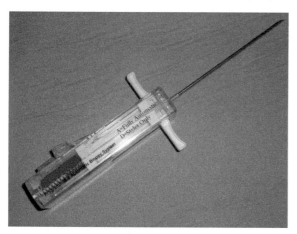

Figure 12.8   Single-use (disposable) spring-activated biopsy needle.

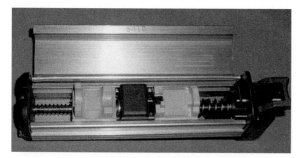

Figure 12.9   Re-usable spring-loaded biopsy device.

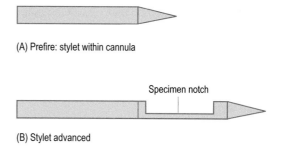

(A) Prefire: stylet within cannula

(B) Stylet advanced

(C) Cannula advanced to cut and cover specimen

Figure 12.11   Diagram to show biopsy needle sampling action. As the needle is advanced into the breast and positioned against the target lesion, the inner sampling stylet is enclosed within an outer cannula (a). On deploying the needle, the stylet advances forward allowing tissue to drop into the sampling notch (b). In rapid succession, the cannula is advanced over the stylet to cut and cover the sample (c) before the needle is withdrawn.

The 'throw' of the biopsy device indicates the distance that the needle tip is propelled forwards when the spring mechanism is activated. Needle throw is typically 22 or 23 mm, but some devices allow a choice of short (15 mm) or long (22 mm) throw. Novice operators are well advised to measure the throw distance using the on-screen electronic callipers prior to taking a biopsy to ensure there is adequate tissue beyond the lesion to accommodate the needle safely (Fig. 12.13). Most devices have a choice of front (or side) and end firing buttons to accommodate user preference. It is good practice to test-fire the biopsy device at the start of every procedure to check correct needle placement and effective device operation, and to demonstrate to the patient the noise it will make when deployed (Duthie 2001).

The technique for preparation and deployment of a typical multiuse device is summarized in Box 12.4.

At the end of biopsy procedures, disposable equipment is discarded and multiuse devices should be cleaned in accordance with local infection control guidelines and the device manufacturer's instructions. Cleaning regimes may include initial cleaning with mild detergent and warm water, hot water rinsing and thorough drying, followed by autoclave, ethylene oxide or Cidex steriliza-

> **Box 12.4 Operation of biopsy device and cutting needle**
>
> 1. Remove biopsy device from storage box and disinfect
> 2. Remove cutting needle from sterile packaging
> 3. Pull back actuator handle twice to prime ready for deployment—this action may automatically engage the safety button
> 4. Open device's hinged top cover to expose needle carrier blocks
> 5. Install needle onto carrier blocks ensuring correct location of spacer guide
> 6. Remove spacer guide
> 7. Close hinged top cover
> 8. Remove safety catch and test deploy Re-prime and disengage safety catch
> 9. Insert needle into patient and localize into prefire position (see text)
> 10. Release safety button
> 11. Deploy needle by pushing either front or rear trigger button
> 12. Withdraw needle from breast
> 13. Pull actuator handle back once to draw back outer cannula and reveal tissue sample in biopsy notch of stylet
>
> Adapted from Manam (no date)

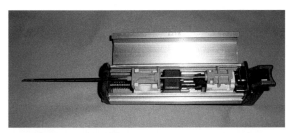

Figure 12.12 Correct loading of a disposable biopsy needle into the re-usable device is facilitated by the provision of 'spacer' clips.

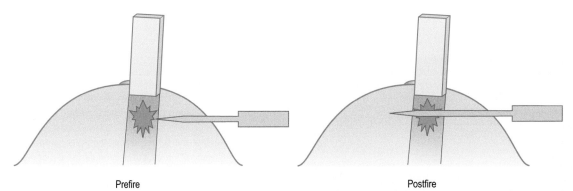

Prefire Postfire

Figure 12.13 Diagram to show how the 25 mm 'throw' distance of a biopsy needle on deployment means that the needle goes through and beyond the majority of lesions.

tion, and periodic lubrication of internal moving parts to maintain efficient function (Manam® Medical Products, no date).

ULTRASOUND-GUIDED NEEDLE CORE BIOPSY TECHNIQUE

Special needle guides that couple to the transducer and allow one fixed needle path, the position of which can be overlaid on the ultrasound image display, are available to assist operators performing ultrasound-guided needle interventions. In the breast, however, it is difficult to achieve a safe needle path parallel to the chest wall with such devices, and a freehand technique is almost universally adopted. The freehand technique (Fig. 12.14) requires no special transducer adaptor, gives greater flexibility of the needle pathway for safe and successful core biopsy of lesions throughout the depth of the breast and is more accurate for smaller lesions. This is the technique that will be described.

Choice of an appropriate skin entry site is crucial to the success and safety of the procedure. In the standard breast ultrasound examination position, the antero-posterior thickness of breast tissue is minimized and reduced to approximately 2–3 cm in most patients. Care must be taken when inserting and advancing needles to ensure they do not traverse the intercostal spaces and enter the pleural cavity or pericardial sac (Madjar 2000, p. 188). Wherever possible, biopsy needles should be

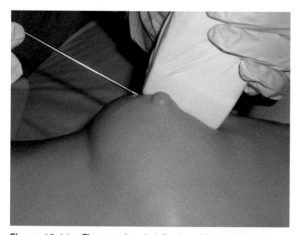

Figure 12.14 The two-handed freehand breast biopsy technique requires the operator to hold the transducer in one hand whilst manipulating the biopsy needle with the other. Good hand, eye and sensory coordination is required, and operators are well advised to practice the technique so that they can confidently perform a biopsy with the transducer and the biopsy device in either hand.

inserted at a short distance from the edge of the transducer, more peripherally in the breast, so that they can be advanced towards target lesion at the correct depth in a plane near parallel to the chest wall (White 1997, Harvey & Moran 1998). Not only is this the safest technique, but breast curvature and tissue compliance usually allow the transducer face also to be aligned parallel to the chest wall to give good sonographic visualization of the needle shaft. Effective skin entry sites will be very close to the edge of the transducer in most patients, with deeper lesions requiring slightly more separation to give greater positioning flexibility (Fig. 12.15).

Care also needs to be taken to ensure there will be adequate breast tissue distal to the target lesion so that the skin on the opposite side of the breast is not breached when the needle is automatically advanced on deployment of the biopsy device.

In view of the presence of dense connective tissue, nerve fibers and increased vascularity in the subareolar region, needle pathways traversing directly behind the nipple and areola are associated with increased risk of bleeding and greater patient discomfort, and should be avoided.

Administration of local anesthesia

Once the skin entry site has been chosen, the breast should be cleaned with a preinjection medicated swab prior to intradermal infiltration of local anesthetic (Duthie 2001). Local anesthetic can be combined with a vasoconstrictor (adrenaline 1:200 000); this significantly reduces bleeding and extends the rate of absorption, prolonging duration of neural blockade. Multiple 2 ml doses may be drawn from a single 20 ml bottle for sequential procedures using separate sterile needles, with the surplus discarded at the end of each session.

Local anesthetic infiltration technique is summarized in Box 12.5.

Local anesthetic administration should be performed under sonographic guidance; care must be taken to ensure that the anesthetic is free from small air bubbles and does not obscure the area of interest (Heywang-Kobrunner 2001, p. 140; AIUM 2002). The anesthetic should be administered slowly with regular aspiration to avoid accidental intravascular injection, and care taken not to exceed the maximum safe dose, particularly when multiple biopsies are performed on the same patient (20 ml of 1% lidocaine with adrenaline 1:200 000).

Preparation of the transducer

The ultrasound transducer should be cleaned with a compatible antiseptic wipe, acoustic coupling gel applied to the scanning surface and then it should be covered

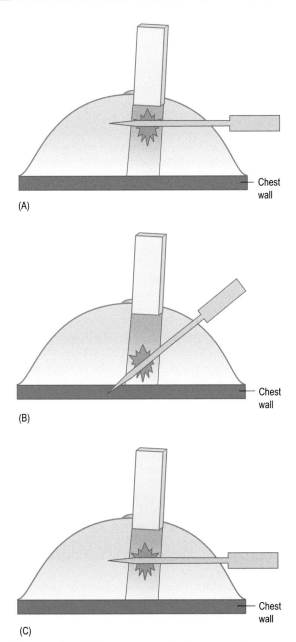

(A)

(B)

(C)

Figure 12.15 Diagram to show the importance of ensuring the biopsy track is parallel to the chest wall (A). Use of an acute angle will increase the risk of breaching the chest wall (B) a more peripheral entry site is required for deeper lesions (C).

Box 12.5   Technique for injection of local anesthetic

- Ensure patient is comfortable and positioned for biopsy.
- Explain what you are about to do
- Wash hands with antibacterial soap and warm running water, and dry
- Clean the skin incision site with an alcohol swab and allow it to dry
- Check local anesthetic type, dose and expiry date.
- Using 21G (green) needle draw up 2 ml of local anaesthetic into a 2 ml syringe
- Attach 25G (orange) needle to syringe
- Approach patient, taking care not to touch anything
- Reassure patient and warn that injection will be sharp and sting initially
- Puncture skin at angle of approximately 20–30° to depth of 2–4 mm
- Aspirate to check tip is not intravascular—if blood aspirated, withdraw, change needle and try again
- Slowly inject 2 ml of local anesthetic into subcutaneous tissues (a small white weal should form)
- If required, further intradermal and deeper injections around the lesion can be made (using a 21G green needle)
- Monitor patient for signs of adverse reaction
- Allow 2 min for neural blockade before performing skin incision

with a sterilized single-use cover. Sterile coupling gel is applied to the outer aspect of the transducer cover over the scanning surface (Fig. 12.16).

Making the skin incision

A small skin incision is required to facilitate passage of a biopsy needle of 14G or larger. Once loss of neural sensation has been established, using the tip of a sterile size 11 scalpel blade, a linear 3–5 mm cut is made through the skin and immediate subcutaneous connective tissue at the intended site of needle entry. Care must be taken not to rotate the scalpel blade to widen the incision; this

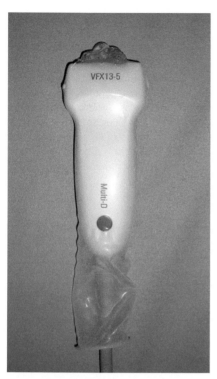

Figure 12.16 The transducer should be covered with a sterile sheath and prepared with sterile coupling gel when performing biopsy and localization techniques.

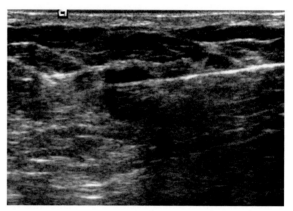

Figure 12.17 Good visualization of the whole shaft of the biopsy needle should be obtained when the needle is parallel to the transducer footprint and aligned with the scan plane.

is unnecessary and can be associated with poor healing and granuloma formation.

Obtaining the tissue sample

The transducer is applied to the patient's skin and its long axis aligned with the target lesion and the skin incision (Harvey et al 2000). The biopsy needle is inserted through the skin and subcutaneous tissue layer and must then be confidently located on the ultrasound image. The biopsy needle should remain in line with the scan plane during the procedure so that the operator has continuous visualization of the needle shaft and tip throughout (Madjar et al 1999, Harvey et al 2000).

If the needle cannot be visualized, transducer alignment with the target lesion and skin incision should be checked and corrected before slowly sweeping the needle from side to side through the breast, keeping the shaft parallel to the chest wall, until it is seen to coincide with the scan plane. The transducer itself should not be moved to 'find' the needle since this will invariably result in loss of the target lesion from the scan plane and thus from the image, necessitating complete relocation of the lesion.

When the needle is aligned with the acoustic scan plane, the whole length of the shaft should be visible as a hyper-reflective (white) line (Fig. 12.17). If the needle is not fully aligned with the scan plane, only a cross-section of the shaft is visible (as a white dot); in such cases, the operator does not know at what position along the needle length the scan plane is positioned, in particular the operator has no idea where the end of the needle is.

The angle between the needle and transducer contact surface should be kept as small as possible to give optimal needle visualization, and parallel to the chest wall to minimize risk of violating the thoracic cavity; this is particularly critical for deep-seated lesions and in patients with small breasts (Jackson et al 1996). If the needle is initially advanced towards the lesion at an oblique angle, breast curvature and compliance will usually allow pivoting of the biopsy device handle towards the chest wall to give a parallel trajectory when the biopsy is taken. This maneuver can also be employed to try to lift deep-seated lesions slightly anterior from the chest wall (Harvey & Moran 1998, Heywang-Kobrunner et al 2001, pp. 141–142).

When lesions are located in the anterior two-thirds of the breast, or the breasts are relatively large, an angle between 30 and 60° (to horizontal) may be used if there is sufficient depth of breast tissue between the lesion and chest wall to accommodate the needle throw (Jackson et al 1996).

Once the lesion and biopsy needle are visible in the scan plane and the needle has been advanced until its tip is just touching the edge of the lesion—the prefire position—the patient is encouraged to keep very still and warned that they will hear a loud clicking sound as the biopsy device takes the tissue sample; potentially alarming terminology such as 'fire' and 'gun' should be avoided (Harvey et al 2000). The biopsy device is then deployed, maintaining gentle pressure of the needle tip against the lesion. Deployment advances the needle and cutting sheath in rapid succession through the lesion. Care must be taken to make sure the safety catch is released prior to inserting the biopsy device into the patient; failure to do this will not be apparent until an attempt to deploy the device fails; once the safety catch has been released, a further attempt at accurate needle positioning will be required.

The operator can be confident and satisfied that a representative tissue sample has been obtained by observing the needle passing through the target abnormality on the ultrasound image (Fig. 12.18). The transducer can be rotated through 90° to check that the needle is centrally located within the lesion (Madjar 2000, p. 25) or a confirmatory three-dimensional volume obtained (Fig. 12.19). Following needle withdrawal, air bubbles visible within a solid lesion also provide evidence of accurate sampling location.

Pressure is maintained over the biopsy site as the needle is withdrawn and the tissue sample retrieved, inspected and stored.

The likelihood of obtaining an adequate sample of tissue, and thus a definitive diagnosis, increases with the volume and quality of tissue retrieved; a minimum or four or five intact specimens is recommended from a variety of locations within the area of abnormality (Brenner et al 1996, Harvey et al 2000, Fishman et al 2003). The retrieved tissue should be examined with the naked eye to assess its quality and quantity (Fig. 12.20); a 14G biopsy needle typically yields a 2 × 20 mm cylindrical core of tissue (Heywang-Kobrunner et al 2001,

p. 132). A good non-fragmented sample of diagnostic tumor tissue will look firm and creamy-white, and will sink when placed in formalin solution (Harvey et al 2000, Fishman et al 2003); non-diagnostic fatty tissue appears gelatinous and clear, and it floats.

Although a malignant diagnosis is achievable with a scanty tissue specimen, a decent volume of uncrushed tissue is required for full assessment of grade and other prognostic factors; an accurate assessment of the presence of a DCIS component is more likely if some samples are taken from the periphery of infiltrating masses (Badoual et al 2005)

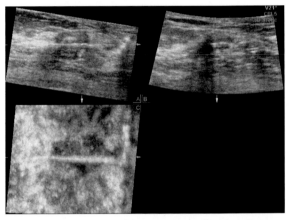

Figure 12.19   Ultrasound images obtained with a three-dimensional probe demonstrate the biopsy needle position within the lesion in three orthogonal planes.

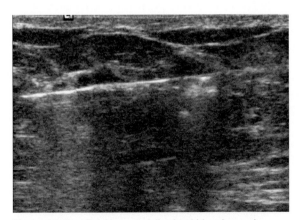

Figure 12.18   The biopsy needle should be observed passing through the lesion in 'real time', and an image recorded to document the sampling location.

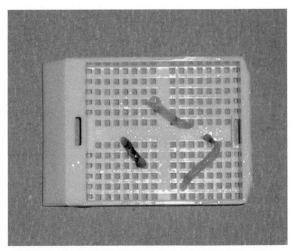

Figure 12.20   Using a 14G needle, at least two or three passes are required to ensure that a good quality specimen is retrieved.

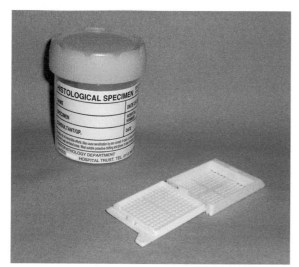

Figure 12.21   Needle core biopsy specimens should be transferred to plastic cassettes and placed in histology pots containing formalin for transport to the pathology laboratory.

Table 12.6   Minimum data set for receipt of pathology specimens

Request form	Specimen container
Full name of patient	Patient identification
Patient's date of birth, hospital identification or NHS number	Family name Given name Date of birth Hospital number
Location of patient— ward or out-patients	
Destination for report— name of consultant	
Nature of specimen (what)	Specimen details
Anatomical location of sampling site (where)	Type Site (including laterality)
Relevant clinical information (why)	
Date of sampling procedure	Procedure information Type of sampling Date of tissue collection

Storage, documentation and processing of tissue samples

Tissue samples may be washed off the biopsy needle using sterile saline (Harvey et al 2000) or may be lifted with the non-sharp edge of the scalpel blade or a hypodermic needle; they should be placed into a histology specimen pot containing non-coagulant additive fixative such as 10% formalin (Fig. 12.21). The sample container should be accurately labeled with patient and procedure identification, and a histology request form completed; a minimum data set may be required for receipt of specimens in the pathology department (Table 12.6). Care must be taken to ensure that there is no possibility of transposition of samples or documentation between patients. This risk will be minimized if container preparation and form completion are integral components of each individual procedure and are not prepared in advance or at the end of multipatient sessions; it is good practice, and reassuring for the patient, to invite them to verify their identification details as the samples are placed in the histology containers.

The pathology processing procedure is summarized in Table 12.7.

At the end of the biopsy procedure, direct pressure should be applied to the skin entry site for approximately 5 min (Duthie 2001) or until hemostasis is achieved to minimize bruising and hematoma formation (Harvey et al 2000). Following a routine 14G needle puncture, a simple adhesive dressing can be applied. Hypoallergenic and pressure dressings should be available if required.

All equipment should be cleaned or disposed of and the facilities cleared and restored ready for the next procedure.

VACUUM-ASSISTED BIOPSY

The technique of directional vacuum-assisted biopsy (VAB) was developed in the late 1990s and is increasingly being used for stereotactic-, ultrasound- and MRI-guided breast biopsy. It is a feasible and effective alternative to conventional NCB and is also useful for the percutaneous excision of benign and low risk lesions (Parker & Klaus 1997, Fine et al 2003).

The procedure is undertaken with special instrumentation that utilizes mechanical vacuum suction to draw tissue into the collection chamber of the biopsy needle; a high speed rotating coaxial cannula is then advanced to cut a core of tissue (Fig. 12.22). Continuous vacuum suction results in the specimen being transported out of the breast into an external collection chamber from where it can be retrieved using forceps (Heywang-Kobrunner et al 2001, pp. 137–138).

The technique for inserting the VAB probe is similar to that used for a conventional NCB, but the biopsy probe is positioned just below the area of abnormality, activating the vacuum tissue retrieval process suctions tissue down into the needle chamber (Parker & Klaus 1997, Heywang-Kobrunner et al 2001, p. 141). Since the device is directional, additional sampling can be

Table 12.7 The histology process

Specimen receipt	Unique pathology department identification number given

Fixation	In order to:
	    Preserve tissue, inhibit autolysis and putrefaction
	    Prevent diffusion
	    Harden the tissue to facilitate handling and sectioning
	    Protect tissue for subsequent processing
	    Aid staining

Dissection	Ascertain dimensions and macroscopic appearance (all dissected tissue retained for 6 months) Blocks cut from (larger) specimens and transferred to color-coded cassets
Processing: embedding in paraffin wax	Dehydration to remove water Cleaning with organic solvent (xylene) to replace alcohol Impregnation of tissue with molten wax to dissolve xylene Cooling—tissue cast into solid wax block (all blocks retained for at least 10 years)
Section cutting into paraffin spares	Microtome used to cut 4 μm paraffin wax sections from wax block into a water bath Collected onto glass slides Washed, heated (to melt wax) and dried
Staining of paraffin spares	Some stained with hematoxylin, eosin and saffron to demonstrate cell nuclei, red blood cells, cytoplasm and connective tissue; Some saved for immunochemistry; estrogen receptors, progesterone receptors, Cerb$_2$ antigen retrieval Optional staining for fungi, microorganisms
Reporting	Paraffin spares viewed under microscope Appearances described and diagnoses documented Findings communicated to Consultant Breast Surgeon and discussed at multidisciplinary clinical meeting

Jackson (2005).

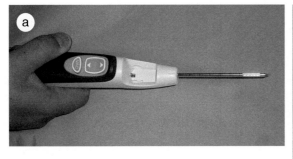

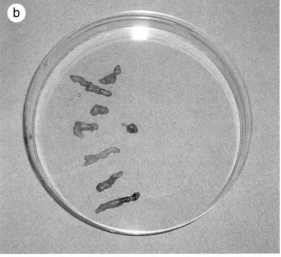

Figure 12.22 (a) The vacuum-assisted breast biopsy device is of similar overall size to a spring-loaded device but takes a larger gauge (8 or 11G) sample and is only inserted into the breast once. (b) Larger specimen cores obtained with a vacuum-assisted biopsy device increase sampling accuracy.

performed adjacent to the initial biopsy site by simply rotating the device. The biopsy probe itself remains at one location in the breast throughout, allowing multiple cores to be extracted without having to traverse the breast repeatedly for each successive sample.

Commercially available VAB devices use either 8G or 11G (or 14G) needles and are able to retrieve higher quality and greater quantity of tissue compared with 14G spring-loaded biopsy devices. This results in greater diagnostic accuracy with lower false-negative rates and less risk of disease underestimation (Burbank et al 1996, Jackman et al 1997, Parker et al 2001, RCR 2003). Small lesions (<15 mm) can be effectively excised using 11G equipment, and larger ones (15–30 mm) using an 8G probe (Parker et al 2001, Fine et al 2003, March et al 2003).

If the biopsy procedure completely removes the area of abnormality such that it is no longer apparent clinically or on the postbiopsy images, small marker clips (Fig. 12.23), it can be inserted through the VAB device to localize the biopsy site for follow-up and subsequent treatment (Parker & Klaus 1997). Clip migration can occur over time; early clip migration, immediately after the biopsy, has been attributed to hematoma formation, but more commonly with stereotactic procedures due to expansion of breast tissue on release of compression— the 'accordion' effect (Burnside et al 2001, Philpotts & Lee 2002, Harris 2003, Birdwell & Jackman 2003).

VAB is a more expensive procedure than conventional NCB but, because the instrumentation is of larger caliber, it yields a greater volume of tissue; in experienced hands, procedure duration is not extended and the technique is gaining popularity as a safe, acceptable and well-tolerated procedure with low overall complication rates (1–7%) and mild, short-lived side effects (Burbank et al 1996, Fine et al 2003, Huber et al 2003, March et al 2003, Philpotts et al 2003).

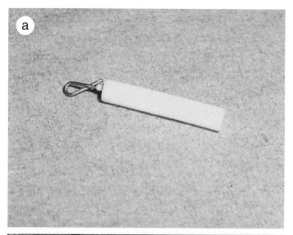

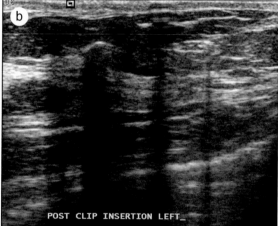

Figure 12.23   (a) Marker clips can be positioned in the breast with the vacuum-assisted biopsy device to localize the tissue sampling site on subsequent mammograms or ultrasound images. (b) Ultrasound images show acoustic shadowing at the site of the marker clips.

PRESURGICAL LOCALIZATION OF FOCAL LESIONS

Ultrasound-guided localization can be used prior to surgical biopsy or excision to localize small impalpable lesions that can be confidently visualized on ultrasound (Jackson et al 1996, Madjar 2000, p. 25, Heywang-Kobrunner et al 2001, pp. 152, 155). When clinically occult abnormalities are detected at mammography, it is worth performing an ultrasound examination since a sonographically guided localization is quicker and more comfortable for the patient compared with a stereotactic mammography-guided procedure and does not involve further radiation exposure.

A variety of localization techniques are suitable for ultrasound guidance; choice depends upon lesion posi-

tion and type but is also determined by local surgical and radiological expertise and preferences, and by the logistics of coordinating the scheduling of localization and surgical procedures (Heywang-Kobrunner et al 2001, p. 158, RCR 2003).

Skin marking

Simple marking of the patient's skin with semi-permanent ink directly over the lesion and sonographic measurement of vertical lesion depth may be adequate to localize a relatively superficial abnormality (RCR 2003). As with other localization techniques, it is important that this is done with the patient in a position similar to that adopted at surgery.

Dye injection

A small amount (0.2–0.3 ml) of patent or methylene blue dye may be injected into the center or periphery of a lesion to give the surgeon a visible guide for dissection (Madjar 2000, p. 195, Heywang-Kobrunner et al 2001:1, p. 8). The dye remains localized for approximately 2–3 h, but after this becomes disperse throughout the breast and thus ineffective as a localization aid.

Carbon tracking

Biopsy sites and needle tracks can be marked using activated charcoal; approximately 1–1.5 ml of a sterile solution of 4 g of charcoal in 100 ml of 0.9% saline may be injected into a lesion and continuously along the needle track as it is withdrawn (Heywang-Kobrunner 2001, p. 158). This is a well tolerated and safe alternative to wire localization and, since it is done at the time of biopsy, it obviates the need for two preoperative interventions (Mullen et al 2001).

Wire localization

Placement of an anchored thin wire through a lesion is the most accurate, and therefore the recommended and most widely used technique for localization of small and deep-seated abnormalities (RCR 2003, Wilson 2003, p. 101). A variety of localization wires are available and, again, choice depends on local radiological and surgical preference (Wilson 2003, p. 101). The technique for placement of localization wires is initially similar to that for a needle biopsy but, because the localization device is of smaller caliber (20G) no skin incision is required. In addition, the distance from the target lesion to the wire skin entry site must be as short as possible to minimize surgical track length (Jackson et al 1996). For wire localization, the transducer should be positioned with the target lesion at the edge of the field of view *nearest* the skin entry site and the wire introduced as close to the transducer as possible (Fig. 12.24); this will mean the wire pathway is at a relatively acute orientation to the chest wall and will require transducer angulation to optimize visualization (Jackson et al 1996).

The localization device, consisting of a thin central wire and a coaxial outer cannula (Fig. 12.25), is prepared for insertion by withdrawing the proximal end of the wire away from the hub of the cannula until the distal 'anchoring' elements of the wire are fully within the distal tip of the cannula; often there is a visible marker on the wire to show the correct position. The cannula and enclosed wire are then inserted into the breast and advanced to pass through the area to be excised. The wire is then advanced through the cannula so that

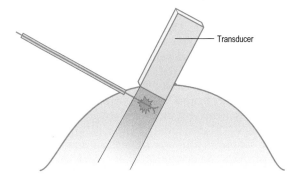

Figure 12.24 Diagram showing the correct technique for ultrasound-guided hookwire placement—note that the wire is inserted as close to the transducer as possible and the lesion is at same end of transducer as the wire insertion site and the transducer face is parallel to the wire shaft.

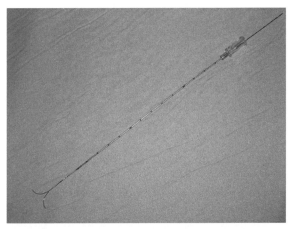

Figure 12.25 Photograph of a typical hooked localization wire.

anchoring elements become fixed in the tissue slightly beyond the target area (Fig. 12.26); surgeons will invariably be able to locate lesions when the wire actually passes through, but may struggle if the wire tip lies short or only adjacent to it (Wilson 2003, p. 101). The outer cannula is then carefully withdrawn to leave the inner wire in situ. Care must be taken to avoid dislocation of wires, particularly in fatty breasts, in the interval between localization and surgery. An adequate length of wire must extend beyond the skin so that the wire can be securely taped (Heywang-Kobrunner et al 2001, p. 159); patients should be advised to restrict arm movement on the affected side.

The majority of lesions for presurgical localization will, by nature of their small size, have been detected through the screening program. Even though the wire may be visualized within a focal lesion sonographically (Heywang-Kobrunner et al 2001, p. 157), lateral and

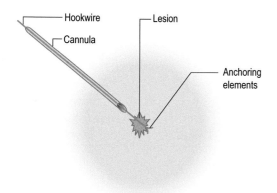

Figure 12.26 Diagram showing the optimal position of the anchoring elements of a hookwire localization device just beyond the lesion.

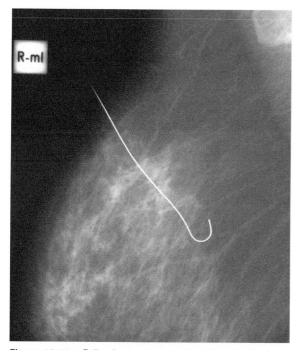

Figure 12.27 Following an image-guided localization procedure, mammography should be performed to confirm the position of the hookwire in relation to the lesion position—it is good practice for such images to accompany the patient to surgery.

cranio-caudal radiographs (Fig. 12.27) are required for surgical planning and to ensure the wire is localized at the original mammographic abnormality and lies at least within 10 mm of it (RCR 2003). Some devices allow the cannula to be re-inserted over the wire and the locking elements to be retracted for re-positioning if required.

The procedure should be documented in sufficient detail to guide the surgical procedure (Madjar 2000, p. 25); diagrams are often helpful, but direct verbal discussion with the surgeon may be necessary.

Surgical specimens should be imaged to confirm accurate and complete excision (Heywang-Kobrunner et al 2001, p. 160); this may either be specimen ultrasound or specimen mammography depending upon which method was used to make the original diagnosis (Fig. 12.28). Contact scanning of excised tissue can be undertaken by applying coupling gel to the outside of the plastic specimen bag or by placing the tissue specimen in a saline-filled transducer cover. Care should be taken to avoid contaminating the ultrasound equipment and the operator's hands; the operator should wear gloves during the examination and wash their hands and the transducer with an antibacterial cleanser at the end of the examination.

PATIENT AFTERCARE AND FOLLOW-UP

Patients should be monitored after an interventional procedure in order to identify and treat procedure-related complications.

Complications are rare and, once immediate hemostasis has been achieved and the puncture wound dressed, most patients are well enough to leave the imaging department. Immediate complications should be apparent at the time of the procedure or if the wound is examined a few days later when the patient returns to be informed of their histology results. Serious and delayed complications are exceptional and present clinically either through routine breast care follow-up or through primary care referral.

It is important that continuity of care is established so that relevant information about the procedure is passed on to appropriate members of the multidisciplinary breast care team. Patients need to know how to access the next stage of their care pathway; in particular, patients should know when and where they will get their biopsy results.

Postprocedure information should be given to patients in both verbal and written format. A typical patient information leaflet (Fig. 12.29) will include a summary of the procedure performed and its purpose, in addition to information on common side effects (pain and bruising) and recommendations for 24 h restriction of strenuous activity, non-aspirin-based analgesia and wound care (Duthie 2001); patients should be made aware of who to contact and how to do this should they have any concerns once they have left the imaging department.

The person responsible for performing the biopsy should retain some responsibility for checking the results of the biopsy to ensure that an adequate and representative sample has been obtained and that the diagnosis is in keeping with both clinical and imaging evaluation

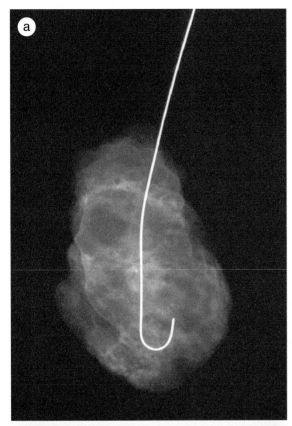

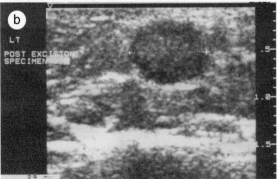

Figure 12.28   (a and b) Following excision, confirmation that the lesion has been successfully removed and is within the surgical specimen can be established with mammography (a) or ultrasound scan (b) .

(Britton and McCann 1999, Heywang-Kobrunner et al 2001, p. 149, Vargas et al 2004). Results must also be communicated to the referring clinician, and effective communication is achieved with regular multidisciplinary clinical case management meetings which key members of the imaging team attend.

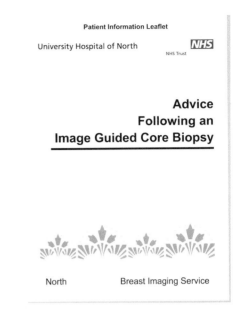

Figure 12.29   Patients should be given written information following image-guided interventional procedures.

A second needle core procedure may be indicated when the initial biopsy fails to obtain sufficient material for analysis or when there is discrepancy between the histology and clinical or imaging assessments (Hauser et al 2000). Since percutaneous biopsy has low (<2%), but nevertheless finite false-negative and disease underestimation rates, surgical excision biopsy is indicated when biopsy results are discordant with clinical and/or imaging findings or when histology shows atypical ductal hyperplasia or radial scar (Harvey et al 2000, Heywang-Kobrunner et al 2001, p. 149, Vargas et al 2004).

Responsibility for informing patients of their results lies with the referring clinician, and this is often done with the support of specialist breast care nurses.

IMAGE-GUIDED PROCEDURE-RELATED COMPLICATIONS

All interventional procedures that breach the integrity of the patient's skin with a sharp object carry inherent risks to both patients and the staff performing the procedures.

Staff risk is essentially limited to inoculation by patient-contaminated sharps and contamination of mucosal surfaces with patient body fluids; with both there is potential for acquisition of blood-borne infections such as hepatitis and HIV/AIDS (SoR 1998). Careful adherence to local and professional body infection control, sharps disposal and needle-stick injury policies will minimize this risk to a negligible level.

In the event of sharps injury or blood contamination, the area should be washed with warm water and blood samples taken from the recipient and, if possible, the donor. The incident must be recorded and reported, and prophylactic antiviral drugs considered if the source is high risk or serologically confirmed to be an HIV carrier (Bradford Hospitals NHS Trust 2005).

The incidence of patient-related complications following ultrasound-guided breast intervention is low; clinically significant complications are rare, and those requiring surgical management exceptional (Parker et al 1993, Frazee et al 1996, Yim et al 1997, Meyer et al 1999, Smith et al 2001). Fine needle aspiration procedures are rarely associated with complication, the complication rate for 14G needle core biopsy being around 2% and the rate for larger bore vacuum-assisted procedures slightly higher at 3–6% (Philpotts et al 2003, Liberman et al 2005). Information given to patients as part of the informed consent process need only include the most common complications (Harvey et al 2000).

Pain and bleeding

Fine needle aspirations are relatively painless and do not require local anesthesia or postprocedure analgesics. Hemostasis is usually achieved within a few minutes; a simple adhesive dressing is applied to the puncture site and can be removed after a couple of hours.

Reversible neural blockade is achieved using intradermal local anesthetic for large bore (8–14G) NCB procedures; the effect persists for approximately 90 min and patients are advised they may require commercially available analgesics for up to 24 h. Periprocedural bleeding is minimized if a combination of local anesthetic and vasoconstrictor (adrenaline) is used; hemostasis is usually achieved with 5–10 min direct compression of the puncture site, depending on needle caliber and procedure duration. A simple adhesive dressing is applied and should remain in place for 24 h.

Bruising, hematoma and pseudolesion formation

Although occasionally profuse bleeding does occur, fine needle aspiration procedures are not usually associated with significant bruising or hematoma formation; hematoma formation, however, is inevitable with core biopsy procedures. Bruising invariably resolves spontaneously within 7–14 days; early subsequent imaging may demonstrate small asymptomatic hematomas, oil cysts and fat necrosis, but these rarely persist or result in clinically significant sequelae (Harvey et al 2000, Huber et al. 2003).

Increased risk of postprocedure bleeding (>10 min) has been noted in stereotactic-guided VAB and attributed to lack of breast compression compared with that possible between successive passes of a conventional biopsy needle (Simon et al 2000). Pain and bleeding can be minimized with the use of more local anesthetic (3–6 ml intradermally and 8–12 ml in the deeper tissues), the application of longer (10 min) post-procedure compression and the use of ice bags (Huber et al 2003).

A small amount of bleeding from the nipple may follow centrally located biopsies that have traversed larger ducts.

Vaso-vagal reactions

Vaso-vagal reactions are less likely with ultrasound-guided procedures than with erect stereotactic procedures since the patient will be lying down. VAB takes longer and is slightly more traumatic than conventional NCB and may therefore have a higher risk (Simon et al 2000, Liberman et al 2005).

Signs and symptoms of impending faint include tinnitus, nausea, perspiration and yawning; the patients become quiet and pale. Severe reactions may cause bradycardia, collapse and twitching, although this is usually rapidly reversed by lowering the patient's head and raising their legs.

Hyperventilation can be treated with simple reassurance and encouragement of diaphragmatic breathing; re-breathing techniques are no longer recommended.

Epithelial displacement (tumor seeding)

Potential for seeding of malignant cells along needle tracks is well recognized and may occur in up to 50% of large bore (14G larger) percutaneous biopsies; tumor seeding is not believed to be clinically significant since the incidence and quantity of tumor cells detected in relation to interval since biopsy suggest that the cells do not survive displacement (Diaz et al 1999, Hoorntje et al 2004). Although most patients with premalignant and invasive disease will undergo mastectomy or breast conservation with chemo- or radiotherapy anyway, a restrained approach with sampling restricted to the minimum amount of tissue necessary for a definitive preoperative diagnosis is recommended (Tot et al 2002, p. 101).

Tumor cell displacement is noted to be less likely with VAB, presumably because there is only one episode of needle insertion during the procedure (Diaz et al 1999, Liberman et al 1999, Parker et al 2001).

Local skin reactions

Very occasionally, patients will suffer localized inflammation, granuloma formation or cosmetic scarring at the skin puncture site; true post-biopsy infection is rare (Meyer et al 1999)

Pneumothorax

Arguably the most significant procedure-related risk to the patient undergoing an ultrasound-guided needle intervention is that of needle violation of the chest wall and puncture of thoracic contents. Pneumothorax is rare but has been reported when needles have traversed the parietal pleural membrane during positioning or deployment of automatic devices (Gately et al 1991, Meyer et al 1999). Risk is greatest with inexperienced operators and in the axillary tail of thin women (Bates et al 2002). Risk is minimized with continuous real-time visualization of the needle in the patient, careful attention to ensure the whole shaft of the needle is kept in the scan plane and ensuring that the needle pathway is parallel to the chest wall.

Pseudoaneurysm

Pseudoaneurysm is a recognized complication of percutaneous diagnostic intervention, and there have been several reported cases following image-guided breast biopsy (Smith 1996, Beres et al 1997, Chorny et al 1997, McNamara & Boden 2002, Dixon & Enion 2004).

Often, arterial trauma is evident in view of brisk bleeding at the time of biopsy, but the diagnosis can be confirmed using color flow mapping and spectral Doppler (Fig. 12.30) with delayed presentation (Smith 1996, Chorny et al 1997, Dixon & Enion 2004). Attempts at

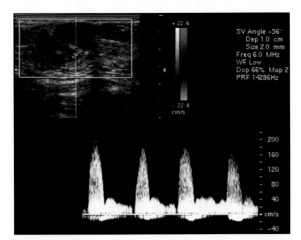

Figure 12.30 Color flow mapping and spectral Doppler appearances of a pseudoaneurysm which formed as a result of a needle core biopsy 3 months earlier.

external compression-induced repair have not met with success (Smith 1996, Beres et al 1997, Chorny et al 1997, McNamara & Boden 2002). Sonographically guided mechanical and pharmaceutical embolizations are feasible (Beres et al 1997, McNamara & Boden 2002) and reduce the need for surgical management.

Anesthetic toxicity and allergic reactions

Occasionally patients will suffer allergic reactions or other side effects after local anesthetic infiltration. Particular care must be taken to avoid toxicity in patients with a history of asthma, epilepsy or cardiovascular, respiratory, thyroid and liver impairment (Astra Zeneca 2001). Doses used for image-guided tissue sampling procedures are usually well below maximum permitted doses, although care must be taken to avoid intravascular injection and when multiple and/or bilateral biopsies are performed. Toxic effects are usually limited to cardiovascular and central nervous system effects; patients should be monitored for at least 30 min after anesthetic administration, even if the tissue sampling procedure is abandoned or completed earlier.

There is a potential risk for anaphylactic reaction to sterile gloves and probe covers in patients with a latex allergy. Whenever interventional procedures are performed, resuscitation equipment and drugs should be readily accessible since, if recognized and treated early, outcomes of adverse reactions are usually good. Personnel should be trained and ready to undertake ABC life support.

IMAGE RECORDING

A visual record of ultrasound-guided procedures should be made using a selection of *still* images, and these should be retained and retrievable in accordance with normal archiving protocols. The images should be labeled to correlate them with a specific examination of an individual patient as described in Chapter 7 (Table 7.2).

A standard set of images of a biopsy procedure (Fig. 12.31) should include:

- A 'control' image of the abnormality/lesion at the start of the examination before the interventional procedure
- A *prefire* image to show the orientation of the needle to the lesion and the chest wall
- Images to show the needle in situ at the point of aspiration/tissue sampling and annotated with the number of needle 'passes' performed
- A final image to show the appearances of the lesion at the end of the procedure.

(Heywang-Kobrunner et al 2001, p. 141)

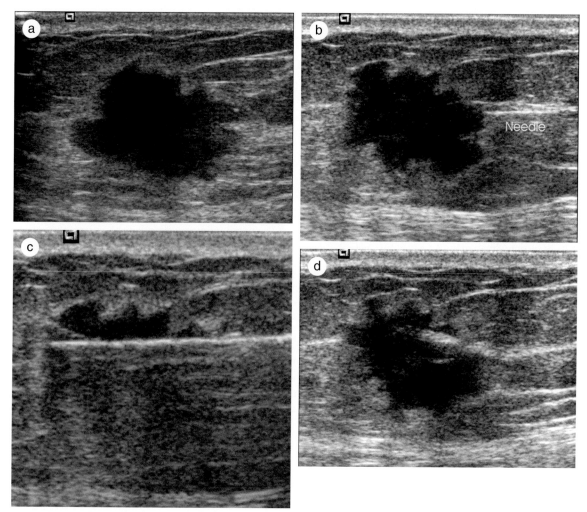

Figure 12.31 (a–d) As a minimum, images recorded during a needle core biopsy should include (a) the lesion to be sampled, (b) the needle in the prefire position abutting the lesion and parallel to the chest wall, (c) the deployed biopsy needle passing through lesion and (d) the air track that can be seen in the lesion following needle removal.

If the purpose of the procedure was to retrieve some tissue containing microcalcification, the success of the procedure should be documented by obtaining a specimen radiograph (Heywang-Kobrunner et al 2003, RCR 2003).

PROCEDURE REPORTING

A departmental record of all interventional procedures should be maintained to facilitate personal and service audit, and risk management. In addition to patient and operator identification, this record should include details of clinical aspects of the procedure and histological and patient outcomes (Box 12.6). The record should be regularly and periodically reviewed within an overall quality assurance program to evaluate success and complication rates so that areas for service improvement may be identified.

Close attention should be paid to rates for:

- Diagnosis, including where appropriate
  - Benign to malignant ratio
  - False-positive and false-negative rates
- Complications
- Inconclusive results
- Re-biopsy/excision rates and outcomes.

Box 12.6   Information to be included in departmental record of interventional procedures.

- Date of procedure
- Patient identification
    name, date of birth, hospital number
- Location of lesion
- Image-based diagnosis
- Pharmaceuticals used
    local anesthetic—type, dose and expiry date prophylactic antibiotics
- Personnel involved
    radiographer, radiologist, nurse
- Referring clinician
- Number of passes
- Immediate complications and associated treatment
- Histological result
- Further action/patient management decision as appropriate

Box 12.7   Procedure-specific information to be included in the report of an ultrasound-guided interventional procedure

- Laterality of breast and location of lesion within breast
- Procedure performed
- Approach used
- Type and amount of local anesthetic used
- Skin incision if made
- Complications and any treatment, if appropriate
- Specimen radiography, and results, if indicated (microcalcification)
- Clip placement if performed
- Postprocedure mammography/sonography, and results, if performed (hookwire localization)

Examination reporting should be in keeping with the general guidance given in Chapter 7. Reports related to interventional procedures, however, require additional information about the procedure (Box 12.7).

SUMMARY

A wide range of image-guided interventional procedures are used to assist in the diagnosis and management of breast disease. Performance of these under ultrasound control has many advantages over clinical guidance or guidance with other imaging techniques. Ultrasound-guided breast intervention is cost-effective, accurate and well tolerated by patients, but is technically demanding; its safe practice requires considerable operator knowledge and skill.

References

AIUM 2002 Standard for the performance of breast ultrasound examination. Laurel, MD: American Institute of Ultrasound in Medicine.

Arisio R, Cuccorese C, Accinelli G et al 1998 Role of fine-needle aspiration biopsy on breast lesions: analysis of 4110 cases. Diagnostic Cytopathology 18(6):463–467.

AstraZeneca 2001 What you should know about Xylocaine® 0.5%, 1.0% and 2.0% with adrenaline 1:200,000 (product leaflet). Luton, UK: Astra Zeneca.

Badoual C, Maruani A, Ghorra C et al 2005 Pathological prognostic factors of invasive breast carcinoma in ultrasound-guided large core biopsies-correlation with subsequent surgical excisions. Breast 14(1):22–27.

Bates T, Davidson T, Mansel RE 2002 Litigation for pneumothorax as a complication of fine-needle aspiration of the breast. British Journal of Surgery 89(2):134–137.

Beres RA, Harrington DG, Wenzel MS 1997 Percutaneous repair of breast pseudoaneurysm: sonographically guided embolisation. AJR American Journal of Roentgenology 169:425–427.

Beyer T. Moonka R 2003 Normal mammography and ultrasonography in the setting of palpable breast cancer. American Journal of Surgery 185:416–419.

Birdwell RL, Jackman RJ 2003 Clip or marker migration 5–10 weeks after stereotactic 11-gauge vacuum-assisted breast biopsy: report of two cases. Radiology 229(2):541–544.

Bradford Hospitals NHS Trust (no date) Sharps injuries and blood contamination. Bradford, UK: Department of Occupational Medicine, BHNHST.

Brenner RJ, Farjardo L, Fisher PR et al 1996
Percutaneous core biopsy of the breast—effect of
operator experience and number of cores on diagnostic
accuracy. AJR American Journal of Roentgenology
166:341–344.

Britton PD 1999 Fine needle aspiration or core biopsy.
The Breast 8(1):1–4.

Britton PD, McCann J 1999 Needle biopsy in the NHS
breast screening programme 1996/1997: how much
and how accurate? The Breast 8(1):5–11.

Britton PD, Flower CD, Freeman AH et al 1997
Changing to core biopsy in an NHS breast screening
unit. Clinical Radiology 52(10):764–767.

Burbank F, Parker SH, Fogarty TJ 1996 Stereotactic
breast biopsy: improved tissue harvesting with the
Mammotome. American Surgeon 62(9):738–744.

Burnside ES, Sohlich RE, Sickles EA 2001 Movement of
a biopsy site marker clip after completion of stereotactic directional vacuum-assisted breast biopsy—case
report. Radiology 221:504–507.

Cabasares HV 1997 Office-based breast ultrasonography
in a small community surgical practice. American
Surgeon 63(8):716–719.

Chorny K, Raza S, Bradley FM et al 1997 Pseudoaneurysm formation in the breast after needle core biopsy.
Journal of Ultrasound in Medicine 16:849–851.

Dennis MA, Parker SH, Klaus AJ et al 2001 Breast biopsy
avoidance: the value of normal mammograms and
normal sonograms in the setting of a palpable lump.
Radiology 219(1):186–191.

Diaz LK, Wile EL, Venta LA 1999 Are malignant cells
displaced by large-gauge needle core biopsy of the
breast? AJR American Journal of Roentgenology
173(5):1303–1313.

Dixon AM 2006 Education and training for advanced
practice: principles of course design and assessment
applied to a stereotactic needle core biopsy of the
breast module. Radiography 12(2):79–87.

Dixon AM, Enion DS 2004 Pseudoaneurysm of the
breast: case study and review of the literature. British
Journal of Radiology 77:694–697.

Duijm LEM, Guit GL, Zaat JOM et al 1997 Sensitivity,
specificity and predictive values of breast imaging in the
detection of cancer. British Journal of Cancer
76(3):377–381.

Duthie S 2001 Stereo core biopsy of the breast. Synergy.
London: Society of Radiographers, pp. 14–19.

Fine RE, Whitworth PW, Kim JA et al 2003 Low-risk palpable breast masses removed using a vacuum-assisted
hand-held device. American Journal of Surgery
186(4):362–367.

Fishman JE, Milikowski C, Ramsinghani R et al 2003
US-guided core-needle biopsy of the breast: how many
specimens are necessary? Radiology 226:779–782.

Frazee RC, Roberts JW, Symmonds RE et al 1996 Open
versus stereotactic breast biopsy. American Journal of
Surgery 172:491–493.

Gately CA, Maddox PR, Mansel RE 1991 Pneumothorax:
a complication of fine-needle aspiration of the breast.
British Medical Journal 303(6803):627–628.

Graf O, Helbich TH, Fuchsjaeger MH et al 2004
Follow-up of palpable circumscribed noncalcified solid
breast masses at mammography and US: can biopsy be
averted? Radiology 233:850–856.

Harris AT 2003 Clip migration within 8 days of 11-gauge
vacuum assisted stereotactic breast biopsy—case report.
Radiology 228:552–554.

Harvey JA, Moran RE 1998 US-guided core needle
biopsy of the breast: technique and pitfalls.
Radiographics 18(4):867–877.

Harvey JA, Moran RE, Hamer MM et al 1997 Use of a
turkey breast phantom for teaching breast core-needle
biopsy. Academic Radiology 4:565–569.

Harvey JA, Moran RE, DeAngelis 2000 Technique and
pitfalls of ultasound-guided core-needle biopsy of the
breast. Seminars in Ultrasound, CT and MRI
21(5):362–374.

Hatada T, Aoki I, Okada K, Nakai T et al 1996
Usefulness of ultrasound-guided, fine-needle aspiration
biopsy for palpable breast tumours. Archives of Surgery
131(10):1095–1098.

Hauser JB, Mendelson E, Shaffer K 2000 ACR practice
guideline for the performance of stereotactically guided
breast interventional procedures. Reston, VA: American
College of Radiology.

Heywang-Kobrunner SH, Dershaw DD et al 2001
Diagnostic breast imaging. 2nd edn. Stuttgart:
Thieme.

Heywang-Kobrunner SH, Schreer I, Decker T et al 2003
Interdisciplinary consensus on the use and technique of
vacuum-assisted stereotactic breast biopsy. European
Journal of Radiology 47(3):232–236.

Hoorntje LE, Schipper ME, Kaya A et al 2004 Tumour
cell displacement after 14G breast biopsy. European
Journal of Surgical Oncology 20(5):520–525.

Huber S, Wagner M, Medl M et al 2003 Benign breast
lesions: minimally invasive vacuum-assisted biopsy with
11-gauge needles—patient acceptance and effect on
follow-up imaging findings. Radiology 226:783–790.

Jackman RJ, Burbank F, Parker SH et al 1997 Atypical
ductal hyperplasia diagnosed at stereotactic biopsy:
improved reliability with 14g, directional, vacuum-
assisted biopsy. Radiology 204(2):485–488.

Jackson P 2005 Histopathology. Lecture notes. Bradford,
UK: Division of Radiography, University of Bradford.

Jackson VP, Reynolds HE, Hawes DR 1996 Sonography
of the breast. Seminars in Ultrasound, CT and MRI
17(5):460–475.

Klijanienko J, Cote JF, Thibault F et al 1998 Ultrasound-guided fine-needle aspiration cytology of nonpalpable breast lesions: Institut Curie's experience with 109 histologically correlated cases. Cancer 84(1):36–41.

Kolb TM, Lichy J, Newhouse JH 1998 The effect of breast density, age and hormonal status upon breast cancer detection and stage: a comparison of sensitivities of screening mammography, ultrasound and physical examination. Radiology 209(P):391.

Laws SAM, McNamara IR, Cheetham JE et al 2002 Fine needle aspiration cytology prior to breast ultrasonography does not alter ultrasound diagnostic accuracy or patient management. The Breast 11:320–323.

Liberman L, Vuolo M, Dershaw DD et al 1999 Epithelial displacement after stereotactic 11-gauge directional vacuum-assisted breast biopsy. AJR American Journal of Roentgenology 172(3):677–681.

Liberman L, Bracero N, Morris E et al 2005 MRI-guided 9-gauge vacuum-assisted breast biopsy: initial clinical experience. AJR American Journal of Roentgenology 185:183–193.

Lister D, Evans A, Burrell H et al 1998 The accuracy of breast ultrasound in the evaluation of clinically benign discrete symptomatic breast lumps. Clinical Radiology 53:490–492.

Litherland J 2002 Should fine needle aspiration cytology in breast assessment be abandoned? Clinical Radiology 57(2):81–84.

Litherland JC, Evans AJ, Wilson AR et al 1996 The impact of core biopsy on pre-operative diagnosis rate of screen detected breast cancers. Clinical Radiology 51(8):562–565.

Madjar H 2000 The practice of breast ultrasound. New York: Thieme.

Madjar H, Rickard M, Jellins J 1999 IBUS guidelines for the ultrasonic examination of the breast. European Journal of Ultrasound 9:99–10.

Manan Medical Products (no date) The ProMag automatic biopsy device. Form 1038 Revision F PM-INS#1. DOC Manam Medical Products.

March DE, Coughlin BF, Barham RB et al 2003 Breast masses: removal of all US evidence during biopsy using a handheld vacuum-assisted device—initial experience. Radiology 227:549–555.

McNamara MP, Boden T 2002 Pseudoaneurysm of the breast related to 18-gauge core biopsy: successful repair using sonographically guided thrombin injection. AJR American Journal of Roentgenology 179:924–926.

Melotti MK, Berg WA 2000 Core needle breast biopsy in patients undergoing anticoagulation therapy. AJR American Journal of Roentgenology 174:245–249.

Meyer JE, Smith DN, Lester SC et al 1999 Large-core needle biopsy of non-palpable breast lesions. Journal of the American Medical Association 281(17): 1638–1641.

Mullen DJ, Eisen RN, Newman RD 2001 The use of carbon marking after stereo-tactic large-core-needle breast biopsy. Radiology 218(1):255–260.

NHS Cancer Screening Programmes 2001 Guidelines for non-operative diagnostic procedures and reporting in breast cancer screening. NHSBSP Publication No. 50. Sheffield: NHS Cancer Screening Programmes.

NHS Cancer Screening Programmes 2003 Quality assurance guidelines for surgeons in breast cancer screening. NHSBSP Publication No. 20. 3rd edn. Sheffield: NHS Cancer Screening Programmes.

NHS Cancer Screening Programmes 2005 Quality assurance guidelines for breast cancer screening radiology. NHSBSP Publication No. 59. Sheffield: NHS Cancer Screening Programmes.

Parker SH 1994 Percutaneous large core breast biopsy. Cancer 74(1 Suppl):256–262.

Parker SH, Klaus AJ 1997 Performing a breast biopsy with a directional, vacuum-assisted biopsy instrument. Radiographics 17(5):1233–1252.

Parker SH, Jobe WE, Dennis MA et al 1993. US-guided automated large-core breast biopsy. Radiology 187(2):507–511.

Parker SH, Burbank F, Jackman RJ et al 1994 Percutaneous large-core breast biopsy: a multi-institutional study. Radiology 193(2):359–364.

Parker SH, Klaus AJ, McWey PJ et al 2001 Sonographically guided directional vacuum-assisted breast biopsy using a handheld device. AJR American Journal of Roentgenology 177:405–408.

Phillips G, McGuire L, Clowes D 1994 The value of ultrasound-guided fine needle aspiration in the assessment of solid breast lumps. Australasian Radiology 38(3):187–192.

Philpotts LE, Lee CH 2002 Clip migration after 11-gauge vacuum assisted stereotactic biopsy: case report. Radiology 222:794–796.

Philpotts LE, Hooley RJ, Lee CH 2003 Comparison of automated versus vacuum-assisted biopsy methods for sonographically guided core biopsy of the breast. AJR American Journal of Roentgenology 180:347–351.

Ralleigh G, Michell MJ 2002 Image guided breast biopsy. International Journal of Clinical Practice 56(8):583–587.

RCN 2005 Hand hygiene. Online. London, Royal College of Nursing. Available at: http://www.rcn.org.uk/resources/mrsa/healthcarestaff/infectioncontrol/handhygiene.php Accessed 22 November 2005.

RCR 2003 Guidance on screening and symptomatic breast imaging. 2nd edn. BFCR(03)2, London: Royal College of Radiologists.

Rubin M, Horiuchi K, Joy N et al 1997 Use of fine needle aspiration for solid breast lesions is accurate and cost-effective. American Journal of Surgery 174(6):694–696.

Schoonjons JM, Brem RF 2001 Fourteen-gauge ultrasonographically guided large-core needle biopsy of breast masses. Journal of Ultrasound in Medicine 20(9):967–972.

Simon JR, Kalbhen CL, Cooper RA et al 2000 Accuracy and complication rates of US-guided vacuum-assisted core breast biopsy: initial results. Radiology 215:694–697.

Skills for Health 2003 M5.0: Undertake biopsy of breast tissue using X-ray guidance. Online. Available at: http://www.skillsforhealth.org.uk/viewcomp.php?id=1165 Accessed 12 August 2005.

Smith DN, Rosenfield Darling ML, Meyer JE et al 2001 The utility of ultrasonographically guided large-core needle biopsy: results from 500 consecutive breast biopsies. Journal of Ultrasound in Medicine 20(1):43–49.

Smith SM 1996 Breast pseudoaneurysm after core biopsy. AJR American Journal of Roentgenology 1996; 167:817.

Smith A, Lodge TD 2004 Can radiographic equipment be contaminated by micro-organisms to become a reservoir for cross infection? Synergy. London: Society of Radiographers, pp. 12–17.

Snead DR, Vryenhoef P, Pinder SE et al 1997 Routine audit of breast fine needle aspiration (FNA) cytology specimens and aspirator inadequate rates. Cytopathology 8(4):236–247.

Sneige N, Fornage BD, Saleh G 1994 Ultrasound-guided fine-needle aspiration of nonpalpable breast lesions. Cytologic and histologic findings. American Journal of Clinical Pathology 102(1):98–101.

Soo MS, Rosen EL, Baker JA et al 2001. Negative predictive value of sonography with mammography in patients with palpable breast lesions. AJR American Journal of Roentgenology 177:1167–1170.

SoR 1998 Control of infection protocol. London: Society of Radiographers.

Stetten G, Chib V, Hildebrand D et al 2001 Real time tomographic reflection: phantoms for calibration and biopsy. Online. IEEE/ACM International Symposium on Augmented Reality. New York. Available at: http://www.stetten.com/george/rttr/ISAR_Stetten_01.pdf Accessed 23 February 2006.

Tot T, Tabar L, Dean PB 2002 Practical breast pathology. New York: Thieme.

Vargas HI, Vargas MP, Gonzales KD et al 2004 Diagnosis of palpable breast masses: ultrasound-guided large core biopsy in a multidisciplinary setting. American Surgeon 70(10):867–871.

Wells CA, Perera CA, White FE et al 1999 Fine needle aspiration cytology in the UK breast screening programme: a national audit of results. The Breast 8(5):261–266..

White FE 1997 Ultrasound-guided biopsy of the breast. RAD Magazine 23(271):28.

Wilkinson LS, Given-Wilson R, Hall T et al 2005 Increasing the diagnosis of multifocal primary breast cancer by the use of bilateral whole-breast ultrasound. Clinical Radiology 60:573–578.

Wilson R 2003 Radiological procedures In Lee L, Stickland V, Wilson R et al (eds) Fundamentals of mammography. Edinburgh: Churchill Livingstone, pp. 91–104.

Woodcock NP, Glaves I, Morgan DR et al 1998 Ultrasound guided Tru-cut biopsy of the breast. Annals of the Royal College of Surgeons of England 80(4):253–256.

Yim JH, Barton P, Weber B et al 1997 Mammographically detected breast cancer. Benefits of stereotactic core versus wire localisation biopsy. Annals of Surgery 223:688–697.

Zardawi IM, Hearnden F, Meyer P et al 1999 Ultrasound-guided fine needle aspiration cytology of impalpable breast lesions in a rural setting. Comparison of cytology with imaging and final outcome. Acta Cytologia 43(2):163–168.

Chapter **13**

Additional diagnostic imaging techniques

Anne-Marie Dixon

INTRODUCTION

Ultrasound is just one of many diagnostic techniques for imaging the breast, and its use and value need to be considered in comparison with other, alternative techniques for producing images of breast tissue anatomy and, in some cases, images that reflect the dynamic physiology of the breast.

In addition to detection and characterization of breast abnormalities, patients with malignant disease also undergo diagnostic imaging procedures as part of the disease 'staging' process to determine the presence or absence of extramammary metastases.

This chapter starts by reviewing those techniques commonly used alongside ultrasound for diagnostic breast imaging, briefly explaining the physical principles underlying image production and illustrating the clinical usefulness of each technique; innovative imaging techniques currently under experimental investigation are then briefly described and the chapter concludes with a short review of the imaging techniques used for staging patients with malignant breast disease.

X-RAY MAMMOGRAPHY

Mammography is well established as the most important diagnostic imaging technique for the detection of breast cancer and forms the mainstay of imaging regimes in diagnostic breast services for screening, surveillance and symptomatic populations.

The mammographic image is essentially a (negative) gray-scale photographic representation of the way the different tissues within the breast attenuate electromagnetic (X) radiation, attenuation being a function of the atomic number of the tissues. Mammographic images are obtained by placing the breast tissue between a source of X-radiation and an image receptor using equipment specially designed for the purpose (Fig. 13.1). Tissues with relatively higher atomic number will attenuate more radiation than those with lower atomic number, the differential attenuation being represented as different degrees of blackening on the image. In conventional photographic film-based imaging, areas of greatest image blackening are associated with tissues of relatively low attenuation such as subcutaneous and retromammary fat, they are said to be radiolucent; conversely radio-opaque tissues, those with higher attenuation such as dense glandular tissue and calcifications, are associated with lighter (whiter) areas of the image (Fig. 13.2). With modern, digital equipment, the gray-scale allocation can be inverted, for example to demonstrate small microcalcifications more conspicuously as 'black dots' on a lighter background (Fig. 13.3).

The mammogram is a two-dimensional anatomical representation of breast tissue that is used to derive clinically useful information about the quantity and density of glandular breast tissue and about the spatial location, shape and dimensions of focal abnormalities—three-dimensional spatial awareness of anatomical relationships is achieved using two projections of each breast, one to give an oblique medio-lateral representation of anatomy and the other to give an supero-inferior 'view'.

Whilst there are many factors that influence the overall success of mammographic imaging, the ability to dem-

onstrate pathology fundamentally relies on the existence of a difference in X-radiation attenuation between abnormal and normal tissues. The main strengths of mammographic imaging are its ability readily to demonstrate solid attenuating tumors in contrast to radiolucent involuted breast tissue in older women (Fig. 13.4), and its ability to demonstrate and characterize the highly atten-

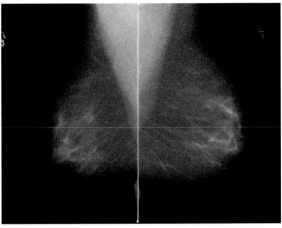

Figure 13.2 Normal mammography appearances of medio-lateral oblique projections. The parenchymal fibro-glandular tissue is more radio-opaque (whiter) than the supporting fatty tissue (mid-gray).

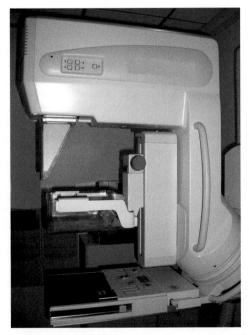

Figure 13.1 Application-specific X-ray equipment used to perform mammography.

Figure 13.3 With digital mammography equipment, the gray-scale polarity can be inverted better to visualize microcalcifications.

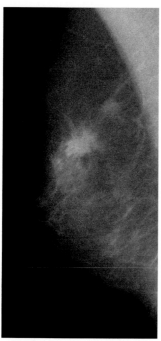

Figure 13.4   A right medio-lateral oblique mammogram showing an obvious focal lesion in a fatty breast—the lesion is more radio-opaque (light gray) in comparison with the radiolucent (dark-gray) fatty tissue.

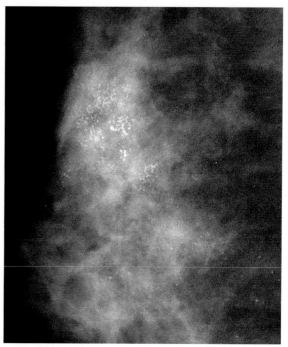

Figure 13.5   On a magnified view of the mammogram the characteristic features of malignant microcalcifications are apparent; they are typically irregular in size, shape and density (pleomorphic).

uating microcalcifications that are associated with preinvasive malignant disease (Fig. 13.5). Its main technical limitations lie in its inability to delineate attenuating tumors surrounded by attenuating normal glandular breast tissue—similar image densities are superimposed and are thus indistinguishable (Fig. 13.6), and the similarity in attenuation of some well-defined cystic and solid lesions potentially renders image interpretation nonspecific (Fig. 13.7).

Since mammographic imaging requires exposure to ionizing radiation, inevitably it comes with an associated, dose-dependent, biological risk of inducing malignancy. It is important to ensure that any mammography examination is 'justified' in radiological protection terms such that the magnitude of its potential benefit, in terms of cancer detection, exceeds the associated radiation risk (Law & Faulkner 2002). Younger women are more likely to have dense breast tissue, are at less risk of malignant breast disease and more likely to have well-defined benign focal lesions. In these women, the likelihood of deriving benefit from a potentially detectable mammography-demonstrated cancer may cease to outweigh the inherent radiation risk. For these reasons, ultrasound is considered a more appropriate first-line imaging investigation in young women and those suspected of having benign disease (RCR 2003).

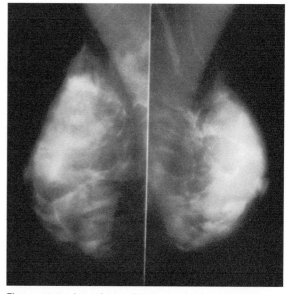

Figure 13.6   In patients with dense glandular breasts, overall mammographic density is increased, making it difficult to appreciate superimposed focal lesions—the invasive carcinoma in this patient is not as readily apparent as in Fig. 13.4.

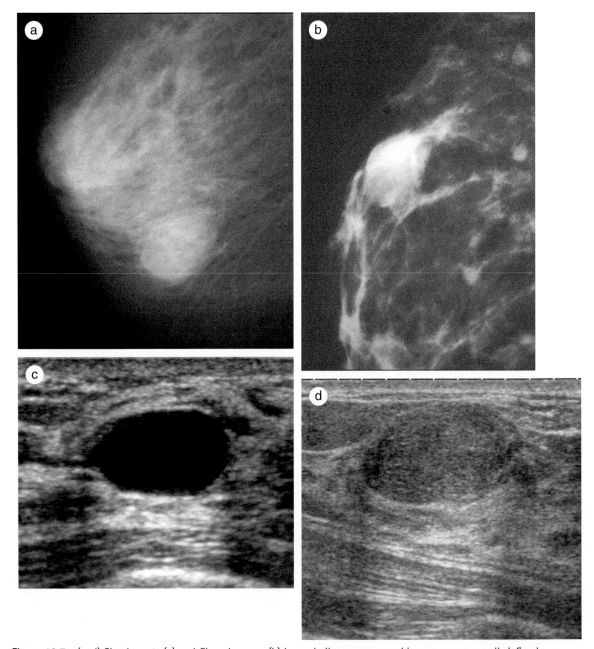

Figure 13.7   (a–d) Simple cysts (a) and fibroadenomas (b) have similar mammographic appearances: well-defined focal areas of increased density. Ultrasound will readily differentiate the fluid-filled anechoic cyst (c) from a solid fibroadenoma (d).

In the majority of cases when mammography has been performed as the first-line imaging investigation and a focal abnormality is detected, it is also useful to perform an ultrasound examination; in addition to providing further information that may assist differential diagnosis, such as assessment of axillary lymph node morphology, ultrasound guidance is preferred for any subsequent interventional procedures as it does not incur radiation hazard, is more cost-effective and is generally more comfortable for the patient. Lesions that are not visible at ultrasound, and in particular microcalcifications, will need to be localized for intervention using a stereotactic mammography technique.

MAGNETIC RESONANCE IMAGING

Magnetic resonance imaging (MRI) is increasingly being used in diagnostic breast services for 'problem-solving' in difficult cases and has also gained some acceptance in screening high risk populations; it has long been accepted as the most sensitive imaging technique for evaluating women with complications following breast augmentation.

Despite its high sensitivity and lack of associated radiation hazard, MRI is a relatively expensive investigation to perform and has limited specificity. With the exception of silicone implant evaluation, MRI is not suitable as a first-line or a sole investigation, and is only indicated in selected cases (Box 13.1). As an additional or 'comple-

---

Box 13.1   Appropriate indications for breast MRI

Primary diagnosis

- Suspected implant failure
- Preoperative assessment of extent of a known tumor
- Determination of multicentric ipsi- or contralateral disease
- Searching for a suspected primary breast tumor when a patient presents with lymph node or distant metastases
- Assessing response to neoadjuvant chemotherapy
- Screening high risk populations, particularly young women, those with dense breasts and genetic (BRCA1, BRCA2) mutation carriers

Postoperative

- Evaluation of potential residual disease
- Evaluation of potential local recurrence at site of wide local excision
- Evaluation of potential local recurrence after breast reconstruction
- Monitoring neoadjuvant chemotherapy

(after Heywang-Kobrunner et al 2001, p. 105, Kneeshaw et al 2003)

---

mentary' imaging technique, MR images should always be interpreted alongside those obtained with conventional mammography and/or ultrasound and with reference to clinical findings (Heywang-Kobrunner et al 2001, pp. 103, 108).

MR-compatible interventional equipment and consumables are available commercially; however, a significant number of MR-detected abnormalities, particularly malignancies, will have a mammographic or sonographic correlate and, although these may not exhibit 'typical' malignant features, identification reduces the need for MRI-guided biopsy (Sim et al 2005).

MR images are generated using information about the behavior of protons in the atoms of bodily tissue, particularly in the hydrogen atoms. Protons themselves have a net positive charge and are constantly in motion; as a moving electric charge, they have an associated magnetic field. The MR scanner contains a superconducting magnet that generates a high strength (0.5–1.5 Tesla) homogeneous magnetic field—it is worth noting here that if patients have any in-dwelling metallic 'foreign bodies', even medical devices such as pacemakers and surgical clips, these are absolute contraindications to the examination.

For breast MRI, the patient is positioned prone on the examination couch so that the breast(s) are suspended and immobilized within the field of radiofrequency (RF) transmission/receiver coils. The patient is then moved into the MR scanner magnet where, in response to the scanner's magnetic field, the patient's protons (and their associated magnetic fields) align with the scanner's magnetic field—this is known as longitudinal alignment. The RF coils are then used to transmit an electromagnetic wave, or RF pulse, across the patient, which results in a net transfer of energy to some of the protons and also displacement of their axis of motion—this only happens when the RF pulse frequency is the same as that of the proton motion—this is the 'resonance' part of magnetic resonance imaging! An electric current, the 'MRI signal', is generated by the magnetization associated with proton movement in the transverse plane; this signal is then picked up by the RF coils. The use of dedicated 'double-breast surface coils' (Fig. 13.8) and good patient immobilization optimize the sensitivity and image resolution (Heywang-Kobrunner et al 2001, p. 106). When the RF pulse is turned off, the protons gradually 'relax' back to their original energy state and 'relax' back to their original direction of movement. The MR image is generated using the proton relaxation times combined with information about the spatial location of the origin of MR signals within the body. Varying the magnetic field strength over the cross-section of the body generates the spatial information; since proton motion varies according to magnetic field strength, so

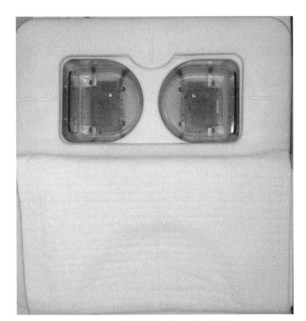

Figure 13.8 Dedicated 'double breast' radiofrequency surface coil device.

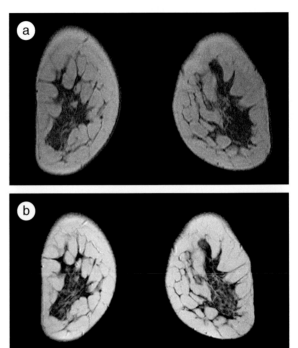

Figure 13.9 (a) T1-weighted sequences are usually used for MRI breast imaging. (Image courtesy of Mrs D. Dambitis, United Leeds Teaching Hospitals, Leeds, UK.)
(b) T2-weighted sequences provide additional information that may help to differentiate benign and malignant disease. (Image courtesy of Mrs D. Dambitis, United Leeds Teaching Hospitals, Leeds, UK.)

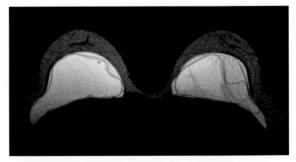

Figure 13.10 MRI is the most accurate diagnostic imaging technique for detection of implant rupture (see Ch. 10). (Image courtesy of Mrs D. Dambitis, United Leeds Teaching Hospitals, Leeds, UK.)

MR signals from protons located at different field strengths will also vary.

Relaxation times are determined by tissue composition and structure, are dependent upon the nature of surrounding structures and are proportional to magnetic field strength. Although MRI does not allow definitive tissue characterization, by varying RF pulse strength, timing and duration it is possible to 'weight' the effects of certain tissue characteristics within the image in order to emphasize different anatomical information (Fig. 13.9). Special silicone-specific sequences (Fig. 13.10) are employed in patients with breast implants to highlight free silicone (Kneeshaw et al 2003).

As on mammography and ultrasound imaging, lesions that are well defined, lobulated, smooth edged and without mass effect on surrounding tissues are likely to be benign, whilst lesions that are spiculate, irregular or poorly defined are more likely to be malignant (Reddy & Rankin 2002).

Contrast-enhanced MRI (ce-MRI) involves the intravenous administration of paramagnetic substances, the most common one being gadolinium bound to di-ethylene-triamine-penta-acetic acid (Gd-DTPA); this has the effect of shortening proton relaxation times and is predominantly used to 'enhance' visualization of tumor angiogenesis. Although MR imaging without the use of contrast is appropriate when silicone implant rupture is suspected, ce-MRI is used for all other referrals, with comparison of pre- and postcontrast (subtraction) images

an important component of image interpretation (Fig. 13.11). In addition to providing extra morphological information about the presence and distribution of enhancement, ce-MRI gives physiological information about the rate of enhancement (uptake and washout)

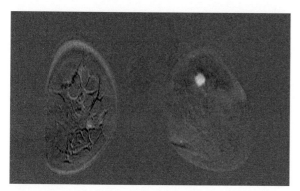

Figure 13.11 This MRI subtraction image highlights the contrast enhancement in a focal lesion in the left breast. (Image courtesy of Mrs D. Dambitis, United Leeds Teaching Hospitals, Leeds, UK.)

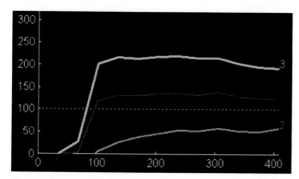

Figure 13.12 MRI time intensity curves. Malignant lesions tend to have rapid contrast uptake and early washout (turquoise line); the red line tracing would be categorized as suspicious for malignancy; benign lesions tend to show more gradual, continuous or delayed contrast enhancement (orange line). (Image courtesy of Mrs D. Dambitis, United Leeds Teaching Hospitals, Leeds, UK.)

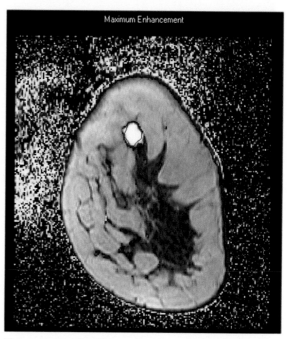

Figure 13.13 An MRI maximum intensity projection showing peripheral contrast enhancement—this feature is associated with malignant lesions. (Image courtesy of Mrs D. Dambitis, United Leeds Teaching Hospitals, Leeds, UK.)

through quantitative evaluation of variation in signal enhancement over time, i.e. the time–intensity curve (Fig. 13.12). The additional information is used in conjunction with anatomical MRI tumor features to improve differentiation of benign and malignant lesions and to assess tumor activity during neoadjuvant chemotherapy.

Although a degree of overlap in appearances precludes absolute differentiation in some cases, typically, malignant tumors show strong focal enhancement, particularly at their periphery (Fig. 13.13), and exhibit rapid contrast uptake and early washout (Fig. 13.14) whilst diffuse, delayed and well-circumscribed enhancement with a gradual progressive uptake and slow washout profile is more likely to be associated with benign disease

(Heywang-Kobrunner et al 2001, pp. 110–111, Reddy & Rankin 2002, Kneeshaw et al 2003).

With some patients, careful attention must be paid to the scheduling of MRI examinations as false-positive diagnoses may occur in the early postoperative/post irradiation period due to scar tissue formation, in women on hormone replacement therapy and at various stages of the menstrual cycle (Kuhl et al 1997, Muller-Schimpfle et al 1997, Heywang-Kobrunner et al 2001, p. 108, Kneeshaw et al 2003).

RADIONUCLIDE IMAGING

Radionuclide imaging (RNI) is a sensitive, primarily physiological, imaging technique that demonstrates biochemical tissue characteristics and gives information about functional changes associated with disease processes (Elgazzar 2001, Bombardieri et al 2003). The technique involves the intravenous administration of a pharmaceutical product that preferentially accumulates in the tissues of interest, to which has been added a radionuclide tracer substance, most commonly technetium[99m]. The clinical information gained from RNI is derived from the differential distribution of this *radiopharmaceutical* throughout the body, the radioactivity

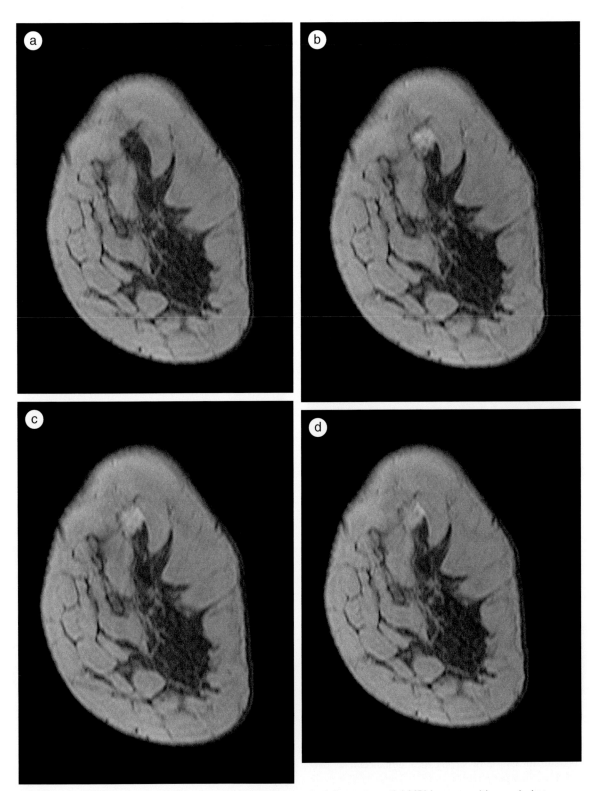

Figure 13.14 (a–e) Contrast uptake and washout data are acquired from sequential MRI images—a 'time series' at (a) 5 min 10 s after injection; (b) 5 min 44 s after injection; (c) 6 min 53 s after injection; (d) 9 min after injection. Sequential slice data are then combined to generate a time–intensity curve (e). (Images courtesy of Mrs D Dambitis, United Leeds Teaching Hospitals, Leeds, UK.)

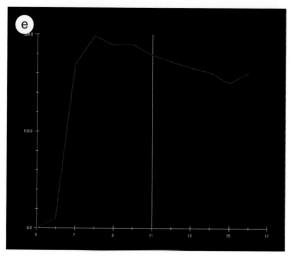

Figure 13.14 *Continued*

allowing it to be detected by non-invasive means using a gamma camera to give both pictorial anatomical representations and quantitative measurements (Sharp 1998, p. 1).

The gamma camera contains a scintillation crystal that detects gamma radiation emitted from the patient as the radionuclide tracer decays and converts it to photons of light; photomultiplier tubes then convert the light energy into an electronic signal from which spatial location and intensity of radioactivity are derived (Sharp 1998, p. 3). It should be noted that this a radiation-based imaging technique and thus careful consideration is required before performing the examination, particularly on a pregnant or lactating woman.

Scintimammography

RNI has been suggested as an alternative to ultrasound or MRI, when an additional imaging investigation is required in patients at high risk, or with a high index of suspicion for breast malignancy in whom clinical and/or mammographic findings are negative, inadequate (scarring, dense breasts, implants) or indeterminate (previous radiotherapy, some calcifications and parenchymal deformities) (Waxman 1997, Murray & Brooks 2000, Bombardieri et al 2003, Brem et al 2005). In addition, scintimammography is considered to have a role similar to that described above for MRI, in the identification of multicentric or contralateral disease and in assessing tumor response to chemotherapy (Bombardieri et al 2003), and is considered more sensitive than mammography and ultrasound for detection of disease recurrence (Buscombe 2002).

In breast imaging, the radiopharmaceutical used is usually technetium^{99m} sestamibi (^{99m}Tc-MIBI)—a product that has an affinity for mitochondrial activity; although faint homogeneous physiological uptake can be seen generally in the breasts (particularly the nipples) and in the axilla, preferential accumulation is markedly evident in breast (amongst other) neoplasms (Bombardieri et al 2003).

The scintimammography technique involves a peripheral intravenous injection of the radiopharmaceutical before placing the patient in close proximity to the gamma camera; the patient is then sequentially repositioned to acquire right and left prone lateral and supine anterior images of both breasts and axillae (Fig. 13.15)—the whole examination taking approximately 40 min (Murray and Brooks 2000, Bombardieri et al 2003).

As with MRI, RNI information can be displayed as either an anatomical gray-scale representation or as a time–intensity curve—this latter is also known in RNI as a time–activity curve. On a gray-scale image, the amount of film 'blackening' is proportional to the amount of radiation emitted at the corresponding anatomical location—areas of increased activity, known as 'hot spots', may be displayed either as darker areas against a 'normal' white background (Fig. 13.16), or as whiter areas against a 'normal' black background (Fig. 13.17). The time–activity curve shows how the amount of radioactivity corresponding to a particular (operator determined) anatomical area of interest varies over time (Fig. 13.18).

Similar to X-ray and ultrasound breast imaging, a lexicon of semi-quantitative terminology has been proposed to categorize radioactivity patterns (Table 13.1) (Brem et al 2005). Image interpretation should be performed in the light of findings from a clinical examination and with reference to the appearances demonstrated at X-ray mammography and ultrasound; menstrual phase is worth noting but, to date, no clear influence on scintimammographic appearances has been noted (Bombardieri et al 2003). False-positive results can occur with recent iatrogenic breast trauma, i.e. needle aspiration and needle or surgical biopsy, in those patients who have had recent radiation therapy or chemotherapy and with some benign proliferative conditions (Bombardieri et al 2003, Brem et al 2005).

RNI is essentially a physiological imaging procedure with relatively poor spatial resolution, as such its sensitivity for small (<10 mm) breast lesions is low, and thus its use as a routine investigation is limited (Bombardieri et al 2003). Improved sensitivity, and the ability to detect subcentimeter lesions, has been demonstrated with prototype dedicated breast-specific gamma cameras that also allow imaging in anatomical planes directly comparable with those used for conventional X-ray mammography (Brem et al 2002, 2005). As was the case, however, with

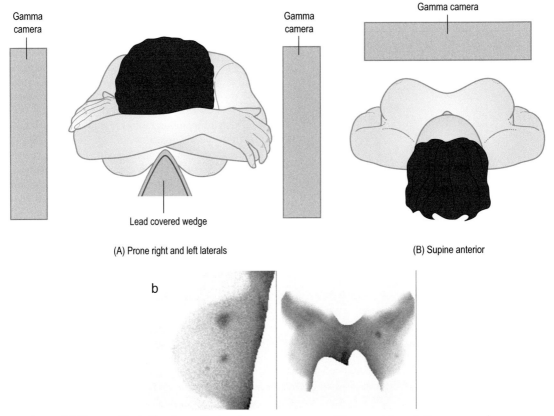

Figure 13.15 (a) Diagram illustrating the patient and gamma camera positions used for scintimammography. (b) Scintimammography images demonstrating multiple tumors in the left breast—note masking of radiotracer activity in the thyroid gland, liver and heart. (Image courtesy of Dr A. Mackie, University Hospital of North Durham.)

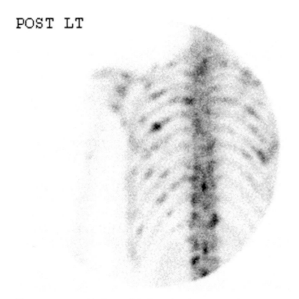

Figure 13.16 Radionuclide imaging bone scan image showing bony metastases as black 'hot spots'.

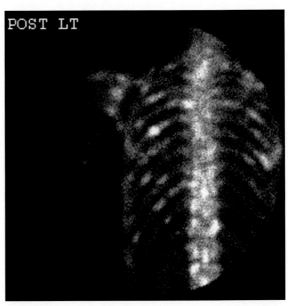

Figure 13.17 Reversed polarity RNI image showing bony metastases as white 'hot spots'.

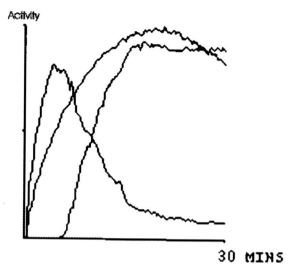

30 MINS

Figure 13.18 Examples of 'time–activity curves' generated from RNI data.

Table 13.1 Scintimammography lexicon for disease classification

Score	Classification	Scintigraphic pattern
1	Normal	Diffuse/no focal uptake
2	Benign	Minimal patchy (physiological) uptake
3	Probably benign	Scattered patchy uptake
4	Probably abnormal	Mild focal uptake
5	Abnormal	Marked focal uptake

Brem et al (2005).

early breast MRI, the clinical usefulness of RNI as a screening tool is likely to be limited until the capability to perform gamma camera-guided localization techniques is developed, and its clinical potential is shown to outweigh its associated biological risk.

Single photon emission computed tomography (SPECT)

The conventional radionuclide image is a planar image demonstrating three-dimensional distribution of radio-activity in two dimensions and thus inherently superimposing information about structures at different depths within the patient; SPECT imaging involves the collection of radionuclide activity information in multiple planes around the patient and the mathematical recon-struction of this information to produce images that represent discrete cross-sectional slices of the patient (Gemmell & Staff 1998).

The improved contrast resolution, and removal of overlying structures, renders SPECT a more sensitive technique than planar imaging (Mathieu et al 2005).

Positron emission tomography (PET)

The technique of PET requires either a modified dual-headed gamma camera, or a dedicated PET imager, to allow the simultaneous detection of pairs of gamma rays (traveling in opposite directions) produced during the annihilation process when positrons (positively charged electrons) combine with (negatively charged) electrons (Sharp 1998, p. 325). With multiple detectors arranged in rings around the patient, the detection of truly coin-cident pairs of gamma rays allows the location of an originating (positron-emitting) radionuclide within the patient to be determined to within approximately 3 mm (Sharp 1998, p. 326). The positron-emitting radiophar-maceutical fluorine-18 fluorodeoxyglucose (FDG) is a glucose analog that demonstrates areas of increased metabolic activity, a process that is enhanced in malignant cells.

FDG-PET imaging results for primary breast cancer detection are inconsistent across published studies and, although sensitivity is independent of breast density, the technique may yield false-negative results for very small lesions, lobular carcinoma and in situ disease; as it is also associated with high cost and a radiation dose, it is not recommended for screening in preference to conventional X-mammography (Rostrom et al 1999, Bombardieri et al 2003, Mustafa et al 2004). However, FDG-PET has an accepted role in breast cancer staging, re-staging and in monitoring response to treatment—the technique is able to demonstrate tumor recurrence more accurately than mammography and is unique among diagnostic imaging investigations in that it reliably dem-onstrates local, regional and distant metastatic disease during a single whole body examination (Rostrom et al 1999, Mustafa et al 2004).

PET is nevertheless a physiological technique that somewhat lacks spatial precision; however, recently developed PET-CT (computed tomography) systems allow fusion of (functional) PET and (anatomical) CT images and enable improved tumor localization and identification and permit more accurate disease staging and treatment planning (Wechalekar & Sharma 2004).

Sentinel node localization

The presence or absence of tumor in regional lymph nodes is an important prognostic indicator in patients with breast cancer. Failure to remove diseased regional lymph nodes surgically will result in disease understaging, suboptimal treatment and a poorer prognosis (Krasnow and Elgazzar 2001). Conversely, extensive excision of all, including disease-free, lymph nodes is undesirable since it carries an increased risk of postoperative complication, debilitating long-term upper limb lymphedema, parasthesia and movement restriction, and also potentially removes a filtering mechanism that may inhibit tumor cell migration (Krasnow and Elgazzar 2001). Selective excision and histological examination of small numbers of lymph nodes has the potential to reduce the need for radical axillary clearance and reduce associated morbidity in patients with node-negative disease (Madjar 2000, p. 182).

The lymph nodes that receive the initial lymphatic drainage from a tumor site are known as the sentinel nodes. It is not unusual for there to be multiple sentinel nodes and in multiple locations—in the breast sentinel nodes are usually in the axillary bed but may be in the internal mammary chain or, very rarely, interpectoral, intramammary or elsewhere (Krag et al 1998, Krasnow & Elgazzar 2001). Routine surgical axillary clearance is inherently associated with a risk of understaging patients with disease-containing nodes at other locations.

The technique of RNI sentinel node biopsy (SNB) involves injection of saline-buffered 99mTc labeled with nanocolloid into the breast. Current practice is to use a periareolar intradermal injection technique, as opposed to subdermal or direct peritumoral infiltration, as this appears to give more rapid visualization and significantly higher sentinel node detection rates (Motomura et al 2003, Bury 2005 personal communication). During their course of passage along the lymphatic drainage pathways, the large (radiotracer-labeled) colloid molecules become trapped in the reticuloendothelial cells of the lymph nodes during the phagocytosis process, and this renders the area a 'hot spot' on RNI images (Fig, 13.19). Dynamic imaging allows mapping of the lymphatic drainage pathways from the tumor site (Fig. 13.20) with a small hand-held gamma probe used subsequently to localize the first nodes to receive lymphatic drainage—the sentinel nodes—for surgical excision and histological analysis. Where the sentinel nodes are disease free, the patient can be spared further lymph node dissection, positive sentinel nodes directing the surgeons to continue with more extensive lymphadenectomy.

SNB is a minimally invasive procedure that may be carried out under local anesthesia using out-patient or day-case facilities, and was initially thought to be an attractive alternative to full axillary clearance. However, the technique has proved to be technically challenging

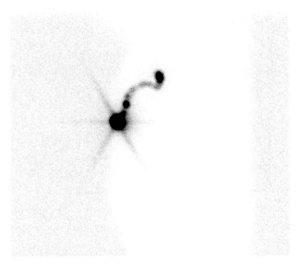

LAT 30 MINS TR

Figure 13.19   Sentinel node mapping. Radionuclide image showing the lymphatic drainage pathway tracking from the breast injection site to the sentinel node in the axilla.

and operator dependent; it assumes that all tumor metastasis occurs in a systematic and orderly fashion—which may not be the case—and it is subject to both false-negative and false-positive diagnoses (Krag et al 1998, Murray & Brookes 2000). Currently, sentinel node localization and biopsy is considered to have most potential for staging small malignant lesions that are likely to be node negative but may have micrometastatic lymph node involvement (Heywang-Kobrunner et al 2001).

RECENT IMAGING INNOVATIONS

In recent years, technological progress, particularly in relation to digital imaging capability and computer-assisted detection (CAD), has led to development and evaluation of advanced mammographic techniques such as tomosynthesis (Niklason et al 1998). This technique overcomes some of the inherent limitations of conventional mammography and shows promise for improving mammographic sensitivity particularly in the dense breast (Chan et al 2005).

In addition, several new methods for image-based diagnosis of breast cancer have been proposed—those

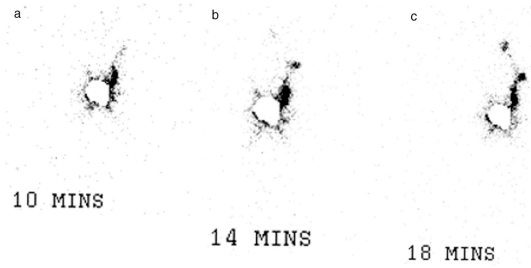

a   b   c

10 MINS

14 MINS

18 MINS

Figure 13.20   (a–c) Sentinel node mapping series. RNI images showing activity at (a) 10 min after injection, (b) 14 min after injection and (c) 18 min after injection. Note that the high activity at the injection site has been masked to improve visualization of the lymphatic drainage pathway.

showing most promising experimental results are based on properties such as tissue elasticity (ultrasound and MR elastography), light transmission (optical tomography/near infrared imaging/laser mammography), electrical impedance and metabolite concentration (electrical impedance spectral imaging, microwave imaging spectroscopy) (Heywang-Kobrunner et al 2001, pp. 129–130, Poplack et al. 2004, IDSI 2005, Zhu et al. 2005).

To be adopted into mainstream clinical use, any new diagnostic imaging technique must demonstrate high sensitivity, particularly for small lesions and preinvasive disease, and high specificity if it is to be used for screening asymptomatic subjects, or it must add a significant amount of important prognostic information in cases of known malignancy. The challenge for any new image-based diagnostic investigation is to surpass the clinical efficacy and cost-effectiveness of the current gold standard 'triple tssessment' approach (Murray 1998).

BREAST CANCER STAGING—DETECTION OF METASTATIC DISEASE

The presence of distant spread of malignant disease has a significant adverse effect on prognosis and requires systemic, in addition to local, measures for disease control and therapy. The most common sites for distant breast cancer metastases are lung, bone and liver (Porter et al 2004). Histological confirmation of breast malignancy

normally triggers referral for chest radiography, bone scintigraphy and liver ultrasound or CT, although in the newly diagnosed asymptomatic patient with a small, low grade tumor the incidence of metastasis is rare and these routine staging tests are not necessarily indicated (Schneider et al 2003, Puglisi et al 2005).

Pulmonary metastases—chest radiography and computed tomography

Plain film chest radiography (Fig. 13.21) is the simplest technique for detecting and monitoring lung metastases, the postero-anterior and lateral projections reliably demonstrating most lesions larger than 10 mm (Armstrong 1992). Increased sensitivity, particularly for smaller lesions, is achieved with CT (Fig. 13.22); however, this is at the expense of reduced specificity, and its use is only recommended in selected cases (Chalmers & Best 1991, Armstrong 1992). On radiography (Fig. 13.23) and CT (Fig. 13.24), pulmonary metastases are evident as discrete, and often multiple solid nodules and, whilst usually spherical and well defined, may also be irregular. Both chest radiography and thoracic CT also have the potential to demonstrate bony metastases, with CT also allowing detection of mediastinal lymphadenopathy.

Bone scintigraphy

Although bony metastases are rare in stage 1 and 2 breast cancers, they are present in up to 50% of patients with

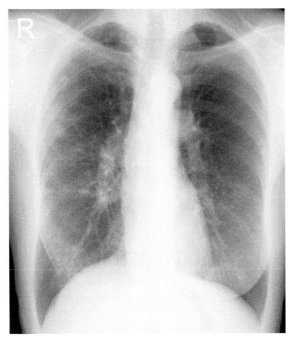

Figure 13.21   The postero-anterior chest radiograph is routinely used to monitor patients with known metastatic breast cancer. A 'normal' examination at presentation is reassuring and makes subsequent disease progression easier to detect.

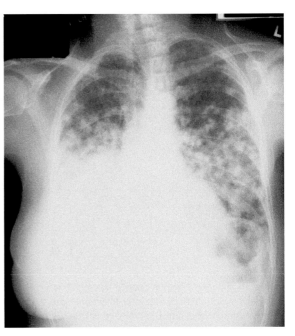

Figure 13.23   Postero-anterior chest radiograph showing lung metastases and malignant pleural effusion in a patient with breast cancer—note the absence of a superimposed breast shadow at left lung base due to the previous mastectomy.

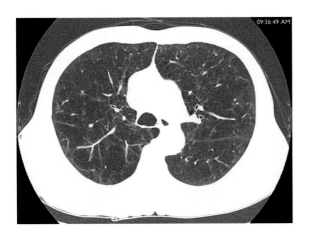

Figure 13.22   Computed tomography images represent axial slices through the body. Manipulation of scan parameters is required to demonstrate different tissue types preferentially. This image has been manipulated to display the lung parenchyma.

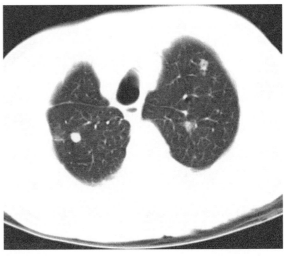

Figure 13.24   CT scan image showing bilateral lung metastases.

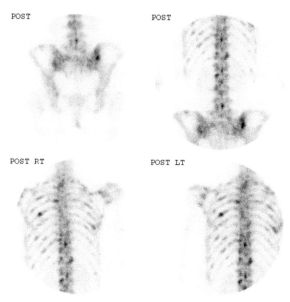

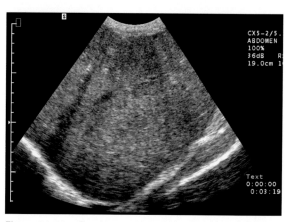

Figure 13.26 On ultrasound images of the liver, multiple diffuse metastases give rise to an overall heterogeneous coarse echo texture with several subtle round focal lesions. (Image courtesy of Dr S. Elliott, Freeman Hospital, Newcastle upon Tyne, UK.)

Figure 13.25 RNI bone scan image series showing widespread bony metastases (black not spots).

stage 3 disease; breast cancer accounts for the majority of bony metastases in the female population (Elgazzar et al 2001). RNI is relatively inexpensive, well tolerated and has high sensitivity, as such it is considered the most appropriate diagnostic imaging investigation for detecting metastatic tumor deposits in the bony skeleton (Murray & Brookes 2000). It is particularly suitable as a routine screening test since early bony metastatic disease is invariably asymptomatic and not apparent at plain film radiography (Elgazzar et al 2001).

Due to a presumed venous hematological mechanism of spread, the most common location for bony metastases is the marrow-rich axial skeleton, particularly the vertebral bodies. After administration of technetium 99m methylenediphosphonate (^{99m} Tc-MDP), metastases are commonly and typically demonstrated on radionuclide images as multiple randomly distributed foci of increased radiotracer uptake (Fig. 13.25).

Liver ultrasound or computed tomography

Liver metastases are less common than either pulmonary or bone metastases. Routine imaging of the asymptomatic patient is rarely of clinical value, and any claims of 'reassurance' value are no more than anecdotal; liver deposits are more likely in those patients with hepatomegaly or altered liver biochemistry (MacVicar 2004). Liver metastases tend to be hyporeflective lesions, often with a 'target' appearance, on ultrasound images (Fig.

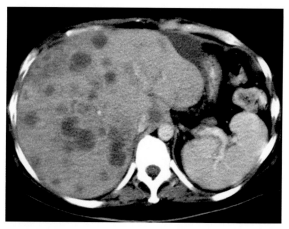

Figure 13.27 Liver metastases are often more conspicuous on CT images.

13.26) and of low attenuation on CT portal phase images (Fig. 13.27) (MacVicar 2004).

SUMMARY

Diagnostic imaging has a vital role in the diagnosis and management of breast cancer, with the imaging specialist having an array of techniques at their disposal. In order that imaging strategies are both cost-effective and clinically efficient, before any test is instigated, careful deliberation is required to assess the relative technical and diagnostic performance characteristics of each investigation, the anticipated diagnostic and therapeutic yield expected, and the overall potential for a positive impact on patient health.

References

Armstrong P 1992 Pulmonary neoplasm. In Grainger RG, Allison DJ (eds) Diagnostic radiology. Edinburgh: Churchill Livingstone, pp. 271–293.

Bombardieri E, Aktolun C, Baum RP et al 2003 Breast scintigraphy: procedure guidelines for tumour imaging. Vienna: European Association of Nuclear Medicine.

Brem RF, Schoonjans JM, Kieper DA et al 2002 High-resolution scintimammography: a pilot study. Journal of Nuclear Medicine 43:909–915.

Brem RF, Rapelyea JA, Zisman G et al 2005 Occult breast cancer: scintimammography with high resolution breast-specific gamma camera in women at high risk for breast cancer. Radiology 237:274–280.

Buscombe JR 2002 Monitoring therapy in breast cancer. Nuclear Medicine Communications 23(7): 619–624.

Chalmers N, Best JJ 1991 The significance of pulmonary nodules detected by CT but not by chest radiography in tumour staging. Clinical Radiology 44(6):410–412.

Chan HP, Wei J, Sahiner B et al 2005 Computer-aided detection system for breast masses on digital tomosynthesis mammograms: preliminary experience. Radiology 237(3):1075–1080.

Elgazzar AH 2001 The pathophysiological basis of nuclear medicine. Berlin: Springer-Verlag.

Elgazzar AH, Shehab D, Malki A et al 2001 Musculo-Skeletal System. In Elgazzar AH (ed.) The pathophysiological basis of nuclear medicine. Berlin: Springer-Verlag, pp. 88–126.

Gemmell HG, Staff RT 1998 Sinngle-photon emission-computed tomography (SPECT) In Sharp PF, Gemmell HG, Smith FW (eds) Practical nuclear medicine. Oxford: Oxford University Press, pp. 13–24.

Heywang-Kobrunner SH, Dershaw DD, Screer I 2001 Diagnostic breast imaging. Stuttgart: Thieme.

IDSI 2005 CTLM® CT laser mammography system—technical description. Florida: Florida Imaging Diagnsotic Systems Inc.

Kneeshaw PJ, Drew PJ, Turnbull LW 2003 MRI imaging of the breast. RAD Magazine 29(337):29–30.

Krag D, Weaver D, Ashikaga T et al 1998 The sentinel node in breast cancer. New England Journal of Medicine 339(14):941–946.

Krasnow AZ, Elgazzar AH 2001 Lymphoscintigraphy. In Elgazzar AH (ed.) The pathophysiological basis of nuclear medicine. Berlin: Springer-Verlag, pp. 330–337.

Kuhl CK, Bieling HB, Gieseke J et al 1997 Healthy pre-menopausal breast parenchyma in dynamic contrast-enhanced MR imaging of the breast: normal contrast medium enhancement and cyclical-phase dependency. Radiology 203:137–144.

Law J, Faulkner K 2002 Two-view screening and extending the age range: the balance of benefit and risk. British Journal of Radiology 75:889–894.

MacVicar D 2004 Breast cancer. In Husband JE, Reznek RH (eds) Imaging in oncology. 2nd edn. London: Taylor and Francis, pp. 559–585.

Madjar H 2000 The practice of breast ultrasound. New York: Thieme.

Mathieu I, Mazy S, Willemart B et al 2005 Inconclusive triple diagnosis in breast cancer imaging: is there a place for scintimammography? Journal of Nuclear Medicine 46(10):1574–1581.

Motomura K, Komoike Y, Hasegawa Y et al 2003 Intradermal radioisotope injection is superior to sub-dermal injection for the identification of the sentinel node in breast cancer patients. Journal of Surgical Oncology 82:91–97.

Muller-Schimpfle M, Ohmenhauser K, Stoll P et al 1997 Menstrual cycle and age: influence of parenchymal contrast medium enhancement in MR imaging of the breast. Radiology 203:145–149.

Murray AD 1998 Magnetic resonance imaging in patients with breast cancer. RAD Magazine 24(278):35–36.

Murray AD, Brooks ME 2000 Nuclear medicine in oncology. Journal of the Royal College of Surgeons of Edinburgh 45(1):110–119.

Mustafa S, Marshall C, Wheatley DC, et al 2004 Double-headed gamma camera PET imaging of the breast. RAD Magazine 30(350):21–22.

Niklason LT, Kopans DB, Hamberg LM 1998 Digital breast imaging: tomosynthesis and digital subtraction mammography. Breast Diseases 10(3–4):151–164.

Poplack SP, Paulsen KD, Hartov A et al 2004 Electromagnetic breast imaging: average tissue property values in women with negative clinical findings. Radiology 231:571–580.

Porter GJ, Evans AJ, Pinder SE et al 2004 Patterns of metastatic breast carcinoma: influence of tumour histological grade. Clinical Radiology 59(12):1094–1098.

Puglisi F, Follador A, Minisini AM et al 2005 Baseline staging tests after a new diagnosis of breast cancer: further evidence of their limited indications. Annals of Oncology 16(2):263–266.

RCR 2003 Guidance on screening and symptomatic breast imaging. 2nd edn. BFCR(03)2, 2003. London: Royal College of Radiologists.

Reddy M, Rankin S 2002 MRI of benign breast disease. RAD Magazine 29(326):35–36.

Rostrom AY, Powe J, Kandil A et al 1999 Positron emission tomography in breast cancer: a clinicopathological correlation of results. British Journal of Radiology 72:1064–1068.

Schneider C, Fehr MK, Steiner RA et al 2003 Frequency and distribution pattern of distant metastases in breast cancer patients at the time of primary presentation. Archives of Gynecology and Obstetrics 269(1):9–12.

Sharp PF 1998 Nuclear medicine imaging. In Sharp PF, Gemmell HG, Smith FW (eds) Practical nuclear medicine. Oxford: Oxford University Press, pp. 1–12.

Sim LSJ, Hendriks JHCL, Bult P et al 2005 US correlation for MRI detected breast lesions in women with familial risk of breast cancer. Clinical Radiology 60:801–806.

Waxman AD 1997 The role of (99m)Tc methoxyisobutyl-isonitrile in imaging breast cancer. Seminars in Nuclear Medicine 27(1):40–54.

Wechalekar K, Sharma B 2004 PET-CT in oncology. RAD Magazine 30(349):4 and 36

Zhu Q, Cronin EB, Currier AA et al 2005 Benign versus malignant breast masses: optical differentiation with us-guided optical imaging reconstruction. Radiology 237:57–66.

Further recommended reading

Elgazzar AH 2001 The pathophysiological basis of nuclear medicine. Berlin: Springer-Verlag.

Heywang-Kobrunner SH, Dershaw DD, Screer I 2001 Diagnostic breast imaging. Stuttgart: Thieme.

Husband JE, Reznek RH (eds) 2004 Imaging in oncology. 2nd edn. London: Taylor and Francis.

Morris EA, Liberman L (eds) 2005 Breast MRI: diagnosis and intervention. New York: Springer.

Schild HH 1990 MRI made easy. Berlin: Schering.

Chapter **14**

Breast imaging service provision, education and training

Jacqui Lee and Anne-Marie Dixon

INTRODUCTION

The use of the terminology *breast imaging* implies, and in reality does involve, a fully integrated approach to the diagnosis of breast disease using a range of image-based techniques alongside other clinical and pathological examinations; this is known as the *triple assessment* approach (Khalkhali & Vargas 2005). The traditional X-ray mammogram remains the primary technique for imaging the breast (Jackson et al 1996) but mammography is now often supplemented by further imaging investigations most commonly ultrasound, a readily available non-invasive technique, magnetic resonance imaging (MRI) and radionuclide imaging (RNI) (Khalkhali & Vargas 2005).

Thus the focus of the modern breast imaging service is much more than the traditional dedicated mammography room within a general X-ray Department. Breast imaging is now appropriately recognized as an imaging subspecialty in its own right, and the present-day breast imaging service is identified as a facility that invariably offers routine access to diagnostic medical ultrasound examinations in addition to conventional X-ray mammography. The ability to offer both these imaging investigations on demand for the majority of referrals is most commonly achieved by locating the service outside the main radiology department as an integral component of a dedicated clinical consultation suite—the Breast, or Breast Screening, Unit (Houssami et al 2005). The less frequently used additional imaging services such as MRI and RNI are more likely to be provided centrally in a main imaging department, and are usually accessed by prearranged appointment.

The aim of any Breast Unit is to provide high quality care to those clients/patients who attend screening and assessment services and symptomatic clinics. In order that a breast service is judged to be of high quality, it needs to provide a seamless diagnostic and patient management pathway that balances the needs of both service providers and service users. The general public is increasingly well informed and, quite rightly, expects to have confidence in the quality of clinical care and be assured that professional standards are high. However, in potential conflict with this is a need to provide an evidence-based service that is clinically and cost effective but has the patient as its central focus.

Dedicated screening and 'one-stop' symptomatic units are now well established in the UK, as breast services have undergone a major restructuring in response to the Calman–Hine report of 1995 (DH 1995). The Calman–Hine report outlined a strategy for improving overall outcomes for patients with cancer through the establishment of national standards of practice and care. Breast cancer was highlighted as one of the most important malignant pathologies that required high quality diagnostic and treatment services as part of a national framework for streamlined early diagnostic and treatment pathways. The responsibility for local implementation of the Calman–Hine recommendations is invested in multidisciplinary teams of healthcare professionals where senior staff members are identified as clinical leads within their individual disciplines, and the team is under the overall leadership of a Clinical Director, usually a consultant surgeon with an interest in breast disease (Table 14.1) (BASO 2005).

Realization, to a large extent, of the Calman–Hine recommendations in screening and symptomatic breast services across the UK has brought encouraging results; breast cancer mortality rates are falling and 5-year survival for invasive disease is increasing at a faster rate in the UK compared with other countries with similar screening and treatment programs (DH 2000a).

Subsequent to the Calman–Hine reforms, publication of the NHS Cancer Plan (DH 2000b) initiated expansion of the National Health Service Breast Screening Programme (NHSBSP) and a requirement to reduce referral to diagnosis and treatment times for all cancers in order to improve cancer outcomes. These ambitious plans had a major impact on diagnostic imaging services in that the increased demand for more timely diagnostic investigations placed great pressure on the radiology and radiography professions (RCR 2002). This led to innovative skills-mix programs to try to increase capacity and recruit and retain adequate numbers of skilled staff in these professions.

The increased demand for ultrasound examinations is a result of technological advances in equipment; smaller and less expensive ultrasound machines are now widely available and this has increased the awareness of both the general public and medical clinicians of the diagnostic

Table 14.1 Constituent members of the breast multidisciplinary team

Diagnostic team	Cancer treatment team
Breast specialist clinician and team	Members of diagnostic team
Consultant surgeon	Consultant clinical oncologist
Associate specialist	Consultant medical oncologist
Breast clinicians	Plastic and reconstructive surgeon
Staff grade surgeons	Medical geneticist
SpR trainees	Data management personnel
Specialist radiologist and radiographer	Research nurse
	Lymphedema specialist
Pathologist	Medical prosthetist
Cytopathologist	Clinical psychologist
Histopathologist	Palliative care team
Laboratory support staff	
Breast care nurse	
Clinical staff	
Administrative staff	

After BASO (2005).

capabilities of this radiation-free investigation. Breast ultrasound, in particular, is a good example of how an imaging technique can rapidly develop from a secondary test used in a minority of patients into an essential and often first-line test for the diagnosis and management of a clinically important disease.

In addition to the demands of the NHS Cancer Plan, several other important factors are contributing to an effective increase in demand on radiology departments and radiologists; these factors are also driving the need for further service expansion and innovative skills-mix across the professional boundaries of the involved healthcare professions (Box 14.1).

In order to meet demand, non-medical allied health professionals, i.e. radiographers, have been encouraged to extend their scope of practice to include tasks previously undertaken by their medical colleagues, advance their practice by taking responsibility for clinical decision making and take on autonomous membership of the multidisciplinary healthcare team (White & MacKay 2004).

RADIOGRAPHER ROLE DEVELOPMENT AND ROLE EXTENSION

Radiographers have always acknowledged the potential for developing and refining their skills; thus, role development and role extension are not new concepts. As long ago as 1971, Swinburne highlighted an anticipated shortage of radiologists and the need to think beyond traditional professional boundaries in order to address this (Swinburne 1971). Radiographers have always been encouraged to provide albeit a verbal, professional opinion in respect of a radiographic image but, by suggesting that radiographers were capable and prepared to take on some of the radiologists' responsibilities, Swinburne broke new ground and championed both a change in the status of the radiographer and recognition of their developmental potential for formal radiographic image interpretation and reporting.

Medical ultrasound was one of the first areas in diagnostic imaging where non-medical personnel, i.e. the ultrasound qualified radiographer, sometimes termed ultrasonographer or sonographer, was allowed formally to generate the official report for a diagnostic imaging examination. Although initially restricted to obstetric ultrasound examinations, this practice was accepted with very little resistance from other healthcare professionals and was subsequently shown to be effective for a wide range of clinical applications. The formal role of 'reporting radiographer' finally became a reality in the latter part of the 1990s, and such role extension is now recognized across many specialized imaging techniques in addition to plain film radiography (including mammography) reporting (Paterson et al 2004, Price 2005).

Radiographer role extension is now incorporated into a framework of formally delegated professional responsibility (GMC 1998, RCR 1998, CoR 2005). Role delegation is currently properly defined, and many duties and responsibilities previously held by a medical doctor are now included in job descriptors for radiographers and ultrasound practitioners who have developed their area of practice, particular examples being reporting and issuing reports, injection of contrast media and undertaking aspiration and biopsy procedures (Price 2005).

The Society and College of Radiographers currently defines the scope of practice of the radiographer as 'that which she/he is educated, competent and authorized to perform' and thus makes it clear that there are effectively no absolute boundaries to practice and that local Schemes of Work and job role descriptions can be developed to meet local individual and service needs (Pollard & Paterson 2005).

The need to modernize the UK health service, and in particular improve delivery of cancer services, has prompted a change in the traditional role of the radiographer, and the last 10 years have seen significant changes in role development and role expansion of non-medical ultrasound practitioners and breast imagers.

In breast imaging, this means that the scope of practice of suitably trained and educated radiographers may now include performance of mammography and ultrasound examinations, responsibility for image interpretation and reporting, and performance of image-guided minimally invasive tissue sampling and preoperative localization procedures. These developments have required innovative programs of study to provide the underpinning education and training and promote the concepts of lifelong learning and continuing professional development (CoR 2003).

As X-ray mammography and breast ultrasound examinations are increasingly performed, interpreted and reported by non-medical healthcare professionals who have undertaken formal postregistration training, these highly skilled healthcare professionals have become identifiable in their own right as Clinical Breast Imaging Specialists. They are integral and autonomous members of multidisciplinary breast care teams alongside their medically qualified radiology colleagues, team membership being defined in terms of an individual's skills and knowledge rather than professional background (White & MacKay 2004).

EDUCATION AND TRAINING FOR THE CLINICAL BREAST IMAGING SPECIALIST

Historically, education and training in general radiography and subsequent training in specialist imaging techniques such as mammography and ultrasound, or specific clinical applications such as breast imaging, has been the remit of the professional body. In the UK, the Society and College of Radiographers (SCoR) administered a basic registration qualification—the Diploma of the College of Radiographers (DCR)—and then a postregistration course—the Certificate of Competence in Mammography—for radiographers who wished to specialize in mammography. This postgraduate qualification was well recognized both within the UK and abroad as a valued award, and employers regularly supported staff to undertake it (Lee et al 2003).

The practice of medical ultrasound was recognized by the SCoR as an extension of diagnostic imaging, and this led to the development and delivery of a Diploma in Medical Ultrasound (DMU). This syllabus-based education and training program led to a formal ultrasound qualification for radiographers and was offered for the first time in 1977 (Jordan 1995). It is interesting to note that breast ultrasound was not separately identified in the original syllabus.

The introduction of the DMU was considered innovative since there was, and still is, no statutory requirement in the UK for any healthcare professional to obtain a qualification in order to practice medical ultrasound. The SCoR restricted applications for the DMU to DCR-qualified radiographers and thus prohibited access to a formal ultrasound qualification to other healthcare professionals who might have wished to engage with accredited medical ultrasound training.

Over the last 15 years, there have been a number of changes in the provision of radiographer education and training programs, the most significant being in response to the 1989 government white paper 'Working Paper 10: Working for Patients (DH 1989). Working Paper 10 took responsibility for the provision of allied health professional education and training away from the professional bodies and transferred it into the higher education (HE) arena, with professional bodies retaining stakeholder status for validation and accreditation processes. The responsibility for commissioning professional education and training provision in line with workforce planning was devolved from national level at the Department of Health to NHS Regional Executives and regional Workforce Development Confederations (WDCs) that were stablished in April 2001 (DH 2000c).

The shift of radiography education into the HE sector was welcomed by the profession and seen as a positive move towards enhancing the professional status of the state-registered radiographer and providing an opportunity for formal recognition of postregistration skill and knowledge development (CoR 1998). The HE model of provision saw existing preregistration diplomas essentially converted into undergraduate Bachelor of Science degrees and specialist postregistration Certificate and Diploma courses, such as mammography and ultrasound, incorporated into modular postgraduate Master's Degree frameworks (Table 14.2).

In the UK, the knowledge, skills and attributes required for the practice of medical ultrasound have been readily aligned at postgraduate level (CoR 1997, CASE 2000). However, this academic ranking is not replicated for international ultrasound education programs despite recognition of the practice of medical ultrasound as a separate profession in the USA, Canada and Australia (Aitken 2005).

The modular nature of HE provision has meant that a wide range of healthcare professionals can now access education and training in medical ultrasound. Most specialist professional qualifications, including ultrasound and mammography imaging and other, clinically focused breast diagnosis programs of study, are now all offered at postgraduate level. These can be accessed either as fully integrated pathways leading to specified named postgraduate awards, i.e. postgraduate certificate in breast imaging, or as stand-alone modules for continuing professional development and extension of individual scope of practice. The multiprofessional nature of such programs promotes interprofessional understanding and awareness, and enables individual healthcare professionals to learn about other professionals' roles and responsibilities. An interprofessional educational approach allows students to share their learning, whilst all students acquire the same complex skills and abilities for the practice of high quality diagnostic medical ultrasound or image reporting for example, irrespective of their individual professional identities. The multiprofessional nature of these learning experiences promotes and facilitates skills-mix across the different professional boundaries and therefore helps to achieve enhanced quality of care for the patient.

Table 14.2 Typical structure of modular postgraduate award

Award	Credit value	Typical module titles
Postgraduate Certificate (PGC)	30	Science & Technology
	15	Professional issues
	15	Clinical–breast ultrasound
Postgraduate Diploma (PGD)	15	Interventional techniques of the breast
	15	Research methods
	30	Mammography image interpretation
Master of Science (MSc)	60	Dissertation

CAREER DEVELOPMENT FOR THE CLINICAL BREAST IMAGING SPECIALIST

The modern radiographer's role is now defined within a Career Progression Framework that identifies practice at assistant, registered, advanced and consultant practitioner levels (Table 14.3) (CoR 2002). Radiography practitioners recognize the need to undertake continuing professional development in order to meet the demands of the modern NHS, and as a result the HE institutions in collaboration with all clinical service providers are delivering the underpinning education and training to support flexible career development pathways (CoR 2002).

Many experienced radiographers holding postgraduate qualifications in mammography and breast ultrasound will be graded as Advanced Practitioners in Breast Imaging—a role that may encompass mammographic film reading, the performance of ultrasound examinations, image-guided biopsy and clinical examinations (Price 2005). In 2004 and 2005, the first appointments of Consultant Radiographer in Breast Imaging were made in the UK; these expertly skilled practitioners carry professional autonomy for patient caseload management and typically undertake initial clinical assessment, image reporting and image-guided biopsy, and provide follow-up care and support (SoR 2005).

DESIGNING PROGRAMS OF STUDY FOR CONTINUING PROFESSIONAL DEVELOPMENT

Most public bodies, such as the UK Department of Health, actively promote lifelong learning through continuing professional development and, as a consequen-

cem health service providers are encouraging and funding their staff to engage in developing creative and innovative career pathways within the Career Progression Framework.

For radiographers, many of the programs of study offered by HE institutions possess the flexibility to enable individual practitioners to step on and step off, at various academic levels, and thus define their own career pathway in order to realize their full professional and academic potential and obtain appropriate recognition and reward for knowledge and skill development. A complete pathway does exist, for suitably motivated and supported individuals, to progress within the four-tier structure from the assistant practitioner role at level 1 of academic study to Masters' level and Doctorate level as a Consultant practitioner (Price 2005).

Development of such vocational programs of study required specific engagement with the concepts of 'fitness for purpose' and 'competence to practice' in the workplace, and an explicit requirement for teaching, learning and assessment strategies that recognize the importance of integrating theory and practice.

Many HE vocational healthcare programs of study adopt a systematic and 'outcomes-based' approach to teaching and learning. This involves articulating *learning outcomes* to specify 'what the successful student will be able to do' at the end of the program of study, and places emphasis on what students will achieve through the learning process rather than what knowledge the teacher will impart (D'Andrea 1999). This approach readily aligns with the SoR's educational philosophy of a learning process that is guided by explicit outcomes and is undeniably learner centered (CoR 2003). The aims and learning outcomes of HE programs in advanced breast

Table 14.3   Career progression framework in the context of breast imaging

Level of practice/grade	Level of underpinning education required	Scope of practice
Assistant practitioner	NVQ3	Two-view screening mammography
	CHE	
Practitioner	BSc	Mammography trainee
	PGC	Probationer period
Advanced practitioner	PGD	Symptomatic, assessment mammography
	MSc	Film reading, image interpretation and reporting
		Ultrasound and reporting
		Image-guided intervention
		Radiographer-led assessment clinics
Consultant practitioner	MPhil	Radiographer-led assessment clinics
	MRes	Education and training
	PhD	Research
		Service development

imaging are likely to reflect an educational philosophy encompassing the acquisition of knowledge and skills to prepare learners for clinical practice, a commitment to lifelong learning and the need to work with others to support innovation and change in service provision (CoR 2003).

TEACHING AND LEARNING STRATEGIES

In vocational educational programs, the student is expected to meet the learning outcomes by acquiring practical skills and underpinning conceptual knowledge, and then apply these in the workplace. Ultrasound and breast imaging HE programs are considered to be *competency based*, being both vocational and professional.

Public confidence in the quality of educational provision and assurance that academic and professional standards achieved by successful learners correlate with safe and competent clinical practice is demonstrated through objective and independent evaluation and assessment of HE course provision by external professional and statutory regulatory bodies such as the Quality Assurance Agency, Health Professions Council and the professional bodies (CoR 1997, CASE 2000, QAAHE 2001). Therefore, all stakeholders involved with the development and provision of education and training for healthcare professionals bear responsibility for the professional and clinical standards of competence.

Development of competence involves acquisition of the specialist skills and discipline-specific knowledge that enable the healthcare professional to be *fit for purpose* and *fit for practice*. The term and concept of *competence* is increasingly familiar to HE providers as more and more HE institutions offer vocational courses and an increasing number of students access tertiary education (Jessup 1991, Barnett 1994). Historically, a divide existed between (theoretical) education and (practical) training, but the competency-based paradigm merges the two to produce an intelligent and highly skilled practitioner capable of providing high quality, evidenced-based care to clients and patients attending the Breast Unit.

In professional and vocational healthcare education, the explicit requirement to link theory and practice is often achieved using work-based study, with the practice placement recognized as an essential and valuable experiential learning environment. It is very difficult for the healthcare students to learn effectively without the opportunity to apply theoretical knowledge in a real-life practical setting. Typically the student will be required to undertake supervised clinical practice in their normal workplace and make a formal record of their experiences and case-mix, often documenting these in a *log-book* or *portfolio* which can be submitted for subsequent formal academic assessment. In addition to the real workplace,

clinical environments can be simulated for demonstration, practical training and assessment purposes using human actor or patient volunteers or using dedicated tissue-mimicking mannequins and phantoms (Dixon 2006).

ASSESSMENT OF PROFESSIONAL COMPETENCE

Assessment is fundamental to any education or training provision, summative, or final assessment being required to enable judgments on achievement of the learning outcomes to be made. Assessment can guide students in their study, be used to determine what students have learned and can provide evidence to employers that successful students are 'fit to practise' (Brown & Glasner 1999). In order to be effective, any assessment method or tool needs to be fair, reliable and valid, with assessment strategies informed by the learning outcomes (Atkins et al 1993, Race & Brown 2001). A valid overall assessment strategy for a vocational program of study will accurately reflect performance in real-life practice and ensure that assessment is focused around learning, the learner and professional standards of practice.

Assessment is clearly recognized as having a considerable influence on the student learning process and, ideally, assessment methods should reflect and enhance student learning. In vocational healthcare education, assessment methods must be meaningful in terms of conferment of clinical competence and they must recognize the importance of practice-based learning. Whilst the HE sector has leveled criticism at practical performance-based assessment methods, the healthcare professions have been quick to point out inadequacies and the unsuitability of traditional assessment methods—the use of unseen examinations and essay writing clearly does not recognize or measure aspects of student achievement considered necessary for an effective professional performance in the clinical workplace.

The overall assessment strategy for a program of study, be it a single module or a full Master's degree, should be a valid and reliable means of judging performance of the 'can do, can cope' healthcare professional (Atkins et al 1993). The requirements for reliability and validity of assessment can be difficult to achieve in the practice setting. The validity of practice-based assessment might be assured if occurring under as near 'normal working conditions' as possible; however, to ensure 'reliability', and consistency between students, there may also be a requirement for some kind of 'independent' or 'external' judgment of performance (Dixon 2006).

New alternative assessment methods are currently being employed to assess professional capability and competence with the use of clinical profiles, records of achievement, learning portfolios and the objective struc-tured clinical examination (OSCE). These all require demonstration of the practical application of theoretical knowledge and, in addition to incorporating substantial work-based learning components, also include self-assessment and critical reflection.

Generally assessment of competence in the workplace utilizes performance criteria designed to match the expected performance of the student in the work-place setting. Performance can be judged by either direct observation or against documented evidence of practice and skill level recorded in a clinical profile or learning portfolio. Practice-based observation of skills (PBOS) involves observing students working normally in their own clinical environment and seems to be the most valid way of assessing their actual performance.

The assessment of clinical competence is normally a dichotomous (pass/fail) judgment of the student as competent or not competent; however, there is a challenge to recognize and assess capability beyond competence.

It has become apparent over time and with consider-able experience in the assessment of clinical competence that students do have the capability of reaching different levels of professional competence despite the same time span for the program of learning. Students are very famil-iar with marks and grades awarded for differential per-formance in submitted written work, and there is perhaps a need to grade clinical practice to distinguish similarly between competent, very able and exceptionally able levels of clinical performance. The Performance Level Descriptor Grid (Table 14.4) is one tool that can be used during the assessment of clinical competence to recog-nize the performance of a student beyond 'competence' and provide constructive feedback on capability using the performance level descriptor terminology (Lee 2000).

THE REFLECTIVE PRACTITIONER

The current learning climate encourages all healthcare students to self-direct their learning and explicitly link theory and practice using a coherent and reflective approach. Encompassing a philosophy of self-directed learning requires performance criteria to be transparent such that the student can have personal ownership for target setting and actual achievement of the learning outcomes. Performance-based assessment should encour-age student self-assessment and allow for self-evaluation of individual progress; invariably this will mean acquiring and incorporating reflective practice skills and the devel-opment of critical self-awareness.

Healthcare practitioners have always informally con-sidered themselves to be reflective in their practice, but HE courses are now actively and conspicuously promot-ing reflection as an integral and overt component of all professional courses (Atkins et al.1993). The SoR Curriculum Framework descriptors aligned to advanced and consultant practice clearly require high levels of reflective ability if the practitioner is to be effective and autonomous within their own discipline (SCoR 2002).

A reflective practitioner is a healthcare practitioner who engages fully with their professional practice, is critically aware of their own performance and the context within which they practice, and is able to use their pro-fessional experiences as a vehicle for learning and effect-ing change. Development and enhancement of the skills of reflective practice are now incorporated into most healthcare programs of study as this is considered a req-uisite attribute at both undergraduate and postgraduate level (Boud 1999).

The purpose of reflection is to focus on one's own learning needs and progress; this is facilitated by employ-ing non-traditional approaches to learning and teaching using the student's real-life practical experiences as the subject material (Boud 1998). One of the fundamental aspects of reflective practice is the transformational nature that increased knowledge has on future action; using historical activity as a stimulus to seek out new knowledge, reflective practice is about turning new understanding into improved practice in the future.

Many groups of students are now asked to participate in problem-based learning (PBL), often incorporating presentation and discussion of authentic case-based material. These PBL sessions accomplish a platform for student learning to focus on good practice and the sharing of good practice. Therefore, the context of the classroom and the practice placement can merge as one learning environment rather than the academic setting being perceived as remote from practice. PBL encour-ages students to think actively about their professional practice and take responsibility for their own learning and professional progress (Wilkie & Burns 2003).

SUMMARY

There is a recognized need within current breast service provision, for increasing numbers of highly skilled intel-ligent practitioners who can manage their own caseload for diagnosis of breast disease. Traditional professional boundaries are being breached in a very positive fashion, and new roles are being developed and defined in response to the career needs of enthusiastic and commit-ted healthcare professionals who are confident and highly motivated to take on this new dimension in breast imaging (Kelly 2005).

The Breast Imaging Clinical Specialist does not just perform radiography of the breast but takes

Table 14.4   Performance Level Descriptor Grid

No.	Descriptor
	DISTINCTION
1	Excellent underpinning of theoretical knowledge to practice.
2	Consistently organized and professional in attitude to colleagues and patients.
3	Exhibits confidence throughout the assessment.
4	Clear and consistent evidence of initiative and synthesis.
5	Efficient and experienced approach to planning and performing the examination.
6	Full adaptation of technique with excellent and safe use of the equipment.
7	Exhibits full responsibility for management of the session.
9	Fluent and appropriate language style to formulate and write a report communicating the full conclusion of the examination.
10	Demonstrates clear and impressive evidence of reflective and evaluative skills.
	MERIT
1	Good underpinning of theoretical knowledge related to practice.
2	Organized and professional in attitude to both colleagues and patients.
4	Clear evidence of initiative and synthesis.
5	Efficient approach to planning and performing the examination.
6	Full adaptation of technique and safe use of the equipment.
7	Clear evidence of responsibility towards management of the session.
9	Proficient use of appropriate language style to formulate and write a report communicating the conclusion of the examination.
10	Demonstrates consistent evidence of reflective and evaluative skills.
	PASS
1	Demonstrates adequate underpinning of theoretical knowledge related to practice.
2	Professional in attitude both to colleagues and patients.
4	Evidence of initiative and synthesis.
5	Effective approach to planning and performing the examination.
6	Proficient adaptation of technique with safe use of equipment.
7	Evidence of responsibility towards management of the session.
9	Utilises an appropriate language style to formulate and write a report communicating the conclusion of the examination.
10	Demonstrates evidence of reflective and evaluative skills.

Lee (2000).

responsibility for reading, interpreting and reporting the mammogram images, requesting further imaging and/ or performing breast ultrasound and then selecting the most appropriate imaging technique to guide wide bore needle core biopsy, fine needle aspiration and/or hook wire localization. Ten years ago, it was not thought possible that a non-medical practitioner could undertake this role, but the emerging Consultant Radiography Practitioner appointments give testament to the skill and role development of these distinctive non-medical healthcare professionals.

Education programs in medical ultrasound and breast imaging are established such that the prospective student working exclusively within the multidisciplinary breast unit can undertake an individual and specialized clinically defined pathway of study that is tailored to their own developmental needs and those of their local clinical service. Radiographers, breast care nurses, breast surgeons, radiologists and sonographers are all accessing modules or full postgraduate award programs and learning alongside each other; the UK now has a noted resource of award-holding breast imaging practitioners from a variety of professional backgrounds all working within the multiprofessional breast care team (DH 2004).

This multidisciplinary and interprofessional approach to breast imaging service provision recognizes both patient and service provider needs by placing high quality timely care for patients at its center and affording empowering opportunities for the continuing professional development of staff.

References

Aitken V 2005 Sonography: profession, tool or both? Imaging and oncology. London: Society and College of Radiographers, pp. 33–40.

Atkins M, Beattie J, Dockrell W 1993 Assessment issues in higher education. HE 10. London: Department of Employment.

Barnett R 1994 The limits of competence: knowledge, higher education and society. Buckingham: Society for Research into Higher Education and Open University Press.

BASO (Association of Breast Surgery at BASO) 2005 Guidelines for the management of symptomatic breast disease. European Journal of Surgical Oncology 31: S1–S21.

Boud D 1998 Work based learning in HE, can we respond to the challenge? Seminar Presentation, Centre for Policy Studies in Education, University of Leeds.

Boud D 1999 Avoiding the traps: seeking good practice in the use of self assessment and reflection in professional courses. Social Work Education 18(2):121–132. Online. Available at: http://www.education.uts.edu.au/ostaff/staff/publications/db_22_boud_swe_99.pdf Accessed 2 June 2005.

Brown S, Glasner A 1999 Preface. In Assessment matters in higher education. Buckingham: Society for Research into Higher Education and Open University Press pp. vii–viii.

CASE 2000 Validation and accreditation handbook. London: Consortium for the Accreditation of Sonographic Education.

CoR 1997 Occupational standards for diagnostic ultrasound. London: College of Radiographers.

CoR 1998 Radiography education and training for the future: a new policy. London: College of Radiographers

CoR 2002 A strategy for the education and professional development of radiographers. London: College of Radiographers.

CoR 2003 A curriculum framework for radiography. London: College of Radiographers.

CoR 2005 Medical image interpretation and clinical reporting by non-radiologists: the role of the radiographer. London: College of Radiographers.

D'Andrea V-M 1999 Organizing teaching and learning: outcomes based planning. In Fry H, Ketteridge S, Marshall S (eds) A handbook for teaching and learning in higher education. London: Kogan Page, pp. 41–57.

DH 1989 Working Paper 10—Working for patients. London: Department of Health.

DH 1995 A policy framework for commissioning cancer services: a report by the expert advisory groups on cancer to the Chief Medical Officers of England and Wales. London: Department of Health.

DH 2000a Manual of cancer services assessment standards—consultation document. Department of Health, London. Online. Available at: www.dh.gov.uk/assetRoot/04/07/65/04076516.pdf Accessed 20 July 2005.

DH 2000b The NHS cancer plan: a plan for investment, a plan for reform. London: Department of Health.

DH 2000c A health service of all talents: developing the NHS Workforce Consultation document on the review of workforce planning. London: Department of Health.

DH 2004 Job profiles: NHS job evaluation handbook. 2nd edn. Online. Department of Health, London. Available at: www.doh.gov.uk/Publications AndStatistics/Publications/assettRoot/04/09/37/39/04093739.pdf Accessed 13 December 2004.

Dixon AM 2006 Education and training for advanced practice: principles of course design and assessment applied to a stereotactic needle core biopsy of the breast module. Radiography 12(2):79–87.

GMC 1998 Good medical practice. London: General Medical Council.

Houssami N, Irwig L, Simpson JM et al 2005 The influence of knowledge of mammography findings on the accuracy of breast ultrasound in symptomatic women. Breast Journal 11(3):167–172.

Jackson VP, Reynolds HE, Hawes DR 1996 Sonography of the breast. Seminars in Ultrasound, CT and MRI 17(5):460–475.

Jessup G 1991 Outcomes: NVQs and the emerging model of education and training. London: Falmer.

Jordan M 1995 The maturing years—a history of the Society and College of Radiographers, 1970–1995. London: Society and College of Radiographers.

Kelly J 2005 Advanced practice in breast care: a case study approach. Synergy. London: Society of Radiographers, pp. 21–27.

Khalkhali I, Vargas H 2005 Practical use of ultrasound at a dedicated Breast Cancer Center. Breast Journal 11(3):165–166.

Lee L, Stickland V, Wilson R et al 2003 Fundamentals of mammography. 2nd edn. Edinburgh: Churchill Livingstone,

Lee JM 2000 Using competence based assessment, is it possible to distinguish between levels of performance? European Journal of Ultrasound 13(Suppl. 1):S9.

Paterson AM, Price R, Thomas A et al 2004 Reporting by radiographers: a policy and practice guide. Radiography 10:205–212.

Pollard A, Paterson A 2005 Foreword. In: Medical image interpretation & clinical reporting by non-radiologists: the role of the radiographer. London: Society and College of Radiographers.

Price R 2005 Critical factors influencing the changing scope of practice; the defining periods. Imaging & oncology. London: Society and College of Radiographers, pp. 6–11.

QAAHE 2001 The framework for higher education qualifications in England, Wales & Northern Ireland.

Gloucester: Quality Assurance Agency for Higher Education.

Race P, Brown S 2001 The ILTA guide: inspiring learning about teaching and assessment. York: Institute for Learning and Teaching in Higher Education.

RCR 1998 Inter-professional roles and responsibilities in a radiology service BFCR(98)6. London: Royal College of Radiologists.

RCR 2002 Clinical radiology: a workforce in crisis. BFCR(02)1. London: Royal College of Radiologists.

SCoR 2002 Interim guidance on implementing the Society and College of Radiographers career progressions framework. London: Society and College of Radiographers.

SoR 2005 Consultant Radiographers (online) Society of Radiographers, London. Available at http://www.sor.org/members/professional/consultant/index.htm Accessed 15 November 2005.

Swinburne K 1971 Pattern recognition for radiographers. Lancet 589–590.

White P, McKay JC 2004 The specialist radiographer—does the role justify the title? Radiography 10(3):217–222.

Wilkie K, Burns I 2003 Problem based learning: a handbook for nurses. Basingstoke: Palgrave Macmillan.

Glossary

3D ultrasound: technique used to obtain and display information from a 'volume' block—rather than a thin 'slice'—of tissue

absorption: conversion of ultrasound energy into heat in the tissues—contributes to overall attenuation of the ultrasound beam as it passes through tissue

accessory breast tissue: additional (ectopic) deposits of functional breast tissue—usually located along the 'milk line'

acoustic impedance: a measure of the reaction of tissue particles to the passage of sound waves—a characteristic of tissue density and compressibility

acoustic interface: boundary between tissues that have different acoustic impedance values

acoustic shadowing: reduction in brightness in the image (including total loss of information) deep to strongly attenuating (reflecting, refracting or absorbing) structures

adenoma: benign epithelial tumor originating in glandular tissue

adenosis: abnormal development/formation of glandular tissue

adjuvant therapy: treatments (usually radiotherapy and/or chemotherapy) given in addition to surgery

aliasing: inaccurate representation of (high value) Doppler shift frequencies in the image

anechoic: echo-free—totally homogeneous (simple fluid filled) structures that are displayed 'black' in the ultrasound image—they have no changes in acoustic impedance, thus no reflecting interfaces, and thus give rise to no echo signals

angiogenesis: formation of new blood vessels (by a tumor)

antiradial plane: scan plane at a concentric orientation around the nipple (perpendicular to ductal architecture of the breast)

application preset: a pre-programmed 'default' or baseline combination of ultrasound machine settings selected at the beginning of each examination—likely to optimise the image for the majority of patients

artifact: misrepresented, misplaced, absent or spurious appearances in the image that do not correlate with true anatomical structure or relationships

aspiration: removal of fluid/cellular suspension from a cavity (e.g. via suction using a syringe and hypodermic needle)

asymptomatic: apparently healthy and normal—exhibiting no signs or symptoms of disease

attenuation: reduction of energy in the ultrasound beam by virtue of its passage through tissue—mechanisms include reflection, refraction, scattering and absorption

audit: regular monitoring of organisation, procedures and/or outcomes to ensure adherence to quality standards

augmentation: surgical insertion of silicone/saline prosthesis to increase or remodel breast size/shape

axial resolution: spatial resolution along the ultrasound beam axis, i.e. in an antero-posterior direction; the ability to detect separate structures one behind the other

axillary tail (of Spence): triangular extension of breast tissue from upper outer quadrant towards axilla

B mode ultrasound: brightness mode—ultrasound image display consisting of a two-dimensional matrix of small gray tone dots to represent an anatomical cross section—gray-scale value (brightness) of each dot represents magnitude of reflected ultrasound pulse; position of each dot represents anatomical location of reflecting interface

benign: remaining localised and contained, not able to spread to other anatomical locations

benign breast change: non-specific disturbance of normal physiological ductal/lobular proliferation and involution—common cause of full/tender breasts

bilateral disease: concurrent (synchronous) presence of disease on right *and* left sides of the body

biopsy: removal of a tissue sample—may be obtained percutaneously using a 'cutting' needle (needle core biopsy) or via an 'open' surgical procedure (excision biopsy)

breast conservation: surgical technique localising the extent of excision to the tumor and a surrounding margin of disease free tissue

broad bandwidth: ultrasound is generated across a wide range of frequencies to improve spatial resolution

chemotherapy: treatment of disease using pharmaceutical chemicals to induce cell death preferentially in tumor cells

climacteric: time of life at which female reproductive capacity ends—menopause

color box: area on the 2D B mode image over which Doppler information is displayed

color flow mapping: ultrasound technique used to superimpose information about moving structures on the 2D B mode image—gray-scale shade of pixels is replaced with a color hue proportional to the mean Doppler shift value at each corresponding location

complex sclerosing lesion (CSL): radial scar-type lesion generally exceeding 10 mm diameter

compound imaging: ultrasound technique that generates the image from multiple beam directions—reduces the impact of electronic noise and artifacts and reinforces real structures

computed tomography (CT): diagnostic imaging of multiple cross-sectional slices of the body using X-radiation

computer aided/assisted detection: automatic film-reading system that 'prompts' a human observer to further evaluate specific potentially abnormal areas of the image

computed radiography (CR): technique for acquiring digital radiographic images using cassettes containing phosphor plates rather than conventional analog images using photographic film and intensifying screen systems

contralateral: associated with the opposite anatomical side of the body (right or left)

contrast agent: (pharmaceutical) substance introduced into the body to increase ultrasound (particularly Doppler) echo signal strength

contrast enhancement: increase in ultrasound echo signal strength due to presence of ultrasound contrast agent in the insonated tissue volume

contrast resolution: the ability to display subtle differences in tissue characteristics as different shades of gray in the ultrasound image

Cooper's ligaments: fibrous connective tissue bands that anchor and support the breast parenchyma between the skin and deep layer of the superficial fascia

coupling gel: inert aqueous lubricant used between transducer and skin surfaces to ensure efficient sound transmission

cranio-caudal (CC): the second standard mammography view

curvilinear array: ultrasound transducer having a convex skin contact surface (footprint) and giveing a diverging sector-shaped field of view

Cushing's syndrome: condition resulting from over stimulation of adrenal glands and/or excess corticosteroids in the body

cyst: encapsulated collection of fluid—commonest palpable breast mass

cytotoxic: having the ability to cause cell damage or functional impairment

DCIS: proliferation of malignant cells within the lumen of a mammary duct

de novo: new (primary lesion)

depth of view: maximum depth of tissue displayed in the ultrasound image

desmoplastic: development of fibrous tissue

desquamation: shedding of skin

deterministic: dose-dependent threshold (not chance) effects

direct digital radiography (DDR): technique for directly acquiring digital radiographic images using flat panel detectors rather than cassettes and phosphor plates or analog photographic film/intensifying screen systems

Doppler effect: change in frequency of the returned ultrasound pulse (echo) observed when it is reflected by a moving structure

Doppler ultrasound: ultrasound technique using the Doppler effect to demonstrate and evaluate blood flow characteristics

duct ectasia: abnormal widening (dilatation) of ducts

dwell time: time during which ultrasound transducer is stationary and active at any one anatomical location

dynamic range (DR): the number of shades of gray displayed in the image—increasing the DR will improve contrast resolution but produce a 'flatter' lower contrast image

echotexture: the spatial pattern of reflections in the ultrasound image—'graininess' may be fine or coarse, and homogenous when even and uniform, or heterogeneous when patchy and varied

. . . ectomy: suffix indicating surgical removal

edge shadowing: loss of information due to refraction of the ultrasound beam—seen deep to interfaces at acute angles to the beam axis

elastography: technique using tissue stiffness properties to generate the ultrasound image

electronic focussing: technique used to vary the depth of the narrowest part of the ultrasound beam and thus optimise lateral resolution at particular depths of interest

elevation plane: the vertical plane perpendicular to the long axis of the transducer footprint—the slice thickness or short axis plane

empyema necessitatis: spontaneous drainage of infected pleural exudate through the anterior chest wall

endocrine therapy: treatments used to limit tumor cell response to hormonal stimulation and thus reduce risk of disease progression or recurrence

epidemiology: the study of factors affecting disease frequency and distribution (in order to identify strategies for control and prevention)

epidermal inclusion cyst: cyst resulting from overgrowth of skin epithelium encapsulated by connective tissue

etiology: study of the causes of disease

extended field of view: image display using electronic manipulation of ultrasound beam direction or received echo information to generate a display field of view that exceeds the width of a linear array transducer footprint

familial disease: greater disease prevalence in members of one family than would be expected by chance

fat necrosis: breakdown of lipomatous (fatty) tissue into fatty acids and glycerol—usually associated with trauma

fibroadenoma: commonest benign breast tumor—comprises glandular and fibrous elements

fibrocystic disease: benign breast change associated with pain, nodularity and presence of simple cysts

field of view: cross-sectional area of tissue displayed in the ultrasound image

flow velocity waveform: graphical display of Doppler information to show relative velocities throughout the cardiac cycle

focal zone: operator selectable depth at which ultrasound beam is narrowest and therefore lateral resolution is greatest

footprint: active surface of the transducer available for contact with the patient's skin

frame averaging: pre-processing feature that helps to eliminate noise in the image

galactocele: milk retention cyst—associated with pregnancy or lactation, occasionally occurs in neonates

gel bleed: the slow leakage of silicone over time from a macroscopically intact breast implant

genetic predisposition: harboring a genetic mutation that is associated with increased risk

grading: assessing the degree of malignancy/aggressiveness of a malignant tumor

granuloma: soft tissue mass developing in response to local inflammation, infection or foreign body

gray-scale: range of brightness values displayed in the image

gynaecomastia: overgrowth of parenchymal breast tissue—causing breast enlargement—in males

hamartoma: rare benign lesions formed by localised tissue proliferation—specifically named according to tissue of origin

hematoma: localised collection of blood within soft tissues—bruise

hormone receptor status: tumor characteristic indicative of its susceptibility to hormone stimulated proliferation

hyper-reflective: more heterogeneous tissue—giving rise to multiple echo signals—displayed towards the whiter end of the gray-scale spectrum

hypo-reflective: more homogeneous tissue that gives rise to fewer echo signals—displayed towards the darker end of the gray-scale spectrum

impalpable: not detectable at clinical examination—clinically occult

implant: breast prosthesis—silicone and/or saline-filled pouch surgically inserted for breast augmentation or reconstruction

in situ disease: non-invasive stage of malignant disease—cells have malignant phenotype but disease has not breached the basement membrane

incidence: the number of new cases of a disease occurring over a set period of time

increased through transmission: increased brightness in the ultrasound image deep to tissue that attenuates sound less than adjacent tissue—classically seen deep to fluid-filled structures

infarct: area of necrosis in tissue—may occur when metabolic demand outstrips vascular supply or when vascular supply is obstructed

inflammatory carcinoma: aggressive form of breast cancer characterised by presence of tumor emboli in dermal lymphatics—presents with swollen, edematous and hyperthermic breast—has a poor prognosis

informed consent: implied, verbal or written permission given by patient following the explanation of a proposed health-care activity

intensifying screens: fluorescent panels used in conjunction with photographic film to create conventional plain film radiography (mammography) images

intensity: rate of energy flow through unit cross-section area of the ultrasound beam

invasive disease: proliferation of malignant cells that has breached the basement membrane, involves adjacent tissues and is capable of spreading to other parts of the body (metastasising)

invasive ductal carcinoma: most common invasive breast cancer—an adenocarcinoma with less than 50% of the features of any 'special-type' lesion

invasive lobular carcinoma: second most common invasive breast cancer—often clinically and imaging occult and diffuse in nature

ipsilateral: associated with the same anatomical side of the body (left or right)

isoreflective: tissue with similar attenuation/acoustic impedance properties to adjacent tissue—displayed at the same gray-scale level

juvenile papillomatosis: Swiss cheese disease—multiple focal areas of duct dilatation containing papillary overgrowth of epithelial tissue—presents in adolescence

Klinefelter syndrome: collection of symptoms, often associated with a chromosomal abnormality, including gynecomastia

lateral resolution: spatial resolution across the ultrasound beam—ability to visualise separate structures lying closely side by side

LCIS: non-invasive (pre-malignant) epithelial abnormality arising in the blunt ducts of the breast lobules

linear array: ultrasound transducer having a flat skin contact surface and giving a rectangular field of view

lipoma: slow growing benign tumor containing mature fat cells

longitudinal section (LS): anatomical section parallel to the median sagittal plane

lymphadenopathy: lymph node disease—usually causes lymph node enlargement—associated with benign (reactive) inflammatory/immune response, and malignant (metastatic) disease

lymphocele: localised collection of lymph that may accumulate following trauma/surgery

lymphocytic lobulitis: autoimmune condition usually associated with diabetes mellitus—produces a breast mass with clinical and imaging features that mimic malignancy

lymphedema: accumulation of interstitial fluid in the tissues—usually due to impaired/obstructed lymphatic drainage

lymphoma: malignant tumor of lymphatic tissue origin

magnetic resonance imaging (MRI): technique using magnetic fields and radiofrequency signals to obtain images of anatomical cross-sections of the body

malignant: capable of breaching tissue boundaries and spreading to other anatomical sites

mammography: plain film radiography (diagnostic imaging using X-radiation) of the breast

mastectomy: surgical removal of the breast

mastitis: simple benign infection and inflammation in the breast -associated with pain, erythema and swelling

matrix array: ultrasound transducer having more than one row of piezo-electric elements—allows operator adjustment of slice thickness and thus focussing in two planes

medio-lateral oblique (MLO): the first standard mammography view

medullary carcinoma: rapidly growing highly cellular 'special-type' breast cancer often associated with BRCA1 mutations

menarche: onset of menstruation at puberty

menopause: cessation of cyclical menstrual activity around the age of 50 years

metachronous: occurring at a different time—further tumor development subsequent to the initial disease episode

metastasis: a migrated tumor focus at a remote anatomical location to the primary (index) lesion

microcalcification: calcium deposits smaller than 100 microns in diameter—associated with both benign and malignant disease

milk line: anatomical line from axilla to groin along which accessory breast tissue and/or supernumerary nipples may occur

morbidity: condition of being in an unwell state—often used to describe risk/occurrence of complications/side-effects

morphology: physical or structural characteristics

mortality: death rate

mucinous (colloid) carcinoma: rare slow-growing 'special-type' breast cancer often occurring in older women and usually with a good prognosis

multicentric: multiple tumor nodules throughout the breast(s)—presumed to originate from separate (synchronous) primary tumors

multidisciplinary team (MDT): group of representative members from all health-care professions involved in management of specific type of patients who are invested with responsibility for clinical decision-making

multifocal: multiple tumor nodules in close proximity to each other—confined to one quadrant of the breast and presumed to originate from one primary tumor

multiparous: having given birth to more than one child

National Health Service Breast Screening Programme (NHSBSP): UK mammography-based population breast screening programme—invites women aged 50–70 years

needle core biopsy (NCB): non-surgical, usually image-guided, manual technique for obtaining a tissue sample for histological analysis—percutaneous procedure using spring-activated device and 14G needles

neoplasm: a focal area of abnormal and uncontrolled tissue growth

neovascularisation: formation of a new vascular network (angiogenesis)

noise: random fluctuations in the ultrasound signal—results in overall reduction in image contrast

non-invasive malignancy: in situ disease

Nottingham Prognostic Index (NPI): mathematical formula used to estimate breast cancer prognosis (see Box 2.2) and to categorise patients into different treatment groups

objective: more likely to be independent of the observer/operator

occult: not detectable—i.e. clinically occult—cannot be felt, sonographically occult—does not show up on ultrasound images

oil cyst: focal spherical collection of oily by-products of epithelial degeneration

oncology: branch of medicine concerned with tumors

one-stop (symptomatic) clinic: provision of full range of routine diagnostic investigations (ideally with results) at a single patient attendance

overall gain: equipment control allowing the operator to amplify all received echo signals uniformly and thus increase the overall brightness of the displayed image

Paget's disease (of the nipple): chronic 'eczema' type skin lesion around the nipple—associated with malignancy

palpable: detectable at clinical examination

papilloma: focal epithelial tumor growth within a breast duct—may become intracystic with progressive dilatation and fluid accumulation; may remain benign or become malignant (papillary carcinoma)

parenchyma: functional (as opposed to stromal framework) elements of tissue

parity: condition of having borne live children

penetration: maximum depth from which reflected echo signals can be detected and thus displayed in the image

percutaneous: non-operative technique performed through the skin

persistence: pre-processing feature that helps to eliminate noise in the image (frame averaging)

phyllodes tumor: rare, rapidly enlarging mixed epithelial/stromal tumor with varied benign/malignant histology pattern

piezoelectric effect: conversion of electrical to mechanical (or mechanical to electrical) energy

pleomorphic: varying in size and shape and, in the case of radiographic calcification, density

Poland's syndrome: sporadic congenital abnormality characterised by absent breast development, often in association with underlying muscular, cartilaginous and bony anomalies.

post-processing: equipment control that allows manipulation of the display of stored image information

power Doppler: ultrasound image display where information about moving structures is overlaid on the 2D-Bmode image by replacing the gray-scale shade with a color hue proportional to the amplitude (strength) of the Doppler shift signal at each corresponding location

power output: machine control used to vary the amount of energy coming out of the ultrasound transducer

pre-processing: equipment control that allows manipulation of ultrasound echo information before it is stored (and displayed) in the scanning machine

precocious puberty: development of secondary sexual characteristics (including breast development) before the age of 8 years

prevalence: the total number of cases in existence at a designated time

prognosis: a forecast of the probable outcome of a disease

prognostic factors/indicators: features used to estimate/predict likely clinical course or outcome of disease

prophylactic surgery: surgical removal of apparently normal and healthy breast tissue in high-risk individuals in order to prevent (almost inevitable) development of malignant disease

prosthesis: artificial substitute used to enhance-/-restore appearance or function; e.g. silicone and/or saline-filled pouch surgically inserted to increase, remodel or restore breast size and shape

pseudoangiomatous stromal hyperplasia (PASH): benign, progesterone-stimulated abnormal cellular proliferation resulting in focal overgrowth of stromal tissue

pulsatility index: Doppler parameter used to quantify the appearance of the flow velocity waveform

pulse inversion harmonics: technique used to generate harmonic images using phase-inverted pairs of pulses

pulse length: duration of the initial transmitted burst of ultrasound—manipulated to alter bandwidth properties of the ultrasound beam

pulse repetition frequency (PRF)/scale: equipment control that determines the rate at which ultrasound pulses are emitted—in Doppler imaging this control limits the range of flow velocities that can be detected and demonstrated—higher PRFs are needed to prevent aliasing

pyrexia: abnormally elevated body temperature (fever)

qualitative: described using words
quantitative: described using numbers

radial plane: scan plane aligned with the ductal architecture of the breast

radial scar (RS): predominantly benign proliferating epithelial lesion with a central fibroelastic core—may contain malignant elements—mimics malignancy on mammograms—usually excised

radionuclide imaging (RNI): technique using radioactive decay from pharmaceuticals introduced into the body to generate images

radiotherapy: treatment using ionising radiation to induce cell damage

randomised controlled trial (RCT): a high-quality research study used to evaluate the effect of a clinical intervention (e.g. screening) on a group of subjects (population)

reconstruction: surgical recreation of normal external physical appearance of the breast(s) following mastectomy—may be achieved with prosthesis or autologous tissue

recurrence: return of disease at original location following remission/excision

reflectivity: a measure of variation in acoustic impedance in tissue—represented by the monochromatic (grayscale) shading pattern of the ultrasound image

regional lymph nodes: the first main group of lymph nodes receiving lymph drainage—in the breast this is invariably the axillary basin

reproducibility: producing the same result on multiple occasions

residual disease: any remaining disease at the original location—may be due to incomplete excision/regression/resolution

resistive index: Doppler parameter used to quantify the appearance of the flow velocity waveform

reverberation: image artifact resulting in multiple equidistant horizontal parallel lines—particularly seen immediately deep to the anterior surface of a fluid-filled structure, e.g. cyst or implant, when insonated at right angles

sample volume: equipment control used to choose the anatomical location for which Doppler signals are displayed

sarcoma: malignant tumor arising in mesenchymal supporting stromal tissue

scanning time: total time for which the ultrasound transducer is active and in contact with the patient throughout the ultrasound examination

scheme of work: written instructions that specify normal, standard, routine procedures that should be followed

scintimammography: RNI technique using Technetium^{99m} to generate breast images

screening: investigation of a population of apparently 'healthy' and 'low risk' subjects who have no signs or symptoms of disease

sebaceous cyst: encapsulated collection of fluid arising from an obstructed oil-secreting gland in the skin

sensitivity: ability of a diagnostic test to correctly identify as 'test positive', i.e. abnormal, those individuals who truly have the abnormality of interest

sentinel node: first lymph node to receive tumor drainage

seroma: localised collection of the clear fluid portion of blood; may accumulate following trauma/surgery

slice thickness: width of the ultrasound beam perpendicular to the scan plane (in the elevation plane)—operator adjustable only in matrix arrays

sonographer: non-medical health care professional qualified and undertaking ultrasound examinations

sonologist: medical (usually radiology) healthcare professional who undertakes ultrasound examinations

spatial resolution: the ability to display fine anatomical detail in the ultrasound image

specificity: ability of a diagnostic test to correctly identify as 'test negative', i.e. no abnormality, those individuals who do not have the abnormality of interest

spectral Doppler: ultrasound technique used to represent information about moving structures in graphical format—Doppler shift (y-axis) is plotted against time (x-axis)

spectral gain: Doppler equipment control used to amplify (weak) Doppler signals for optimal display

specular reflection echo reflection occurring when the reflecting interface is smooth and large compared to the incident sound wavelength

staging: disease classification according to the total anatomical extent of malignant tumor(s)

stand off: water- or gel-filled pad placed between transducer surface and patient's skin to either improve contact over an irregular surface contour, e.g. around the nipple; or to place a superficial area of interest at the focal depth of the elevation plane

stereotactic technique: (mammography-based) technique using geometric principles to precisely locate an anatomical area (of the breast for biopsy) in three dimensions

subareolar sepsis: dilatation of central ducts and presence of pathogenic microbial infection

subjective: more susceptible to individual interpretation/variation

surgical margin: thickness of disease-free tissue between the edges of a tumor and the surgical incision planes—needs to be adequate to achieve local control of disease and reduce risk of recurrence

surveillance: regular (clinical and/or image-based) monitoring of apparently healthy subjects at high risk of disease occurrence/recurrence

Swiss cheese disease: juvenile papillomatosis—multiple focal areas of duct dilatation containing papillary overgrowth of epithelial tissue—presents in adolescence

symptomatic: associated with the signs and symptoms of a particular disease

synchronous: occurring/present at the same time/detected during same disease episode

target scan: examination restricted to a localised specific area of interest/abnormality

TDLU: terminal duct lobular unit—most distal branch of a mammary duct and its associated (potentially) milk-secreting alveolus

thelarche: onset of breast development at puberty

thermography: technique using infrared cameras to generate images of surface temperature of the body

time base: horizontal scale on the Doppler flow velocity waveform

time gain compensation: equipment control adjusted by operator to progressively amplify echo signals from deeper structures to counteract effect of attenuation

tissue harmonic imaging (THI): generation of ultrasound images using higher frequency harmonic echo signals to improve image quality by suppressing off-axis echoes

transducer: commonly used term for the handheld device applied to the patient's skin surface that generates sound pulses and detects received echo signals during ultrasound imaging examinations

transverse section (TS): scan plane perpendicular to the medical sagittal plane—an axial section

triple assessment: diagnostic approach encompassing a combination of clinical, imaging and histological investigations

tubular carcinoma: well-differentiated 'special-type' breast carcinoma that is usually 'Grade 1' and has a good prognosis

unilateral: limited to one anatomical side—right *or* left

VAB—vacuum assisted biopsy: non-surgical, usually image-guided, technique for lesion excision or obtaining a tissue sample for histological analysis—percutaneous procedure using vacuum suction device and 11G or 8G needles

vocal fremitus: technique used with power Doppler to induce thoracic vibration and demonstrate focal lesion as areas of vibratory defect

whole breast ultrasound: examination of the whole breast and axilla

zoom: operator control that allows magnification of a localised area of the ultrasound image

Index

Note: page numbers in *italics* refer to figures

Printed in the United States
By Bookmasters